Martin Kaltenbach, Ronald E. Vlietstra

# Concise
# Cardiology

Foreword by
Eugene Braunwald

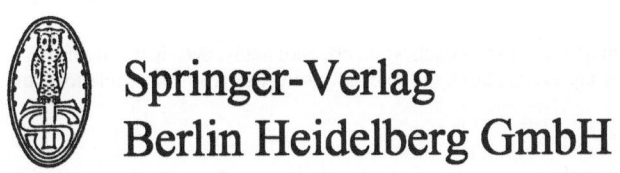 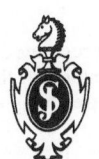

Springer-Verlag
Berlin Heidelberg GmbH

Authors' address:

Martin Kaltenbach, MD
Professor of Medicine
Center of Internal Medicine
Department of Cardiology
Frankfurt University Hospital
Johann Wolfgang Goethe University
6000 Frankfurt/Main 70
FRG

Ronald E. Vlietstra, MB, ChB
Cardiologist
The Watson Clinic
1600 Lakeland Hills Boulevard
Lakeland, Florida 33804-5000
USA

Die Deutsche Bibliothek – CIP-Einheitsaufnahme

**Kaltenbach, Martin:**
Concise cardiology / Martin Kaltenbach ; Ronald E. Vlietstra. –
    Dt. Ausg. u. d. T.: Kaltenbach, Martin: Kardiologie-Information
    ISBN 978-0-387-91394-0      ISBN 978-3-662-30763-2 (eBook)
    DOI 10.1007/978-3-662-30763-2
NE: Vlietstra, Ronald E.:

Copyright © 1991 by Springer-Verlag Berlin Heidelberg
Originally published by Dr. Dietrich Steinkopff Verlag GmbH & Co. KG, Darmstadt 1991
Softcover reprint of the hardcover 1st edition 1991

Medical Editorial: Sabine Müller – English Editor: James C. Willis – Production: Heinz J. Schäfer
Illustrations: P. Lübke, Wachenheim

Printed on acid-free paper

# Preface

This book aims to provide an easily read general account of clinical cardiology. It is primarily designed to meet the needs of medical students, but should be helpful to advanced students in nursing and paramedical fields, as well as providing a review text for medical interns and residents. The book may help to practice modern medicine in a humane way. This means utilizing all possibilities available, but, at the same time, recognizing their limitations. Since progress in the field of cardiology advances rapidly the physician can only keep up with it by understanding diagnostic and therapeutic measures rather than by memorizing multiple facts.

The need for a book such as this one has already been proven by the wide acceptance in Europe of the first two German editions (authored by M.K.). Indeed, this success prompted the collaborative effort represented here. Along with the translation into English, the authors have tried to maintain an international perspective, in tune with the greater global awareness and cooperation of the 1990s.

The book is based on knowledge gained from practical experience and also from lecturing and post-graduate training in a variety of different countries. We wish to express our sincere thanks to our families, our students, and our colleagues in the departments of cardiology of the Johann-Wolfgang-Goethe University Hospital (Frankfurt), the Mayo Clinic (Rochester, Minnesota), and the Watson Clinic (Lakeland, Florida). This work is in no small measure the result of cooperation and teamwork of many years' standing with members of departments of internal medicine, cardiovascular and thoracic surgery, anesthesiology, radiology, pathology, physiology and nuclear cardiology, and we are grateful for these team efforts. We also wish to express our deep appreciation to the publishers for their constant support and guidance.

*August 1991*                                    Martin Kaltenbach
                                                 *Frankfurt, FRG*
                                                 Ronald E. Vlietstra
                                                 *Lakeland, Florida, USA*

# Foreword

Despite recent encouraging trends, cardiovascular disease remains the most common cause of death, disability and hospitalization, and among the most frequent forms of serious illness in the industrialized world. The teaching of contemporary cardiology is a formidable challenge given the striking advances in so many disciplines, both basic and clinical, that have transformed the field in the last two decades. To aid in the education of the specialist a number of detailed, often encyclopedic texts of high quality are now available. In addition, numerous fine monographs on special aspects of cardiology have been published, again for the cardiologist. However, given the sheer magnitude of the problem of cardiovascular disease the vast preponderance of the care of patients with cardiovascular disease is now delivered, not by cardiologists, but rather by internists and family practitioners.

The detailed and the specialized monographs of cardiology are not the appropriate vehicles for the education of medical students, residents, and general physicians in this very important – and by far the largest – subspecialty of internal medicine. Even the fine textbooks of internal medicine that are now available are not quite up to this task, because the practice of clinical cardiology, more than that of any other medical specialty, is dependent on laboratory investigations which provide either graphic tracings or images. Therefore, the teaching and learning of cardiology are heavily dependent on high-quality illustrations, and the space for such material in textbooks of general internal medicine is of necessity quite limited.

*Concise Cardiology* written by Kaltenbach and Vlietstra, two master cardiologists and clinical investigators, thus fills a very special need in cardiologic education. It is, as its title implies, concise, but nonetheless complete. No really important facet of the field is neglected. Difficult concepts are presented with great clarity. The 125 illustrations are clear, judiciously selected, and prepared with care. The emphasis throughout the book is placed on accurate concepts and modern principles underlying the diagnosis and treatment of cardiac patients rather than on details.

A unique strength of the book is its blend of the best of European and North America cardiology. Drs. Kaltenbach and Vlietstra have rendered a most important service to cardiology by preparing this elegant introduction to the field. It is highly recommended to students, residents, and general internists, and will also prove to be of value to cardiovascular specialists who would be well advised from time to time to touch base with the fundamental principles of their field.

*August 1991*                                             Eugene Braunwald, M.D.
                                                        *Boston, Massachusetts, USA*

# Contents

Preface . . . . . . . . . . . . . . . . . . . . . . . . . . . . . . . . . . . . . .   V
Foreword  . . . . . . . . . . . . . . . . . . . . . . . . . . . . . . . . . . . .   VI

**1**         **Importance of cardiovascular diseases for morbidity and mortality** . .   1

**2**         **History taking and physical examination** . . . . . . . . . . . . . . .   4

2.1        History  . . . . . . . . . . . . . . . . . . . . . . . . . . . . . .   4
2.2        Physical examination  . . . . . . . . . . . . . . . . . . . . . .   6
2.2.1      Inspection, palpation, percussion  . . . . . . . . . . . . . . . .   6
2.2.2      Blood-pressure measurement  . . . . . . . . . . . . . . . . . .   8
2.2.3      Auscultation   . . . . . . . . . . . . . . . . . . . . . . . . . .   9
2.2.4      Documentation  . . . . . . . . . . . . . . . . . . . . . . . . .   13

**3**         **Cardiovascular testing** (except exercise testing, see 4.2.2)  . . . . . .   15

3.1        Electrocardiography  . . . . . . . . . . . . . . . . . . . . . .   15
3.2        Phonocardiography, pulse-wave recordings . . . . . . . . . . . .   22
3.3        Echocardiography . . . . . . . . . . . . . . . . . . . . . . . .   22
3.4        Indicator dye dilution method  . . . . . . . . . . . . . . . . . .   25
3.5        Radiologic examination of the thorax  . . . . . . . . . . . . . .   27
3.6        Determination of the heart volume  . . . . . . . . . . . . . . .   27
3.6.1      Diagnostic importance and physiological adaption of the heart
           volume  . . . . . . . . . . . . . . . . . . . . . . . . . . . . .   30
3.6.2      Subtraction angiography  . . . . . . . . . . . . . . . . . . . .   31
3.7        Nuclear imaging techniques (see also 4.2.3) . . . . . . . . . . .   31
3.7.1      Radionuclide ventriculography . . . . . . . . . . . . . . . . . .   31
3.7.2      Thallium scintigraphy . . . . . . . . . . . . . . . . . . . . . .   32
3.8        Computed tomography, positron emission tomography, nuclear
           magnetic resonance  . . . . . . . . . . . . . . . . . . . . . . .   32
3.9        Cardiac catheterization  . . . . . . . . . . . . . . . . . . . . .   33
3.10       Cardiovascular measurements . . . . . . . . . . . . . . . . . . .   34

**4**         **Atherosclerosis**  . . . . . . . . . . . . . . . . . . . . . . . . . . .   36

4.1        Coronary heart disease  . . . . . . . . . . . . . . . . . . . . .   37
4.1.1      Definition . . . . . . . . . . . . . . . . . . . . . . . . . . . .   37
4.1.2      Pathophysiology  . . . . . . . . . . . . . . . . . . . . . . . . .   37
4.1.3      Coronary arteries . . . . . . . . . . . . . . . . . . . . . . . .   39
4.1.4      Collaterals  . . . . . . . . . . . . . . . . . . . . . . . . . . .   39
4.1.5      Development of coronary artery stenoses . . . . . . . . . . . . .   42

| | | |
|---|---|---|
| 4.1.6 | Implications of coronary heart disease, risk factors, progression . . . | 43 |
| 4.1.7 | Prognosis . . . . . . . . . . . . . . . . . . . . . . . . . . . . . . . . | 46 |
| 4.2 | Diagnosis . . . . . . . . . . . . . . . . . . . . . . . . . . . . . . . | 47 |
| 4.2.1 | History and physical examination . . . . . . . . . . . . . . . . . . | 47 |
| 4.2.2 | Exercise ECG . . . . . . . . . . . . . . . . . . . . . . . . . . . . . | 48 |
| 4.2.3 | Nuclear imaging techniques . . . . . . . . . . . . . . . . . . . . . | 54 |
| 4.2.4 | Coronary arteriography . . . . . . . . . . . . . . . . . . . . . . . | 57 |
| 4.3 | Clinical course of angina pectoris . . . . . . . . . . . . . . . . . | 59 |
| 4.3.1 | Stable angina pectoris . . . . . . . . . . . . . . . . . . . . . . . . | 59 |
| 4.3.2 | Unstable angina . . . . . . . . . . . . . . . . . . . . . . . . . . . | 59 |
| 4.3.3 | Angina pectoris at rest . . . . . . . . . . . . . . . . . . . . . . . | 60 |
| 4.4 | Differential diagnosis of angina pectoris, cardiac and non-cardiac chest pain . . . . . . . . . . . . . . . . . . . . . . . . . . . . . . | 62 |
| 4.5 | Therapy of angina pectoris . . . . . . . . . . . . . . . . . . . . . | 63 |
| 4.5.1 | General measures . . . . . . . . . . . . . . . . . . . . . . . . . . | 64 |
| 4.5.2 | Antianginal drug therapy, thrombosis prophylaxis . . . . . . . . . | 64 |
| 4.5.3 | Pharmacodynamics of antianginal agents . . . . . . . . . . . . . | 65 |
| 4.5.4 | Surgical and angioplasty revascularization . . . . . . . . . . . . . | 66 |
| 4.6 | Myocardial infarction . . . . . . . . . . . . . . . . . . . . . . . . | 74 |
| 4.6.1 | Definition, classification . . . . . . . . . . . . . . . . . . . . . . | 74 |
| 4.6.2 | Development of myocardial infarction . . . . . . . . . . . . . . . | 74 |
| 4.6.3 | Pathologic, angiographic and angioscopic findings . . . . . . . . . | 75 |
| 4.6.4 | Clinical manifestations . . . . . . . . . . . . . . . . . . . . . . . | 75 |
| 4.6.5 | Diagnosis . . . . . . . . . . . . . . . . . . . . . . . . . . . . . . | 76 |
| 4.6.6 | Therapeutic interventions and diagnostic procedures in acute myocardial infarction . . . . . . . . . . . . . . . . . . . . . . . . . . . . | 79 |
| 4.6.7 | Complicated myocardial infarction, ventricular aneurysm . . . . . . | 84 |
| 4.6.8 | Cardiac rehabilitation, diagnostic procedures after infarction . . . . | 85 |
| 4.6.9 | Non-transmural myocardial infarction . . . . . . . . . . . . . . . | 87 |
| 4.6.10 | Cardiac rehabilitation . . . . . . . . . . . . . . . . . . . . . . . . | 87 |
| 4.6.11 | Psychologic support of post-infarct patients . . . . . . . . . . . . | 88 |
| 4.6.12 | General lifestyle, chronic drug therapy . . . . . . . . . . . . . . . | 88 |
| **5** | **Inflammatory cardiac disorders** . . . . . . . . . . . . . . . . . . | **89** |
| 5.1 | Endocarditis . . . . . . . . . . . . . . . . . . . . . . . . . . . . | 89 |
| 5.1.1 | Bacterial endocarditis . . . . . . . . . . . . . . . . . . . . . . . . | 89 |
| 5.1.2 | Rheumatic endocarditis . . . . . . . . . . . . . . . . . . . . . . . | 91 |
| 5.1.3 | Rare manifestations of endocarditis . . . . . . . . . . . . . . . . . | 92 |
| 5.2 | Myocarditis, pericarditis . . . . . . . . . . . . . . . . . . . . . . | 93 |
| **6** | **Aortic disorders** . . . . . . . . . . . . . . . . . . . . . . . . . . | **96** |
| 6.1 | Inflammatory diseases of the aorta, luetic, and Takayasu's aortitis . . | 96 |
| 6.2 | Aortic aneurysms . . . . . . . . . . . . . . . . . . . . . . . . . . | 96 |
| **7** | **Cardiac valvular disorders** . . . . . . . . . . . . . . . . . . . . . | **98** |
| 7.1 | Importance, classification, and etiology . . . . . . . . . . . . . . . | 98 |

VIII

| 7.2 | Mitral stenosis | 99 |
|------|-----------------|-----|
| 7.2.1 | Etiology | 99 |
| 7.2.2 | Pathophysiology | 100 |
| 7.2.3 | Clinical manifestations and course | 100 |
| 7.2.4 | Treatment | 105 |
| 7.3 | Mitral insufficiency | 105 |
| 7.3.1 | Etiology | 105 |
| 7.3.2 | Clinical manifestations | 105 |
| 7.3.3 | Clinical course, therapy | 106 |
| 7.3.4 | Anticoagulation in mitral valve disorders | 107 |
| 7.4 | Aortic stenosis | 107 |
| 7.4.1 | Occurrence, etiology | 107 |
| 7.4.2 | Clinical manifestations | 107 |
| 7.4.3 | Clinical course, therapy | 109 |
| 7.4.4 | Indications for surgery and surgical methods | 110 |
| 7.5 | Aortic insufficiency | 110 |
| 7.5.1 | Etiology | 110 |
| 7.5.2 | Clinical manifestations | 111 |
| 7.5.3 | Clinical course, therapy | 112 |
| 7.6 | Pulmonary valve disorders | 113 |
| 7.6.1 | Etiology | 113 |
| 7.6.2 | Pathology, pathophysiology | 113 |
| 7.6.3 | Clinical manifestations | 113 |
| 7.6.4 | Therapy | 115 |
| 7.7 | Tricuspid stenosis | 115 |
| 7.7.1 | Pathology, pathophysiology, occurrence | 115 |
| 7.7.2 | Clinical manifestations, management | 116 |
| 7.8 | Tricuspid insufficiency | 116 |
| 7.8.1 | Occurrence, etiology | 116 |
| 7.8.2 | Clinical manifestations, management | 116 |
| **8** | **Congenital anomalies of the heart and great vessels** | 118 |
| 8.1 | Atrial septal defect | 118 |
| 8.1.1 | Pathology, pathophysiology, occurrence | 118 |
| 8.1.2 | Clinical manifestations, course, management | 119 |
| 8.2 | Ventricular septal defect | 122 |
| 8.2.1 | Pathology, pathophysiology, occurrence | 122 |
| 8.2.2 | Clinical manifestations, course, management | 123 |
| 8.3 | Coarctation of the aorta | 123 |
| 8.3.1 | Pathology | 123 |
| 8.3.2 | Clinical course | 124 |
| 8.3.3 | Clinical manifestations | 124 |
| 8.3.4 | Therapy | 124 |
| 8.4 | Patent ductus arteriosus | 125 |
| 8.4.1 | Occurrence, pathology | 125 |
| 8.4.2 | Clinical manifestations | 127 |

| | | |
|---|---|---|
| 8.4.3 | Therapy | 129 |
| 8.5 | Fallot's tetralogy | 129 |
| 8.5.1 | Pathology | 130 |
| 8.5.2 | Clinical manifestations | 131 |
| 8.5.3 | Therapy | 132 |
| 8.6 | Transposition of the great arteries | 132 |
| 8.7 | Ebstein's anomaly | 132 |
| **9** | **Myocardial diseases** (except myocarditis, see 5.2) | 133 |
| 9.1 | Terminology, etiology, classification | 133 |
| 9.1.1 | Pathology, pathogenesis, pathophysiology | 133 |
| 9.2 | Dilated cardiomyopathy | 134 |
| 9.2.1 | Definition, occurrence | 134 |
| 9.2.2 | Pathology, pathogenesis, pathophysiology | 135 |
| 9.2.3 | Clinical manifestations | 135 |
| 9.2.4 | Therapy | 137 |
| 9.3 | Hypertrophic form of myocardial disease – Hypertrophic cardio-myopathy | 139 |
| 9.3.1 | Definition | 139 |
| 9.3.2 | Occurrence, pathology, pathogenesis | 139 |
| 9.3.3 | Pathophysiology | 140 |
| 9.3.4 | Clinical course | 141 |
| 9.3.5 | Clinical manifestations | 141 |
| 9.3.6 | Therapy | 142 |
| 9.4 | Restrictive cardiomyopathies | 143 |
| **10** | **Systemic and pulmonary hypertension** | 145 |
| 10.1 | Systemic hypertension | 145 |
| 10.1.1 | Definition of high blood pressure | 145 |
| 10.1.2 | Pathogenesis | 145 |
| 10.1.3 | Manifestations of blood pressure elevation | 146 |
| 10.1.4 | Clinical manifestations | 146 |
| 10.1.5 | Therapeutic principles, general measures | 146 |
| 10.1.5.1 | Drug therapy | 147 |
| 10.1.5.1.1 | Calcium antagonists | 147 |
| 10.1.5.1.2 | β-receptor blocking agents | 147 |
| 10.1.5.1.3 | α-blocking agents, peripheral vasodilators | 147 |
| 10.1.5.1.4 | Clonidine and methyldopa | 147 |
| 10.1.5.1.5 | Angiotensin converting-enzyme (ACE) inhibitors | 149 |
| 10.1.5.1.6 | Diuretics | 149 |
| 10.1.5.2 | Management of hypertensive crisis | 149 |
| 10.2 | Pulmonary hypertension | 149 |
| 10.2.1 | Etiology, clinical course | 149 |
| 10.2.2 | Clinical manifestations | 150 |
| 10.2.3 | Treatment | 150 |

| | | |
|---|---|---|
| **11** | **Disorders of circulatory regulation** | 151 |
| 11.1 | Hyperkinetic and hypertensive regulatory disorders | 151 |
| 11.1.1 | Definition | 151 |
| 11.1.2 | Occurrence | 151 |
| 11.1.3 | Pathogenesis | 151 |
| 11.1.4 | Clinical manifestations | 151 |
| 11.1.5 | Differential diagnosis, prognosis | 154 |
| 11.1.6 | Therapy | 154 |
| 11.2 | Hypodynamic and hypotonic circulatory disorders, hypotension | 154 |
| 11.2.1 | Definition | 154 |
| 11.2.2 | Clinical manifestations | 154 |
| 11.2.3 | Therapy | 155 |
| 11.3 | Hyperventilation, pseudo dyspnoe | 155 |
| | | |
| **12** | **Cardiac arrhythmias** | 156 |
| 12.1 | Classification | 156 |
| 12.1.1 | Classification by underlying disease | 156 |
| 12.1.2 | Classification by heart rate | 156 |
| 12.1.3 | Classification by occurrence | 157 |
| 12.1.4 | Classification by need for therapy | 157 |
| 12.2 | Diagnostic procedures | 157 |
| 12.2.1 | Electrocardiography | 157 |
| 12.2.2 | Holter monitoring | 158 |
| 12.2.3 | Ergometry, exercise electrocardiography | 158 |
| 12.2.4 | His bundle electrocardiography | 158 |
| 12.2.5 | Sinus node recovery time | 158 |
| 12.2.6 | Programmed stimulation | 158 |
| 12.2.7 | Intracardiac mapping | 159 |
| 12.3 | Ventricular extrasystoles, ventricular tachycardia, ventricular fibrillation | 159 |
| 12.3.1 | Clinical manifestations | 159 |
| 12.3.2 | Therapy | 159 |
| 12.4 | Supraventricular extrasystoles, atrial fibrillation and flutter, paroxysmal supraventricular tachycardia | 161 |
| 12.4.1 | Therapy | 162 |
| 12.5 | Bradyarrhythmias | 165 |
| 12.5.1 | Definition, occurrence, manifestations | 165 |
| 12.5.2 | Therapy, pacemakers | 166 |
| 12.6 | Intraventricular conduction disorders | 168 |
| 12.7 | WPW, LGL, and long QT syndromes | 169 |
| | | |
| **13** | **Cardiac failure** | 171 |
| 13.1 | Definition, classification | 171 |
| 13.2 | Clinical manifestations | 171 |
| 13.3 | Therapy | 173 |

**14**      **Cardiovascular disorders and sports** . . . . . . . . . . . . . . . . .   174

14.1     Relation between structure and function of the heart, adaptation to
         increased exercise  . . . . . . . . . . . . . . . . . . . . . . . . . . .   174
14.2     Measurement of physical exercise capacity, exercise methods, and
         measurement targets   . . . . . . . . . . . . . . . . . . . . . . . . .   174
14.3     Risk of sport . . . . . . . . . . . . . . . . . . . . . . . . . . . . . .   175
14.4     Sports for the healthy  . . . . . . . . . . . . . . . . . . . . . . . . .   176
14.5     Physical rehabilitation therapy, sport and atherosclerosis, sport in
         modern society  . . . . . . . . . . . . . . . . . . . . . . . . . . . . .   176

**References for further reading**  . . . . . . . . . . . . . . . . . . . . . . .   178

**Subject Index**  . . . . . . . . . . . . . . . . . . . . . . . . . . . . . . . .   179

# 1 Importance of cardiovascular diseases for morbidity and mortality

In past centuries infectious diseases, infant mortality and nutritional diseases were the leading causes of death, whereas in recent times, cardiovascular diseases have become the major killers in developed countries (in 1985 51%, and in 1988 49.7% of deaths in West Germany were due to cardiovascular disease, and in the United States the percentage was 43% in 1988). Cardiovascular diseases are consistently being recognized as the number one cause of death in various countries. There are, however, marked differences between various countries. The mortality rate of coronary heart disease, for example, is much higher in the United States and Europe than it is in Asian countries (Table 1).

Variations are also present within Europe. Finland heads the European mortality list, and there are even significant regional differences between its west and east coasts. In the eastern provinces, mortality rates are very high, whereas in the western regions rates are similar to elsewhere in Europe. These epidemiologic variations are likely caused by different genetic predispositions to coronary heart disease possibly compounded by differences in behavior such as cigarette smoking habits.

The most frequent causes of death due to cardiovascular diseases arise from coronary artery disease and cerebrovascular disease. They are not only the main causes of mortality, but also of morbidity and disability. Unfortunately, death due to cardiovascular disease frequently does not occur at the end of the biologic life span, but often occurs well below the age of 65.

Over past centuries biological life limits have not altered much; there have always been people who have lived to be 90–100 years old. What has changed remarkably is the statistical probability of living to or near to the biological age limit. More and more people are now living into their eighties and nineties. Significant further progress can be achieved only if the main causes for premature death are successfully controlled by prophylaxis and/or therapy.

Cardiovascular diseases have been gaining considerable ground throughout the world since 1940. In a few countries, however, they have declined during the past 20 to 30 years. In the United States, there has been a decrease of some 40% during this time. In Germany this trend is not clearly evident. Figures 1a and 1b show the mortality rates of ischemic heart disease in West Germany for the last 20 years (1968–1988). Mortality rates eventually level off from 1978 onwards, remaining unaltered if referred to total population (Fig. 1a). A considerable change, however, can be found within different age groups (Fig. 1b). Mortality rates are steadily declining in the younger age groups, yet clearly increasing in the higher ages, from 75 years onwards.

The interpretation of all these figures has to be tempered by the fact that diagnosing coronary heart disease has become easier over recent years with the development of new sensitive diagnostic techniques. On the other hand, coronary arteriography, which has

1

**Table 1.** Mortality rate of coronary disorders in several countries after Epstein (from Krayenbühl and Kübler [2])

| Country | Men | | Mortality* (p. 100000, p. year) Women | |
|---|---|---|---|---|
| | 45–54 | 55–64 | 45–54 | 55–64 |
| Finland** | 421 | 1007 | 44 | 222 |
| Scotland | 393 | 929 | 86 | 339 |
| England and Wales | 291 | 723 | 51 | 203 |
| Ireland | 279 | 740 | 65 | 246 |
| Czechoslovakia | 227 | 629 | 40 | 205 |
| Denmark | 214 | 630 | 41 | 179 |
| Norway | 202 | 583 | 24 | 115 |
| Hungary | 198 | 487 | 51 | 193 |
| Netherlands | 194 | 534 | 32 | 122 |
| Belgium | 173 | 476 | 29 | 122 |
| Austria | 161 | 461 | 29 | 117 |
| West Germany | 159 | 496 | 27 | 117 |
| Poland** | 152 | 324 | 22 | 84 |
| Italy** | 128 | 327 | 22 | 92 |
| Bulgaria | 120 | 363 | 32 | 149 |
| Switzerland | 118 | 313 | 17 | 60 |
| German DR | 113 | 323 | 19 | 91 |
| Jugoslavia | 106 | 270 | 31 | 102 |
| Rumania** | 80 | 214 | 25 | 99 |
| France | 78 | 227 | 10 | 52 |
| USA | 292 | 779 | 71 | 253 |
| New Zealand | 287 | 830 | 54 | 255 |
| Australia | 285 | 783 | 74 | 251 |
| Israel | 175 | 561 | 53 | 297 |
| Japan | 30 | 96 | 8 | 39 |

* in 1975 or 1976 except for  ** 1974 or 1975

now been used for 30 years, has refined diagnostic accuracy. Many patients with suspected coronary artery disease have been found to actually have normal coronary arteries and their problems have really been caused by a noncardiac disorder or primary myocardial disease.

Disorders of the coronary arteries with clinical manifestations such as angina pectoris, myocardial infarction, left ventricular dysfunction, and cardiac arrhythmia are the most frequent disease entities, followed by cerebrovascular disorders producing ischemia (transient ischemic attacks) and infarction (stroke). There is a clear correlation between the frequency of strokes and the presence of systemic hypertension, but there is not such a strong association with coronary artery disease. Furthermore, antihypertensive therapy reduces the incidence of stroke, but does not decrease the incidence of myocardial infarction.

For the time being, the fight against coronary heart disease – the "black plague" of the 20th century – must incorporate a variety of elements, including prevention and early diagnosis. With a view to effective prevention, it is essential to address and instruct the

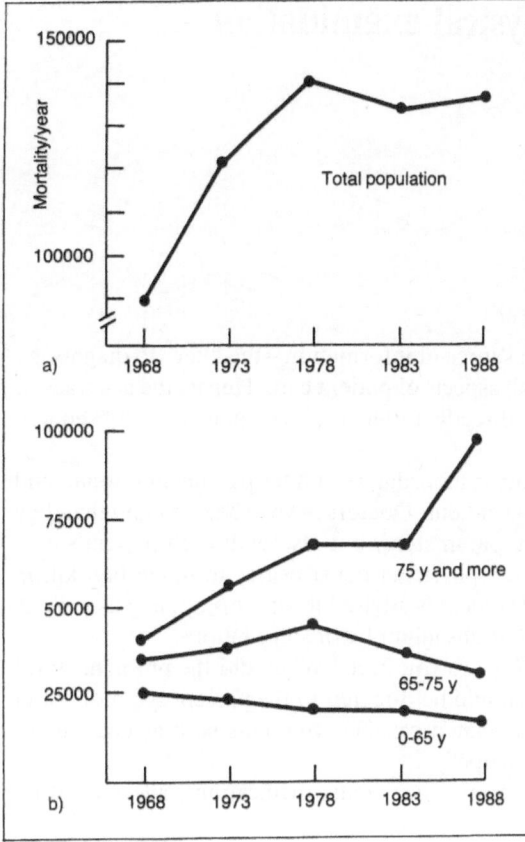

**Figs. 1a, 1b.** Mortality from ischemic heart disease in West Germany 1968–1988. Total mortality has remained unchanged since 1978. There has been, however, a marked shift towards higher age groups with a reduction below 75 and a twofold increase above this age (Statistisches Bundesamt, Wiesbaden, Pos. Nr. 410–414 der ICD).

young and those not yet afflicted. Intimidation and deterrents are not the best approach. They should be abandoned in favor of positively encouraging patients to embrace a healthy lifestyle.

Statistics from the Johns Hopkins University in Baltimore have revealed an optimistic trend among medical staff – doctors themselves have stopped smoking; in 1955, some 60% of doctors were smokers whereas 30 years later (in 1985) only a small percentage (2%) were still smoking. The nursing staff followed this trend with a drop from 60% to 30%, yet still lagging behind the doctors. The decline of doctors' and nurses' smoking habits is now spreading from medical students to students of other disciplines and to the population at large.

People pay particular attention to the personal habits of doctors and medical students, thus allowing them to act as role models. The ancient saying "Iatros gar aner pollon antaxios allon" (meaning: the doctor – and the medical student, must set an example to many people) which guided doctors in antiquity has not lost its inner truth.

3

# 2 History taking and physical examination

## 2.1 History

History taking has remained the richest source of information – the "key" to diagnosis – not only for internal medicine, but for all aspects of patient care. Hence, the accuracy of information provided by the history directly influences the quality of subsequent treatment.

It is essential to develop the case history in accordance with the psychic emotional, and biologic characteristics of each individual patient. Doctors have to bear in mind that they are concerned, not only with objective parameters, but also with each patient's own subjective characteristics. The committed physician never ceases to refine his skill in obtaining the case history. The medical student is advised to start his training as early as possible. The following sequence of questions might be of some help:

1) Referring to the present disease: Why are you here? When did the problem start? How does it affect you? Questions should be directed to the present symptoms and their prior treatment. Are there associated cardiac symptoms such as chest pain, palpitations, shortness of breath, syncope?
2) Past illnesses, hospitalizations, operations, accidents, medications, allergies, drug use.
3) Family history including questions about diseases and cause of death of parents, siblings, cohabitants, the respective husbands and wives, and children; about cardiovascular diseases, metabolic disorders, and known hereditary diseases.
4) Social history with inquiry into the family, home environment, profession, social and financial situation. How a patient views his disease is very often a clue to the psychosocial aspects of his disease. Relating biographical events to the occurrence of specific diseases or symptoms may give hints of possible causes or trigger mechanisms of the disease.
5) Systematic inquiry into vital functions including appetite, eating habits, weight history, bowel movement, micturition, sexual activity, sleep quality, smoking habits, coughing, sputum production.

It is of utmost importance to thoroughly record these findings. The order of the record generally corresponds to the order in which the questions will be asked. A typical example from a German medical center is given in Fig. 2.

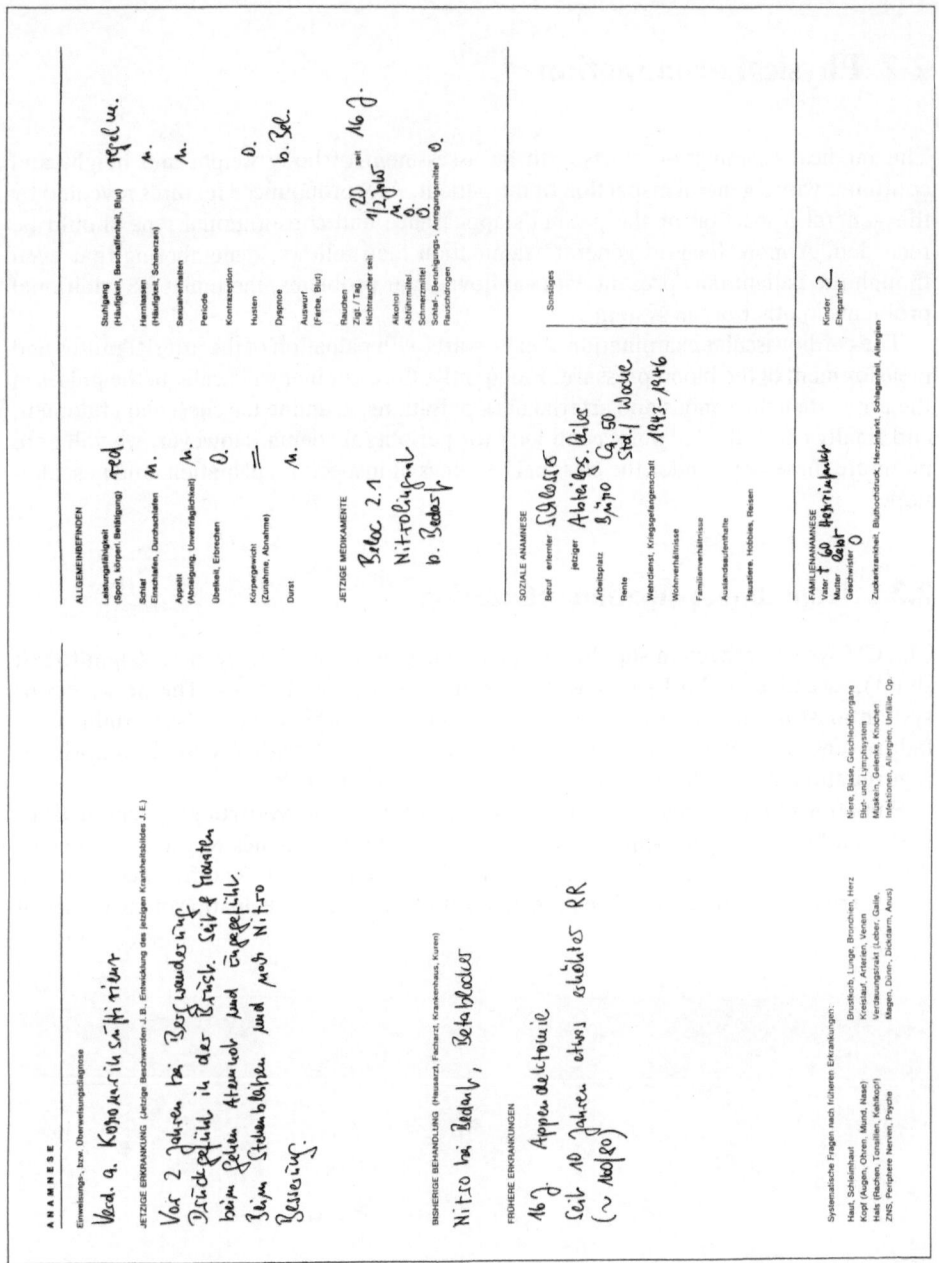

**Fig. 2.** Semi-schematic brief documentation of history taking. The sequence corresponds to the common sequence of history taking, beginning with questions on the present illness and ending with the family history.

5

## 2.2 Physical examination

The medical examination starts with an assessment of body weight and height and continues with a general inspection of the patient. Any pronounced features revealed by the general inspection of the patient's appearance and constitutional type should be recorded. A more focused general examination then follows, remembering that even though the patient may present with cardiovascular problems, there may be additional problems in other organ systems.

The cardiovascular examination usually starts with palpation of the arterial pulses and measurement of the blood pressure. Frequently, the examiner will evaluate the pulses in the arms, then the venous and arterial neck pulsations, examine the chest and abdomen, and finally check the leg pulses and look for peripheral edema. However, we will here integrate these steps under the classical headings of inspection, palpation, and auscultation.

### 2.2.1 Inspection, palpation, percussion

The CV system inspection should include noting pallor (anemia), cyanosis (right to left shunt), sweatiness (shock) or edema (possible right heart failure). The neck venous system must be checked for venous pressure elevation which may indicate right heart failure and for abnormal venous pulsations associated with tricuspid stenosis or regurgitation, pericardial constriction or complete heart block.

Palpation of the peripheral arterial pulses is a vital part of every general examination. It should begin with the upper extremities, and using both hands to check both sides simultaneously, starting with the radial pulses; if there is a doubtful difference between left and right, palpation should be repeated with elevated arms. Palpation of the pulses of

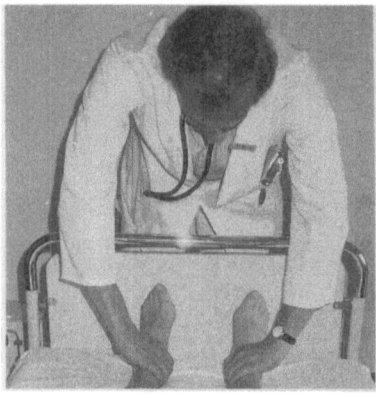 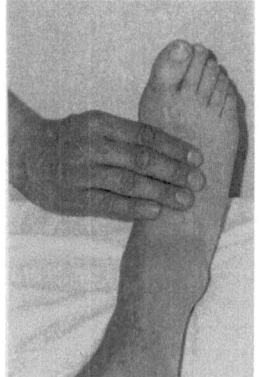 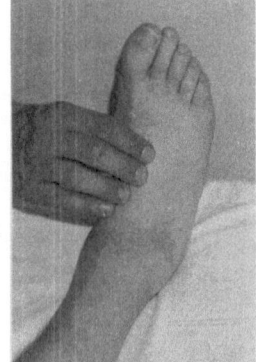

**Fig. 3.** Symmetrical palpation of the posterior tibial artery.

**Fig. 4.** Since the course of the dorsalis pedis artery varies considerably, it is advisable to palpate first with the flat of the fingers (**a**), and only afterwards with the finger pads (**b**).

6

the feet begins with the posterior tibial pulses, because this artery is always palpable at an anatomically fixed position behind the medial malleolus (Fig. 3). The dorsalis pedis artery is quite variable in its course and has to be found by palpating the dorsal aspect of the foot with the flat of the fingers (Fig. 4). Thereafter, the fingertips can be used alone. Palpation of the femoral and popliteal arteries and auscultation of the femoral and iliac arteries is also done. Ratschow's test may be performed to assess the functional effect of a circulatory disorder (Fig. 5). If the radial pulse is not palpable on one or both sides, a similar assessment can be made. The patient lies on his back with elevated arms and rapidly clenches his fists several times.

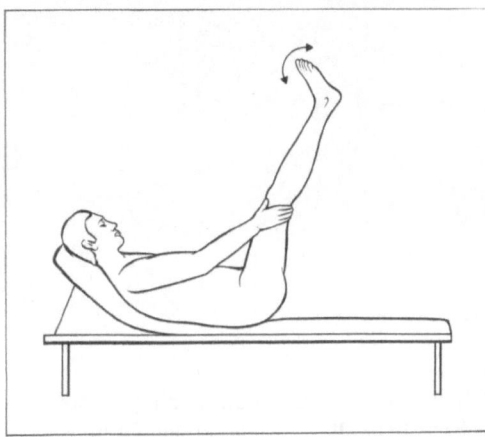

**Fig. 5.** Ratschow's test reveals peripheral circulatory disorders of the legs. The feet are raised as high as possible. A whitening of the foot and its digits (sometimes with concomitant discomfort in the calf) is typical for severe arterial circulatory disorder. A slow refilling of the veins and a dull red coloration (rubor) of the skin after lowering the feet, especially in the presence of clear differences between right and left side, is also pathologic.

Palpation of the abdomen requires a relaxed abdominal wall. Warm hands, short finger nails and gentle examination techniques are prerequisites. First, one palpates with the entire palm for masses or tenderness in all four quadrants. Thereafter, one tries to palpate more deeply below the right costal margin, preferably for multiple respiratory cycles. Palpation pressure should be supported by the second hand. As soon as the fingertips have reached the lower margin of the liver the patient must breathe deeply with an open mouth, and the hand moves upwards in order to avoid reflex respiratory breath holding (Fig. 6). Palpation of the spleen is performed in a similar way, it is often preferable to examine a patient in the right lateral recumbent position and to push the spleen with the left hand from dorsal to ventral. The position of the lower edge of the liver in the midclavicular line is recorded in centimeters below the right costal margin. In the case of liver displacement, caused for instance by a large lung volume with a lowered diaphragm, true liver enlargement can be distinguished by percussing and defining the exact location of the diaphragm.

By palpation, one can usually also recognize any significant enlargement (aneurysm) of the abdominal aorta. Characteristically, an expansile pulsation wider than 3–4 cm in the epigastrium or mid-abdomen represents an abdominal aortic aneurysm. This can be easily confirmed with a B-mode ultrasound scan.

Percussion is used to detect pleural fluid, consolidated lung, and the location of the lung-diaphragm borders. Only rarely, however, can important diagnostic clues be

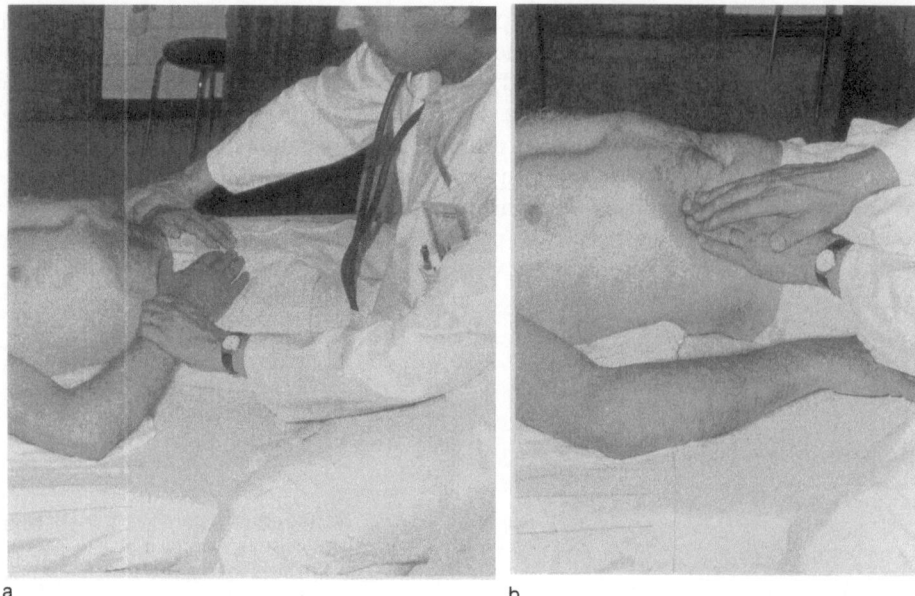

a                                                      b

**Fig. 6.** Palpation of **a** the radial pulse and **b** the liver.

expected from the percussion of the heart. It may be done after determining the position of the diaphragm and the lower border of the liver. Percussing cardiac dullness may sometimes help to recognize pericardial effusion.

## 2.2.2 Blood-pressure measurement

Since Riva and Rocci's invention of the sphygmomanometer and the detection of arterial sounds by Korotkoff, routine blood-pressure measurements have been performed non-invasively with a cuff and a stethoscope. The values obtained noninvasively usually correlate with pressures measured invasively, if certain rules are observed (Table 2).

The upper limit of normal for an adult's systemic artery blood pressure is 140/90, pathologic elevation in blood pressure being above that value. The lower limit of a normal blood pressure is not determined precisely, but it is approximately 90/50. Lower values may be obtained in small healthy persons, in some athletes or during sleep. A borderline elevation in blood pressure can usually be clearly classified as normal or pathological through multiple readings. The physiological variation in blood pressure at rest is up to 50 for systolic and up to 20 mmHg for diastolic pressures. In particular, the diastolic pressure may rise up to 100 mmHg with emotional stress, the systolic value may rise with exercise to over 200 mmHg, and during heavy exercise even up to 300 mmHg. Whereas the systolic blood pressure can be measured relatively well during exercise, measurements of the diastolic pressure with exercise are only reliably done using invasive methods.

**Table 2.** Technique and procedure of blood pressure measurement.

---

**Technique**

- palpate radial pulse on both sides prior to measurement;
- cuff size 12–13 cm;
- calibrated mercury manometer;
- place stethoscope with slight pressure on site of the palpated brachial artery;
- check the systolic value of the first measurement by palpation of the radial artery;
- determine the diastolic pressure by applying only a slight pressure on the stethoscope (disappearance of the Korotkoff sounds).

**Evaluation**

normal 140/90–90/60 mmHg

**Procedure**

Abnormal values or difference between left- and right-sided radial pulse:
- compare left- and right-sided measurement.

In the case of systemic hypertension:
- repeat the blood pressure measurement several times, when the patient is relaxed;
- auscultate right and left renal artery:
  press stethoscope firmly, 5 cm above and lateral to the navel.

The hypertensive patient should be trained in self-measurement. Checking the adequacy of the patient's measurement can be done using a stethoscope with two-fold ear parts, where two examiners may listen at the same time.

---

A suspicion of coarctation of the aorta or arterial stenosis necessitates blood-pressure measurements in all extremities. The measurement at the thigh is done with a larger cuff, whereas measurement at the calf can be done with the normal arm cuff. If peripheral pulses are palpable, the systolic pressure can be determined by palpation, if not, Doppler measurement can be applied for the systolic pressures. The capillary method often allows reliable measuring of systolic blood pressure. For its evaluation, a cuff on the raised thigh is inflated up to 50 mmHg above the value obtained at arm measurement and is kept up until the foot turns pale. Thereafter the foot is lowered to heart level and the cuff pressure reduced until a reddening of the skin is observed. This value corresponds to the systolic arterial pressure.

Blood-pressure measurements may show a decrease in blood pressure in a diseased extremity beyond a narrowed arterial segment. This can only be measured in the event of a vessel narrowing by more than 80% and depends on a number of factors, including the peripheral vascular resistance, blood flow, and presence of collaterals. When in doubt, the measurement should be repeated after decrease of the peripheral resistance by muscular exercise of the diseased area. A Doppler stethoscope may be needed for an accurate assessment of these lower pressures.

## 2.2.3 Auscultation

It is best to use a stethoscope with both a membrane and a bell during cardiac auscultation. The membrane is better for hearing higher pitched sounds and the bell is indispensable in the case of very thin patients, children, and patients with considerable body hair. Low pitched murmurs and gallop sounds are also better heard with the bell.

The following things should be noted on auscultation: heart rhythm, heart rate, general amplitude of heart sounds, any accentuation of the heart sounds, extra sounds and murmurs. Cardiac murmurs can be classified according to intensity or volume, Grade I/VI to VI/VI (Table 3); to the frequency or pitch, varying from low (rumbling) to high (hissing); to the site of maximum intensity, and to the direction of any radiation of the murmur (Fig. 7). Cardiac murmurs should be timed and this may prove rather difficult in cases with tachycardia, often requiring repeated careful auscultation.

**Table 3.** Volume of heart murmurs (from: Zuckermann [7]).

| | |
|---|---|
| **Grade I** | is the faintest that can be detected, often only after several heart beats when the heart "tunes in"; |
| **Grade II** | is a faint but readily recognized murmur; |
| **Grade III & Grade IV** | are intermediate in volume; |
| **Grade V** | is a very loud murmur, but requires a stethoscope to be audible; |
| **Grade VI** | is an execptionally loud murmur that can be heard with the stethoscope just removed from contact with the chest. |

According to another method, the examiner is instructed to place the center of the left palm onto the site of maximum intensity and to determine the volume by feeling the sound vibrations through the hand and travelling along the radius:

| | |
|---|---|
| **Grade I/VI** | is a threshold murmur (pianissimo); |
| **Grade II/VI** | does not cross to the back of the hand (piano); |
| **Grade III/VI** | penetrates to the back of the hand (mezzoforte); |
| **Grade IV/VI** | is auscultated above the radiocarpal joint (forte); |
| **Grade V/VI** | can be heard as far as the upper third of the radius (fortissimo); |
| **Grade VI/VI** | is a distance murmur that can be sensed from a distance of several millimeters or even centimeters. |

It is important to recognize any murmur-free interval before or after the murmur onset and to relate the murmur to the first and second heart sounds and any clicks. Physical exertion such as repeated sitting up of the patient may clarify difficult auscultatory findings, but sometimes the development of tachycardia with exercise further obscures things.

For auscultation of the mitral valve it is helpful to auscultate the patient in the left lateral decubitus position and to listen between the apex and the left anterior axillary line. It is often easier to hear the diastolic murmur of aortic insufficiency when the patient is sitting and bending forward than when he is supine.

The lungs should be ausculted from the top downwards, comparing the findings from the left and right sides. The asymmetry of the lungs and the bronchial system causes, in the healthy, small differences in the right and left findings from percussion and

10

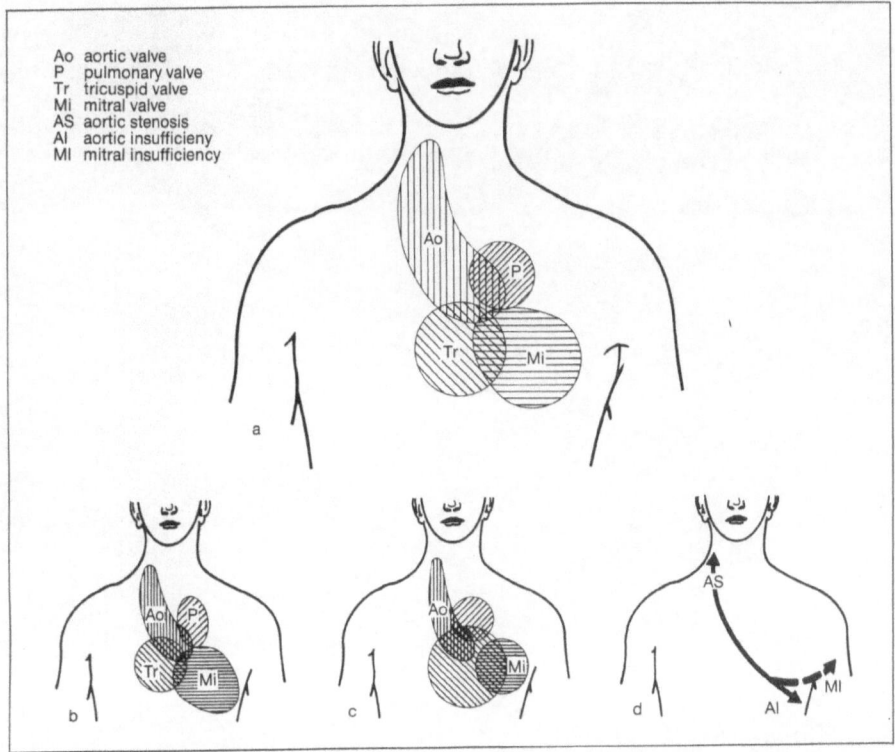

**Fig. 7.** Areas of auscultation for cardiac valve disease: **a** normal extension of sound fields, **b** in left ventricular hypertrophy, **c** in right ventricular hypertrophy, and **d** direction of sound radiation in different valvular disorders (mod. from [1]).

.auscultation. Auscultation of the lungs should include an evaluation of the breath sounds and any additional sounds.

Systemic hypertension necessitates, besides auscultation of the heart and lungs, examination of the abdominal aorta, in particular near the origin of the renal arteries (5 cm above and 5 cm left or right of the navel); and if arterial disease is suspected, auscultation of all great arteries should be performed (Figs. 8, 9). Training in auscultation is facilitated by the use of a double stethoscope, where two examiners auscultate the same position and compare the results. Auscultatory findings may be recorded in writing and then compared with a phonocardiograph.

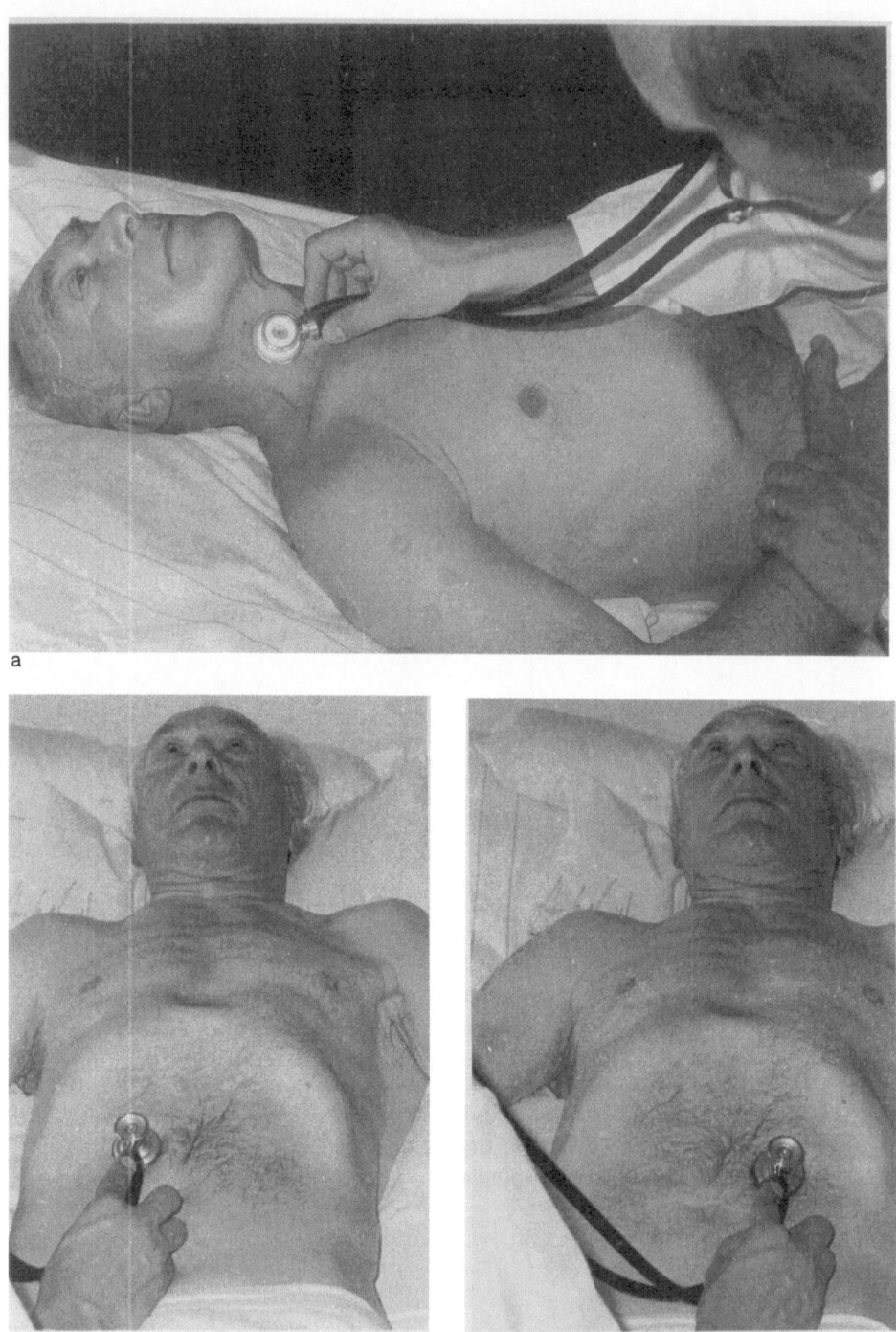

**Fig. 8.** Auscultation of the carotid arteries (**a**), and the right and left renal arteries (**b** and **c**).

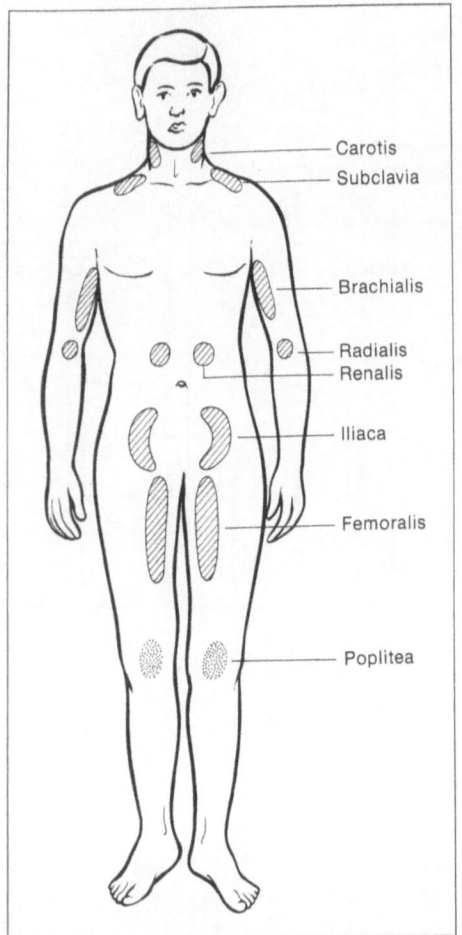

Carotis
Subclavia

Brachialis

Radialis
Renalis

Iliaca

Femoralis

Poplitea

**Fig. 9.** Areas of auscultation for stenotic murmurs of the great arteries. Murmurs of the aorta are audible all the way along the entire length of the aorta, and thus do not appear on the diagram.

## 2.2.4 Documentation

Careful documentation of the history and physical examination is not only the basis for good learning, but it is essential for clinical care. The medical record shown in the example uses a semi-schematic brief documentation which does not require a lot of time (Fig. 10).

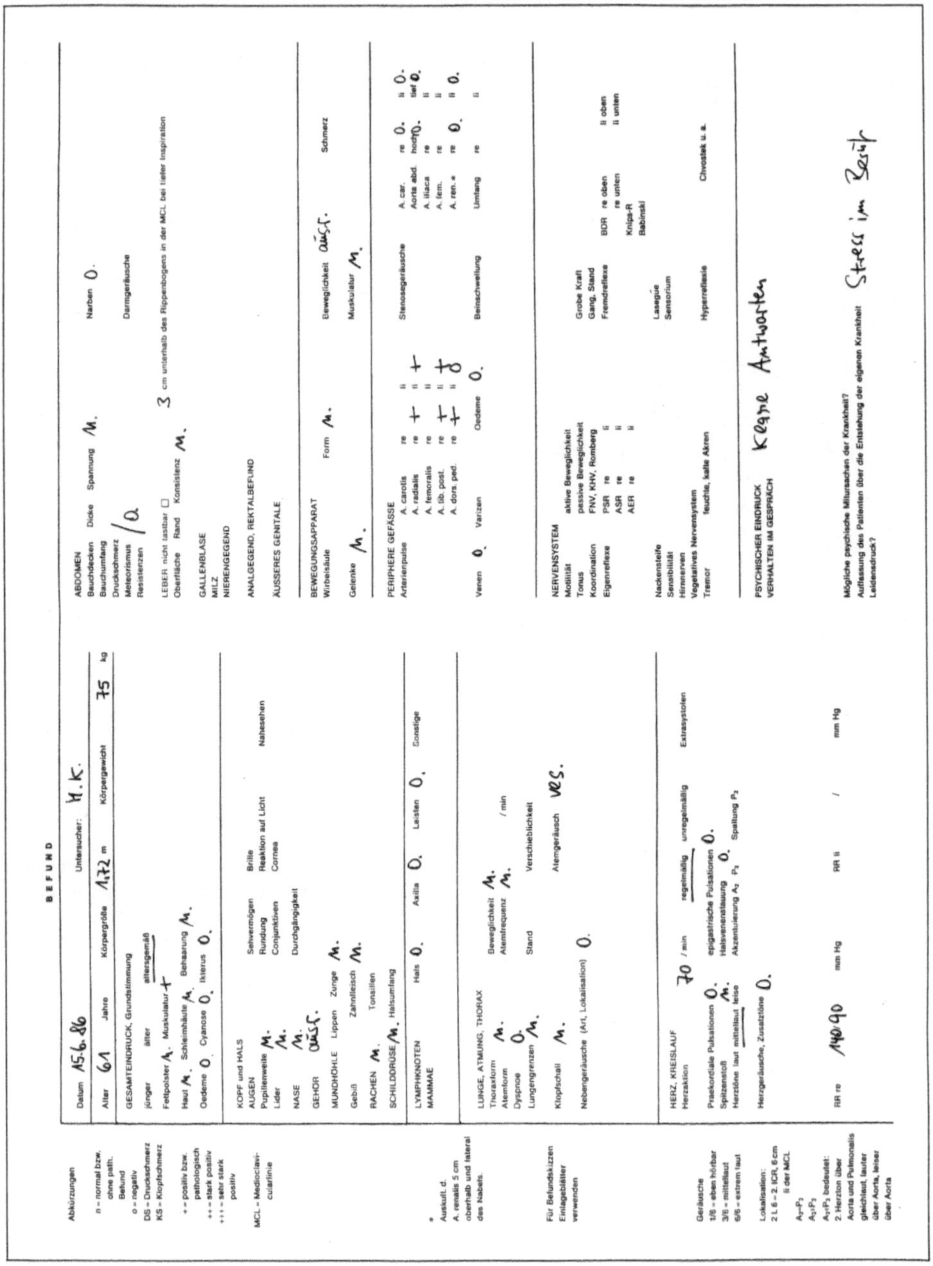

BEFUND

Abkürzungen
n = normal bzw. ohne path. Befund
o = negativ
DS = Druckschmerz
KS = Klopfschmerz
+ = positiv bzw. pathologisch
++ = stark positiv
+++ = sehr stark positiv
MCL = Medioclavicularlinie
* Auskult. d. A. renalis 5 cm oberhalb und lateral des Nabels.
Für Befundskizzen Einlageblätter verwenden
Geräusche
1/6 = eben hörbar
3/6 = mittellaut
6/6 = extrem laut
Lokalisation:
2 L 6 – 2. ICR, 6 cm li der MCL
$A_2$–$P_2$
$A_2$/$P_2$
$A_2$/$P_2$ bedeutet:
2. Herzton über Aorta und Pulmonalis gleichlaut, lauter über Aorta, leiser über Aorta

Datum 15.6.86 Untersucher: H.K.
Alter 61 Jahre Körpergröße 1,72 m Körpergewicht 75 kg

GESAMTEINDRUCK, Grundstimmung
jünger älter altersgemäß
Fettpolster M. Muskulatur +
Haut M. Schleimhäute M. Behaarung M.
Oedeme 0. Cyanose 0. Ikterus 0.

KOPF und HALS
AUGEN Sehvermögen Brille
Pupillenweite M. Rundung Reaktion auf Licht Nahesehen
Lider M. Conjunktiven Cornea
NASE M. Durchgängigkeit
GEHÖR ausr.
MUNDHÖHLE Lippen Zunge M.
Gebiß Zahnfleisch M.
RACHEN M. Tonsillen
SCHILDDRÜSE M. Halsumfang

LYMPHKNOTEN Hals 0. Axilla 0. Leisten 0. Sonstige
MAMMAE

LUNGE, ATMUNG, THORAX
Thoraxform M. Beweglichkeit M.
Atemform M. Atemfrequenz M. / min
Dyspnoe 0.
Lungengrenzen M. Stand Verschieblichkeit
Klopfschall M. Atemgeräusch ves.
Nebengeräusche (Art, Lokalisation) 0.

HERZ, KREISLAUF
Herzaktion 70 / min regelmäßig unregelmäßig Extrasystolen
Praekordiale Pulsationen 0. epigastrische Pulsationen 0.
Spitzenstoß M. Halsvenenstauung 0.
Herztöne laut mittellaut leise Akzentuierung $A_2$ $P_2$ Spaltung $P_2$
Herzgeräusche, Zusatztöne 0.

RR re 140/90 mm Hg RR li / mm Hg

ABDOMEN
Bauchdecken Dicke Spannung M. Narben 0.
Bauchumfang
Druckschmerz
Meteorismus /0
Resistenzen Darmgeräusche
LEBER nicht tastbar ☐ 3 cm unterhalb des Rippenbogens in der MCL bei tiefer Inspiration
Oberfläche Rand Konsistenz M.
GALLENBLASE
MILZ
NIERENGEGEND
ANALGEGEND, REKTALBEFUND
ÄUSSERES GENITALE

BEWEGUNGSAPPARAT
Wirbelsäule Form M. Beweglichkeit ausr. Schmerz
Gelenke M. Muskulatur M.

PERIPHERE GEFÄSSE
Arterienpulse A. carotis re li Stenosegeräusche A. car. re 0. li 0.
A. radialis re + li + Aorta abd. hoch 0. tief 0.
A. femoralis re li A. iliaca re li
A. tib. post. re + li + A. fem. re li
A. dors. ped. re + li 0 A. ren.* re 0. li 0.
Venen 0. Varizen Oedeme 0. Beinschwellung Umfang re li

NERVENSYSTEM
Motilität aktive Beweglichkeit
Tonus passive Beweglichkeit Grobe Kraft
Koordination FNV, KHV, Romberg Gang, Stand
Eigenreflexe PSR re li Fremdreflexe BDR re oben li oben
ASR re li re unten li unten
AER re li Knips-R
Babinski
Nackensteife Lasegue
Sensibilität Sensorium
Hirnnerven
Vegetatives Nervensystem
Tremor feuchte, kalte Akren Hyperreflexie Chvostek u. a.

PSYCHISCHER EINDRUCK
VERHALTEN IM GESPRÄCH Klare Antworten

Mögliche psychische Mitursachen der Krankheit?
Auffassung des Patienten über die Entstehung der eigenen Krankheit Stress im Beruf
Leidensdruck?

**Fig. 10.** German medical record with semi-schematic documentation.

# 3 Cardiovascular testing (except exercise testing, see 4.2.2)

## 3.1 Electrocardiography

Late in the 18th century an Italian, Galvani, used the frog hind limb to demonstrate that living tissues generate electrical activity. Just 80 years ago, Einthoven pioneered studies that showed that the electrical potentials of the heart can be recorded from the body surface. Now, such a recording, the electrocardiogram (Fig. 11), is the most frequently used standard cardiovascular diagnostic test. The recorded changes in field potentials

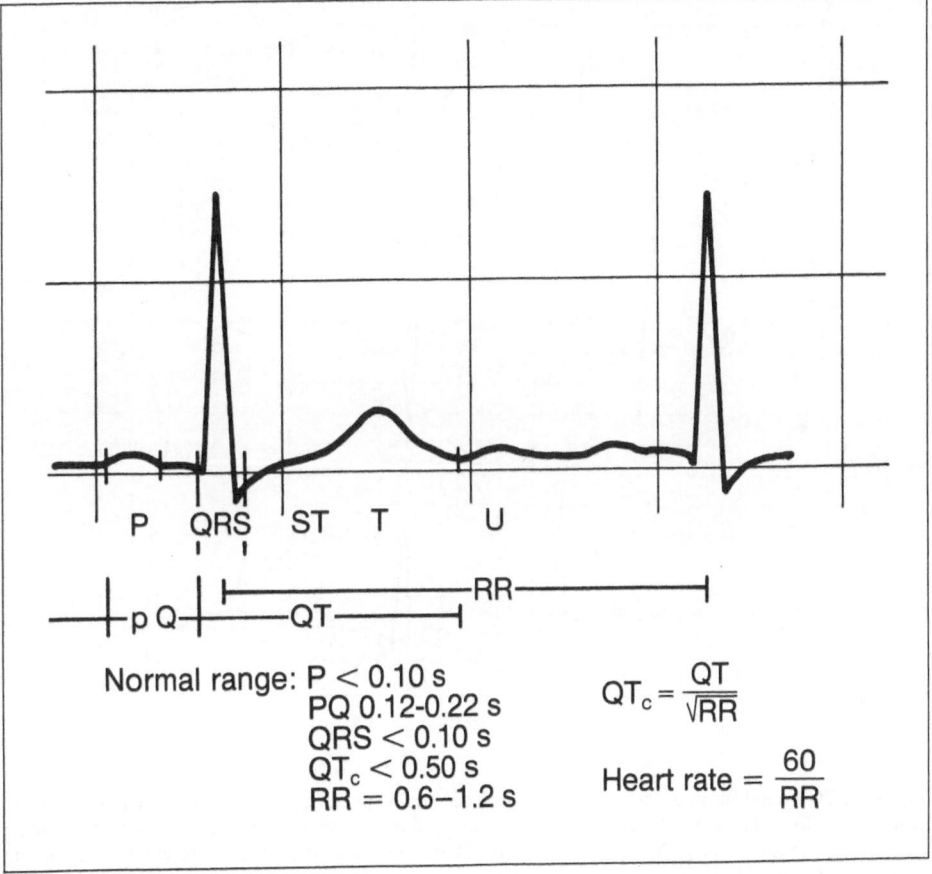

Normal range: P < 0.10 s
PQ 0.12-0.22 s
QRS < 0.10 s
$QT_c$ < 0.50 s
RR = 0.6–1.2 s

$$QT_c = \frac{QT}{\sqrt{RR}}$$

$$\text{Heart rate} = \frac{60}{RR}$$

**Fig. 11.** ECG-abbreviations and normal values

from the body surface are about 100-fold smaller than the potentials recorded in the heart muscle itself, because of conduction disturbance by the air-filled lungs.

The surface potentials obtained are the net instantaneous vectors (summation vectors) of all the electrical forces occurring throughout the cardiac cycle. It should be kept in mind that the surface ECG records electrical phenomena and does not reflect the contractile state of the heart. In certain extreme cases, therefore, a normal ECG can be recorded when the heart is no longer contracting mechanically due to "electro-mechanical dissociation". Despite these limitations electrocardiography has remained a fundamental diagnostic procedure for detecting cardiovascular disorders, ranging in importance immediately after the history and physical examination. This is especially true for the detection of myocardial ischemia (Fig. 12).

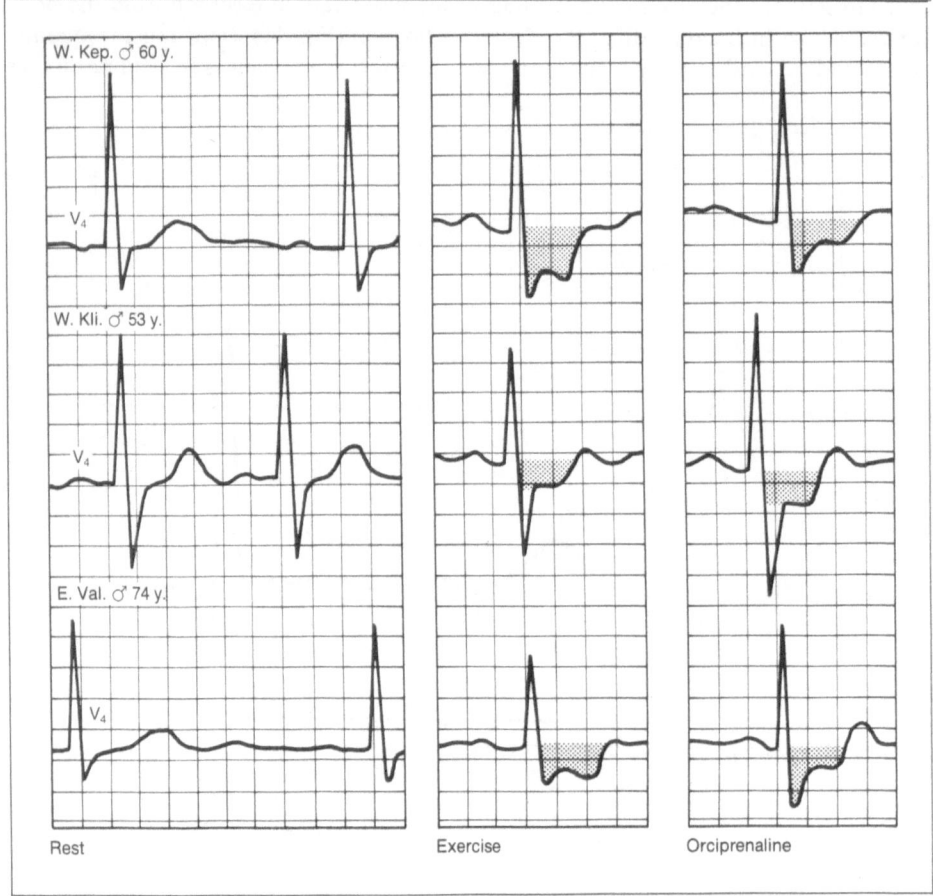

**Fig. 12.** ECG from three patients with exercise-induced angina pectoris. ST-segments were normal on the rest ECG. However, ischemic ST-depression occurred during exercise. The patients reported angina pectoris at that time. The ECGs in the right part of the figure were recorded in a research study during pharmacologic stimulation with the catecholamine-derivative orciprenaline. Symptoms of angina pectoris and ischemic ECG changes were also evident during the infusion.

16

The various components of the electrical activity of the heart are classified using the letters P, Q, R, S, T, U (see Fig. 11). P-waves represent atrial activity and are very important in the evaluation of arrhythmias. Large P-waves may reflect overload of one or both atria. The QRS complexes reflect the sequence of ventricular activation. Changes are seen with hypertrophy and intraventricular conduction disorders. Loss of potentials (loss of R-waves or the occurrence of Q-waves) is often due to loss of viable heart muscle tissue following myocardial infarction. The ST-segment is usually isoelectric. Acute ischemia of the heart muscle usually induces a depression of the ST-segment, but in rare cases ST-elevation is found. A horizontal or descending ST-depression during exercise is of important practical value in the diagnosis of coronary artery disease. It has to be distinguished from ST-segment abnormalities due to hypokalemia, digitalis or hypertension (see 4.2.2).

T-wave changes are caused by many of the same things that are associated with ST-segment changes. However, they are far less reliable in diagnosis because they are sensitively modulated by the autonomic nervous system (Figs. 13, 14). Normal positive T-waves may change into negative T-waves, not only as a result of organic disease, but also of changes in body position, such as changing from the recumbent to the upright position, or by raising the legs while lying down.

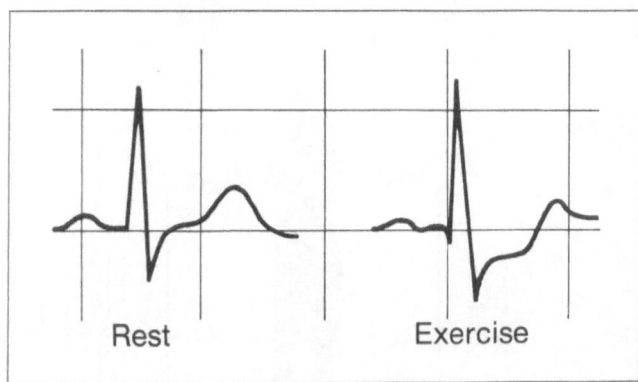

Rest                   Exercise

**Fig. 13.** Typical ST-depression during exercise due to myocardial ischemia produced by coronary artery disease.

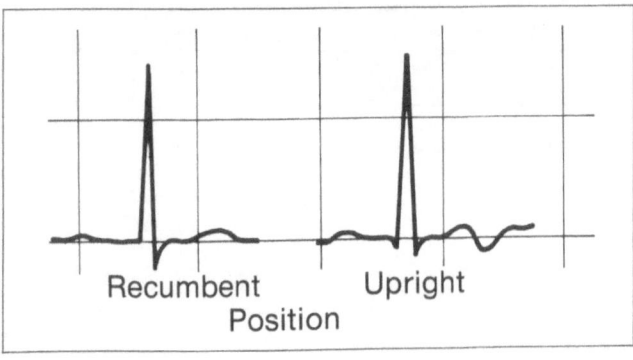

Recumbent     Upright
Position

**Fig. 14.** Change to negative T-wave when standing, modulated by the autonomic nervous system.

17

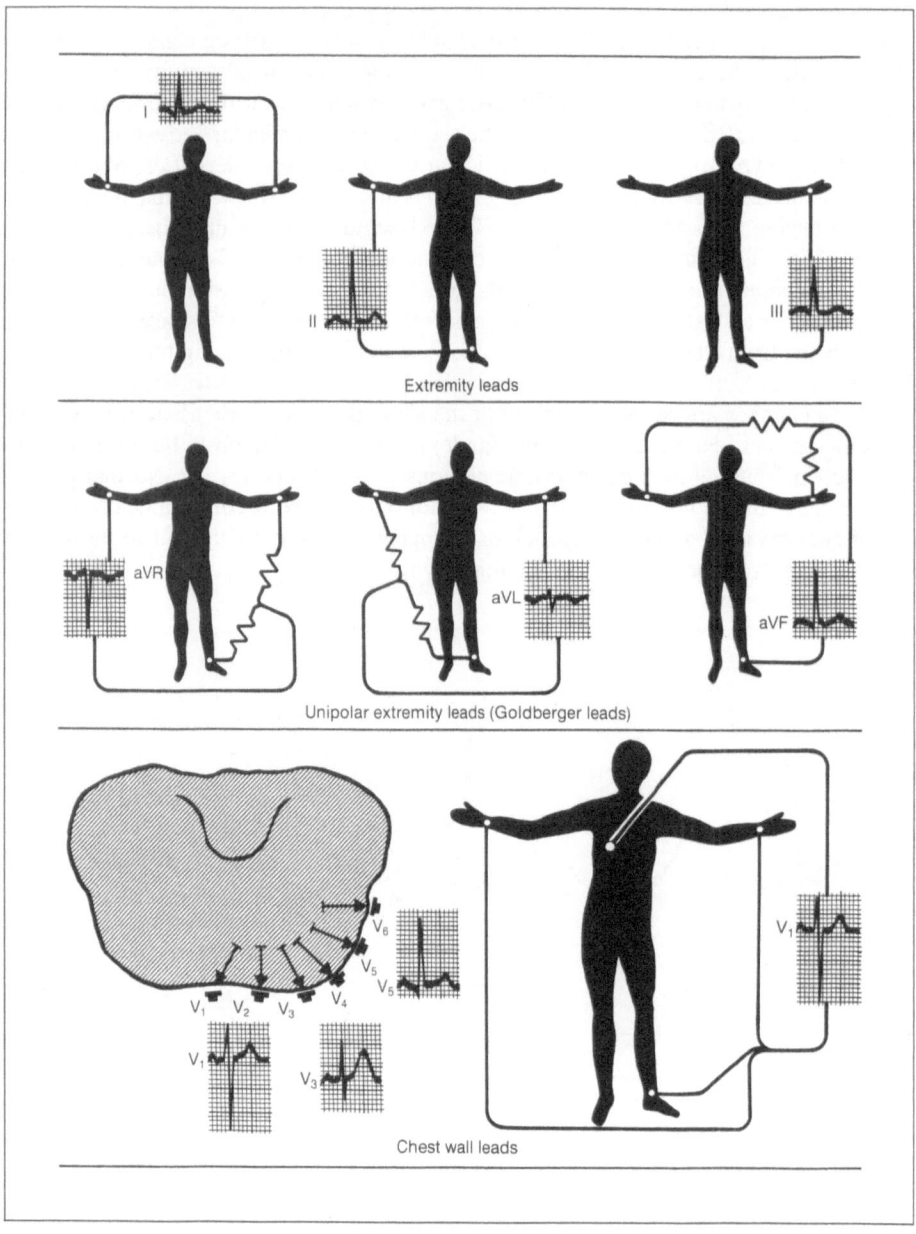

**Fig. 15.** Placement and connection of electrodes for recording of bipolar limb leads, unipolar limb leads, and precordial leads.

The electrical activation waves recorded by the electrocardiogram have defined normal ranges. The PR interval is normally 0.12–0.22 s and the QRS duration 0.07–0.10 s. The pulse rate is determined from the reciprocal of the inter-R-wave distance and at rest is between 60 to 90 QRS complexes per minute; lower when vagal tone is increased and higher during sympathetic stimulation. The exact R-wave interval varies slightly from beat-to-beat. This variation disappears during certain pathologic conditions such as damage to the autonomic nervous system due to diabetic neuropathy.

The electrocardiogram comprises several recordings which measure potential differences between two electrodes fixed at different sites on the body (Fig. 15). Lead I measures the potential difference between the right arm and the left arm, Lead II the difference between the right arm and the left leg, and Lead III the difference between the left arm and the left leg. The same electrodes may be connected to achieve three more recordings, by connecting two electrodes together and measuring versus the third. These leads are called the augmented unipolar leads, aVR, aVL, and aVF. The direction of the largest QRS complex is the "electrical heart axis". A change in the anatomical position of the heart will result in a change of the electrical axis (Fig. 16). During inspiration when the diaphragm falls, the heart also moves, thus inducing the cardiac axis to shift downward and to the right. During expiration the change is upward and to the left. Similar changes can be observed during elevation of the diaphragm due to obesity or

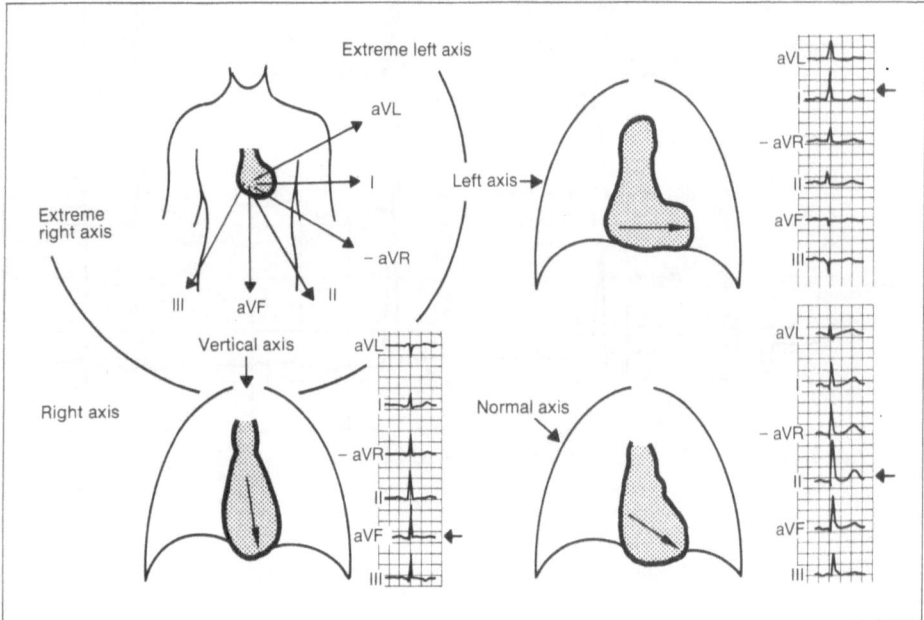

**Fig. 16.** Position of the heart within the chest and determination of the electrical axis of the heart by the ECG. The axis corresponds to the direction of the most positive QRS complex in the bipolar limb leads (I, II, III) and unipolar limb leads (aVL, -aVR, aVF). Schematic drawing (upper left) with ECG examples for horizontal axis, normal axis, and vertical axis. The most positive QRS complex is marked with an arrow in all three ECG examples.

19

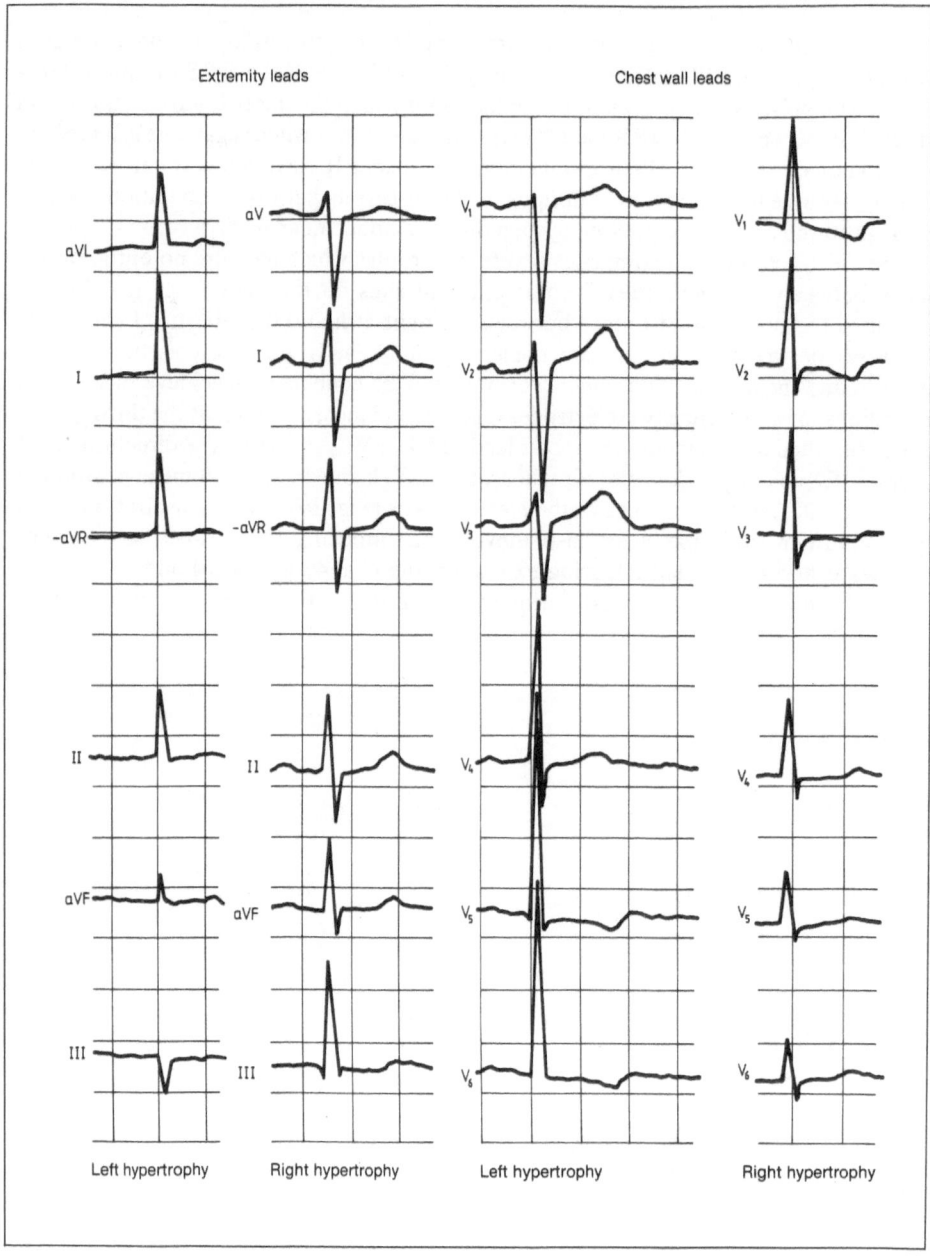

**Fig. 17.** Example of left and right ventricular hypertrophy in limb (extremity) and precordial (chest wall) leads.

when the diaphragm is displaced downward in a tall, thin subject. Many pathological conditions also influence the frontal plane axis.

If the polarity of the recording of aVR is reversed (-aVR), the six frontal plane recordings can be represented such that the axis change between each of them is 30°. The ECG changes continuously from lead recording to recording and the main axis of the QRS complex can then be easily defined (see Fig. 16).

While recording of the extremity leads will show potential differences in the frontal plane, changes in the horizontal plane are recorded with the unipolar precordial chest wall leads. Rotation of the electrical heart axis in the horizontal plane most often occurs with ventricular hypertrophy when the QRS vector moves towards the direction of the hypertrophied ventricle. With left ventricular hypertrophy, the vector moves to the left; with right ventricular hypertrophy, it moves to the right (Fig. 17).

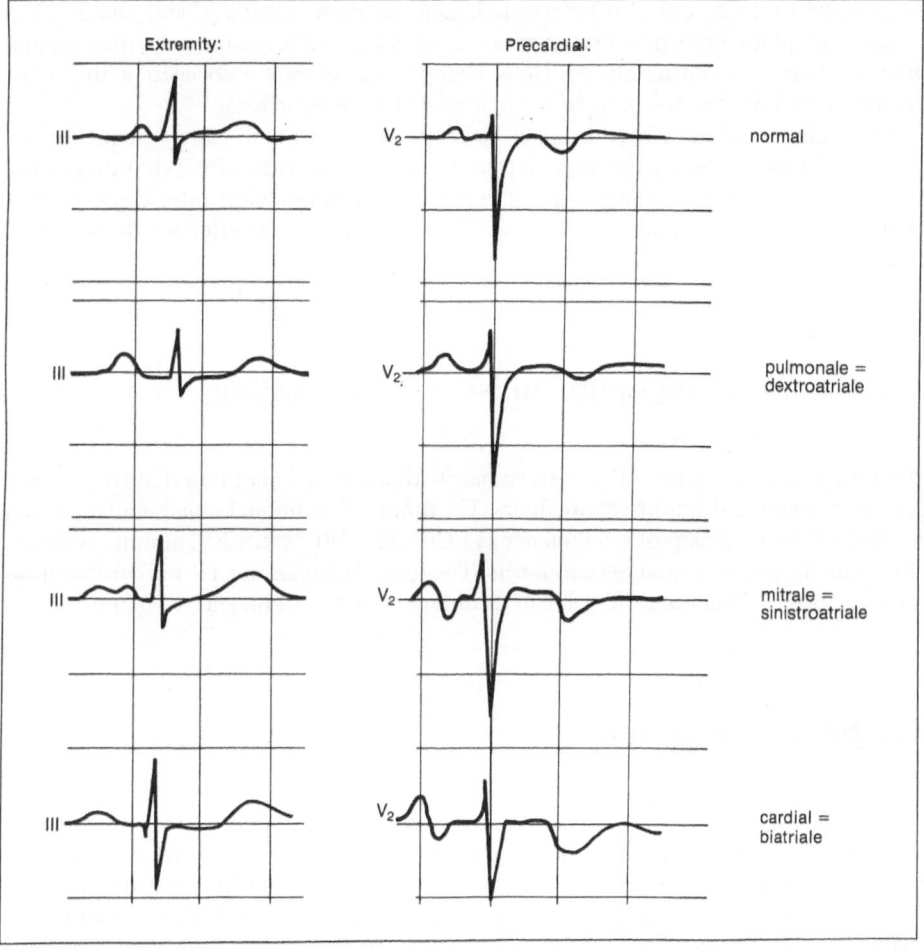

**Fig. 18.** Overload of one or both atria is diagnosed from changes in the P-wave usually best reflected in extremity lead III and precordial lead $V_2$.

The mean electrical axis of the heart corresponds to the largest positive vector of the QRS complex. However, each QRS complex comprises a series of sequential "instantaneous vectors". Sequential changes in the direction of the instantaneous QRS vectors can be displayed as a three-dimensional vector loop. During each heart cycle, these instantaneous vectors change not only in the frontal, but also in the horizontal and sagittal planes. A complete vector representation is therefore only possible with three-dimensional recordings. This is accomplished using three electrodes axes (x, y, and z) at right angles to each other (orthogonal axes). For practical purposes, however a spatial vector cardiogram recording does not routinely provide any definite diagnostic advantage compared to the standard 12 leads mentioned above.

Typical abnormalities of the P-waves due to overload of the atria are shown in Fig. 18.

Exercise electrocardiography is of important diagnostic value. This is especially true for the detection of ischemia which is not present at rest (see 4.2.2). Figure 12 (page 16) shows that in patients with coronary artery stenoses, ischemia can be provoked, not only by physical exercise, but also by catecholamine infusion. Similarly, ambulatory electrocardiographic monitoring often shows ischemic ST-segment depression during regular daily exercise and during stress. These changes are usually associated with angina pectoris (see 4.3), but may also be asymptomatic (silent ischemia).

The diagnosis of an arrhythmia can be established with ambulatory electrocardiographic monitoring using a recorder that can be worn by the patient for 24 h. Intracardiac electrocardiography recordings or recordings with esophageal electrodes allow analysis of the origin of arrhythmias, a step which is often the basis of effective therapy (see 12.2.4).

## 3.2 Phonocardiography, pulse-wave recordings

Phonocardiography records the heart sounds with a microphone; different frequencies can be separated and amplified with filters. The timing of additional sounds and murmurs is achieved with the help of a simultaneous ECG (Fig. 19). Recording of pulse waves is done with the help of pressure transducers. The typical changes seen in the carotid pulse wave in aortic valvular and subvalvular disorders are often of diagnostic value.

## 3.3 Echocardiography

The application of the ultrasonic beam to cardiology was pioneered by Edler and Hertz in Sweden. Originally, the ultrasonic beam gave only a restricted view of cardiac structures. However, today, clinical echocardiography readily allows two-dimensional visualization of all heart structures. Doppler flow-velocity assessments also allow valve stenosis and incompetence and other abnormal flow patterns to be recognized.

The ultrasound impulses are created by piezoelectric crystals which emit ultrasound waves at a frequency range of 2 to 10 MHz. The same crystals also convert the reflected

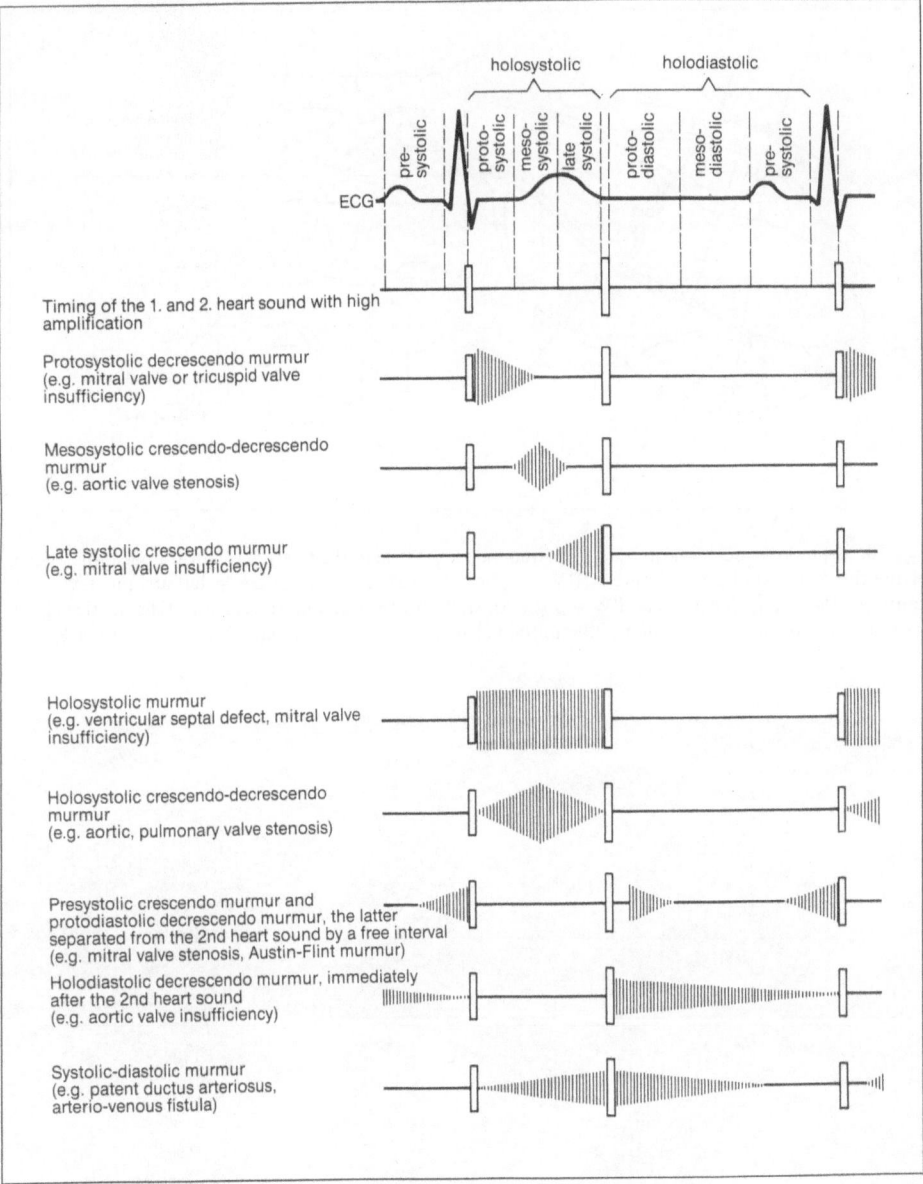

**Fig. 19.** ECG and phonocardiography findings in different cardiac disorders.

ultrasound back to electrical energy. One ultrasonic impulse produces multiple echoes. The time taken for the reflected echoes to return to the transducer changes during a cardiac cycle due to movement of the cardiac structures from or towards the transducer. Those changes are recorded as time-motion tracings on an M-mode echocardiogram (Fig. 20). Two-dimensional echocardiography uses the same principle, but in this case

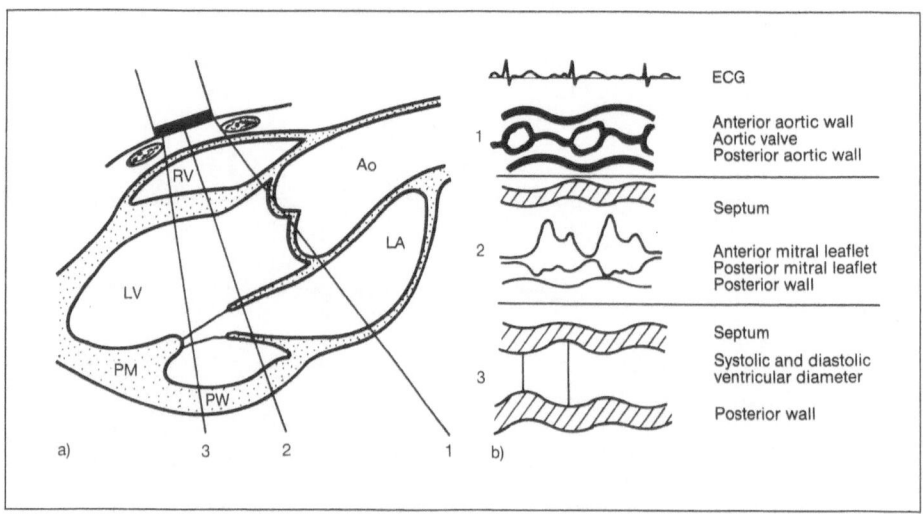

**Fig. 20.** M-mode echocardiography. **a** Longitudinal sector scan of the heart. **b** Echocardiographic images of the three typical planes 1, 2 and 3. RV = right ventricle; Ao = aorta; LA = left atrium; LV = left ventricle; PM = papillary muscle; PW = posterior wall. In 1 the opening and closing of the aortic valve is seen, in 2 the opening and closing of the mitral valve, and in 3 the contraction of the left ventricle.

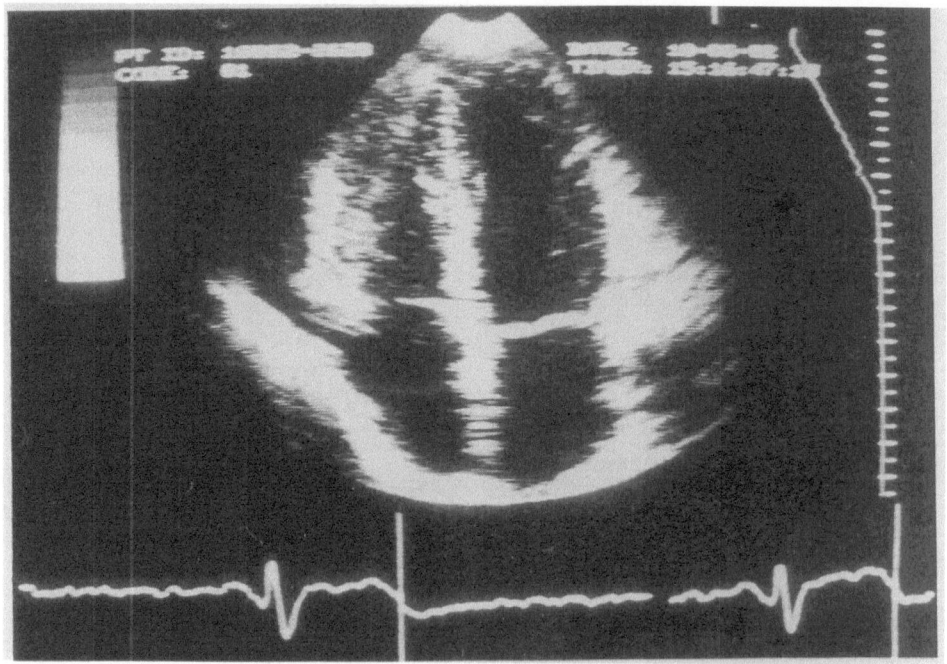

**Fig. 21.** Two-dimensional echocardiogram with visualization of all heart chambers with the "four-chamber-view" during diastole. The transducer is over the apex of the heart. Close to the transducer are both ventricles, below are tricuspid and mitral valves and both atria.

24

the ultrasonic beam moves rapidly within one plane. Thus, a cross-section of the heart can be obtained, where the cross-sectional plane, that is the plane of oscillation of the ultrasonic beam, is oriented to the diagnostically important structures of the heart (Fig. 21). Transducers emit the changing ultrasonic beam, either by mechanical or by electronic means. In the future, three-dimensional imaging is likely, comparable to the ECG recording in vectorcardiography. The ultrasonic beams will then need to oscillate in a number of planes to generate three-dimensional information. Another development is the use of intravascular ultrasound imaging for coronary and peripheral arteries, to visualize atheroma before and after various interventions.

## 3.4 Indicator dye dilution method

If dye is injected into the circulatory system, its flow within the blood stream can easily be traced (Fig. 22). Either the total blood flow velocity or special areas of interest, such as the flow between the peripheral venous system and the lung, or the lung and the peripheral arteries, can be determined. Formerly, circulation times were determined by intravenous injection of ether or decholine, and by measuring the time between the appearance of ether-smell in the breath and the patient reporting a bitter taste on his tongue. Today, measurements are done with indicator dyes. The thermodilution method uses cold fluid as the indicator. Circulation time and cardiac output are reliably measured with small thermistors, which are attached to a catheter. Measurements can be repeated many times. The dye dilution method can be applied during catheterization, but also noninvasively if the arrival of the dye is measured with a photo-electric cell on the ear lobe. The Fick principle and the thermodilution method are especially suitable for measurement of cardiac output. Dye dilution curves are used to determine shunting and pulmonary and systemic blood flows. Figure 22 features typically deformed dye dilution curves as a result of right-to-left or left-to-right shunts. It also shows that the area under the curve increases with decreasing cardiac output. The Fick cardiac output is calculated from the oxygen uptake and arteriovenous difference, using the equation

$$CO \ (l/min) = \frac{\text{oxygen uptake (ml/min)}}{\text{A-VO}_2 \text{ difference (ml/100 ml)} \times 10} \ .$$

The indicator dye dilution cardiac output uses the equation

$$CO \ (l/min) = \frac{I}{c \cdot t} \times \frac{60}{1000} \ .$$

I = dye dose (mg), c = mean concentration (mg/ml), t = duration of unrecirculated dye curve.

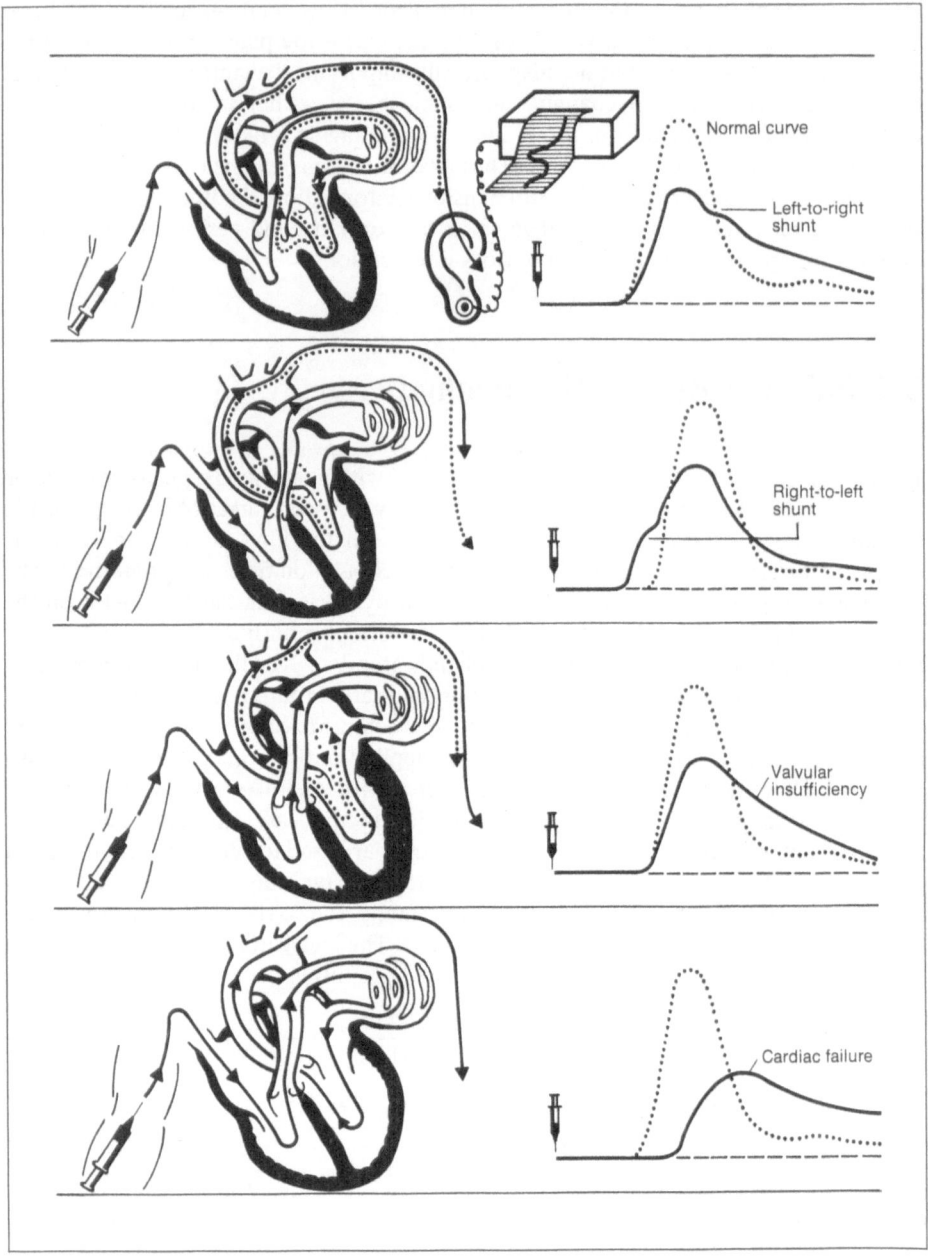

**Fig. 22.** Dye dilution curve with shunts between the pulmonary and systemic circulation (left-to-right and right-to-left shunts), valve insufficiency, and diminished cardiac output due to heart failure (mod. from [1]).

## 3.5 Radiologic examination of the thorax

### The chest roentgenogram

Views are taken in the upright position with a film-focus distance of 2 meters to avoid projection-related distortions. They allow assessment of the cardiac size and silhouette, and possible changes in the venous and arterial pulmonary vessels. Systemic venous congestion leads to an increased distension of the peripheral veins and the right atrium, while pulmonary venous congestion leads to enlarged pulmonary veins, increased interlobular and interalveolar markings (Kerley lines), and if combined with systemic congestion, pleural effusion. Increased pulmonary circulation due to a left-to-right shunt is usually associated with pulmonary arterial and venous engorgement.

### Chest fluoroscopy

Calcification of the cardiac valves, the pericardium, and the coronary arteries can be detected with fluoroscopy. The evaluation of densities, especially those in the mediastinal area may be clarified by rotation of the patient.

## 3.6 Determination of the heart volume

Determination of the heart volume in the recumbent position allows a clearer distinction between a normal and an abnormal cardiac size than does simple measuring of the usual upright chest x-ray. A key reason for the better discrimination of this assessment is that orthostatic changes in venous filling are avoided in the recumbent position. During

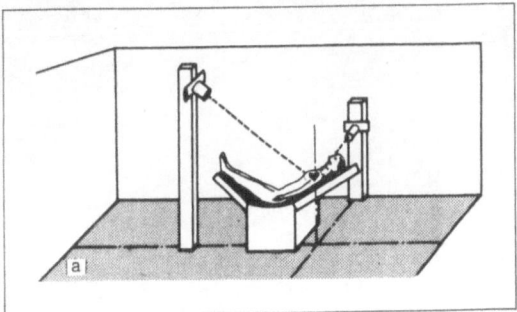

**Fig. 23.** Determination of the heart volume in a partially recumbent (half recumbent) position. Elevation of the legs results in complete filling of the heart, just as in a fully recumbent position, and orthostatic changes in filling are avoided. As opposed to the determination of the volume in the fully recumbent position, a focal distance of 2 meters can be obtained in a standard radiologic room.

recumbency, the heart is being more reliably distended by returning venous blood, thus fully filling the lower pressure system (i. e., the atria). With the upright position there can be a decrease in heart size of up to 50%. This decrease varies from day to day and also varies between individuals.

Due to the reasons given above, a quantitative evaluation of cardiac size is better done with determination of the heart volume than with the usual chest views in the upright position. This method has been used extensively by one of us (MK) for many years; not only is it useful, but it can be done with little extra effort. The two chest views document the cardiac status objectively and are always available for comparison later on.

The exact determination of the cardiac size is done with views of the heart in a recumbent or half-recumbent position (Figs. 23, 24). The half-recumbent position with elevation of the legs up to the cardiac level has the advantage that it will not result in an elevation of the diaphragm and, associated with it, a horizontal movement of the heart. Therefore, not only the heart size, but also changes of the cardiac silhouette can be judged in this position.

The heart volume is calculated using a formula for a rotational ellipsoid, corrected by the roentgenographic magnification (Fig. 25). With a film-focus distance of 2 meters the formula is:

$$\text{Cardiac volume} = \text{length (l)} \times \text{width (w)} \times \text{depth (d)} \times 0.4 \,.$$

Normal values for the cardiac volume are corrected for body weight, or even better, for body surface area. The normal heart volume ranges between 300 and 900 ml.

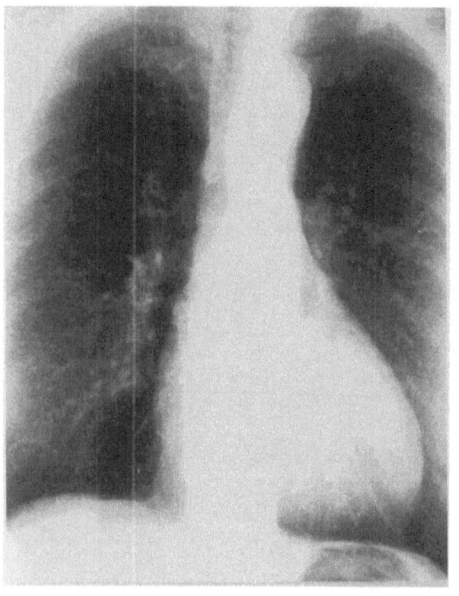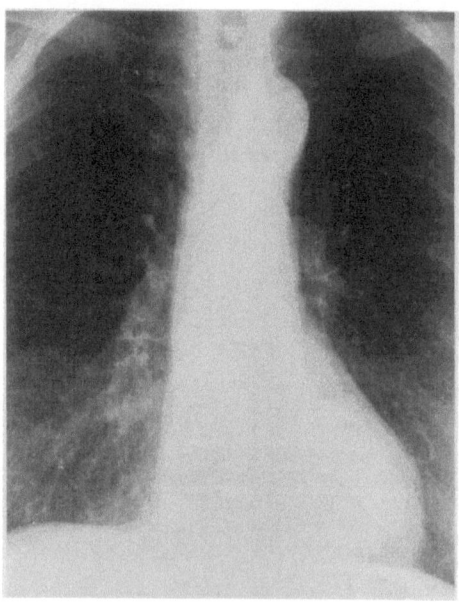

a           b

**Fig. 24.** The view in half recumbent position **a** shows a complete filling, as indicated by the right cardiac silhouette which corresponds to the right atrium; **b** view in the upright position for comparison; the right atrium is not completely filled.

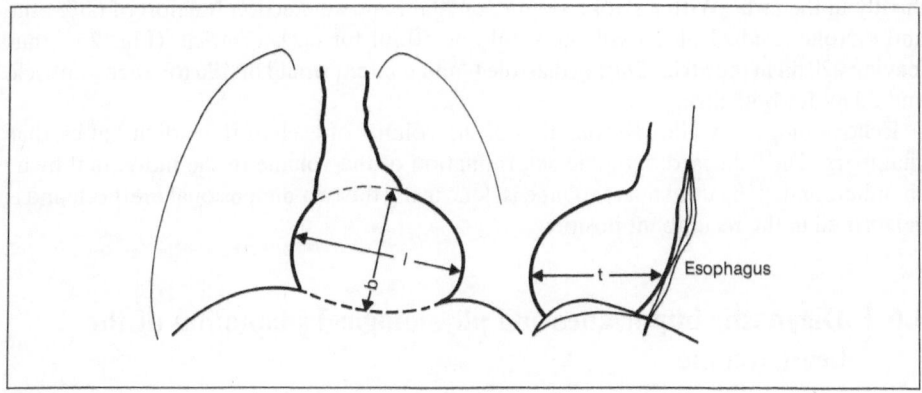

**Fig. 25.** The cardiac volume (cv) is calculated with the three axes (l, w, d) using the formula cv = l × w × d × 0.4.

The average (and upper limit) normal value for a man is 620 (800) ml/1.73 m$^2$. For a woman, it is 550 (700) ml/1.73 m$^2$. The average entire cardiac volume of an adult male of 620 ml corresponds a cardiac weight of 300 grams, this would mean that there would be approximately 320 ml of blood in the heart. This blood volume is distributed in both atria and ventricles. During diastole the volume is mostly in the ventricles, during systole it is

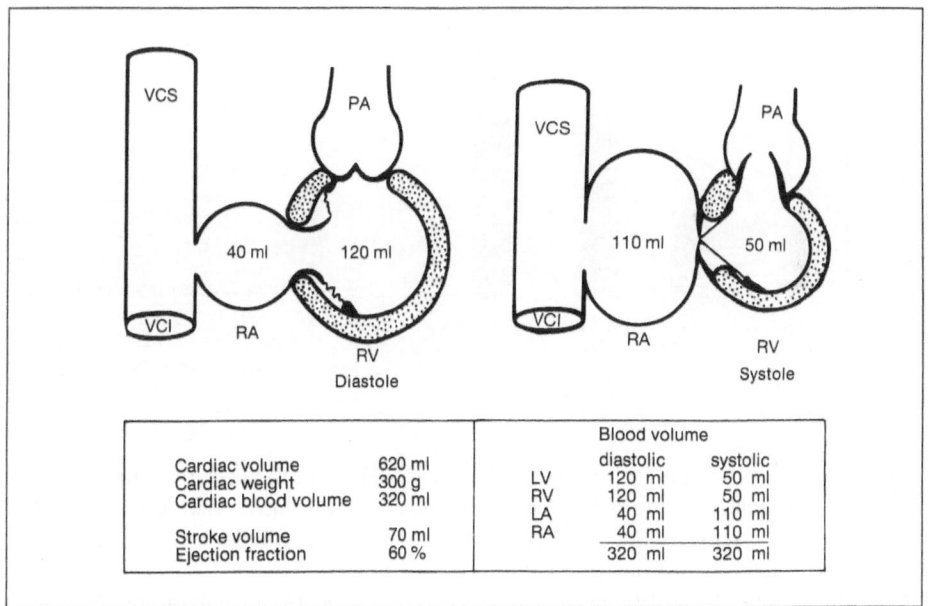

**Fig. 26.** The cardiac volume includes the heart itself (cardiac weight) and the blood within it. The cardiac volume remains constant throughout the cardiac cycle, since the sum of blood content in the ventricles plus atria remains constant during systole and diastole.

29

mostly in the atria. With a stroke volume of 70 ml and an ejection fraction of 60%, the end systolic residual blood volume would be 50 ml for each ventricle (Fig. 26), thus leaving 220 ml in the atria. During diastole blood content would be 120 for each ventricle and 80 ml for both atria.

Echocardiography allows estimation of the volume of each of the individual cardiac chambers. The echocardiographic determination of the volume of the individual heart chambers and of the total heart volume is done using the two-dimensional method, and is performed in the recumbent position.

### 3.6.1 Diagnostic importance and physiological adaptation of the heart volume

Endurance or interval training results in enlargement of the heart with physiological hypertrophy and dilatation of all cardiac chambers (see also 14.1). Pathological enlargement of the heart on the other hand can result, for example, from scar formation and compensatory dilatation of the left ventricle in coronary heart disease. The degree of the cardiac enlargement is a clue to the extent of tissue damage and it is therefore of prognostic importance (Fig. 27). This is also true for primary myocardial diseases, where the degree of the cardiac enlargement is an important parameter of severity and prognosis.

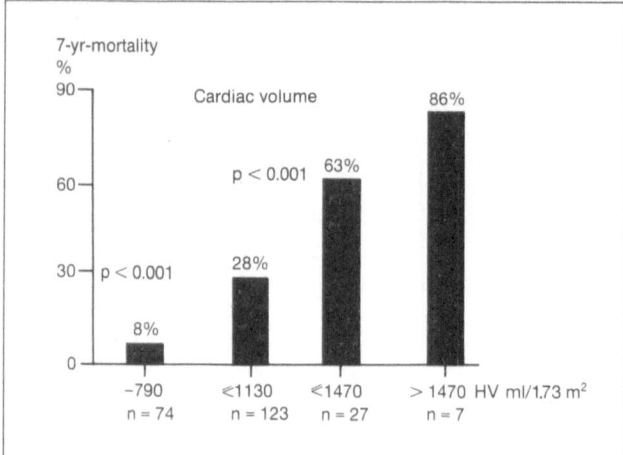

**Fig. 27.** Seven-year mortality rates for patients with coronary heart disease in relation to heart volume determined at the initial examination.

Whereas volume loading of the heart due to valvular insufficiency or shunt quickly leads to cardiac enlargement, pressure loading due to aortic stenosis, pulmonary stenosis or systemic hypertension does not result in early cardiac enlargement. Concentric hypertrophy, however, does occur in these latter disorders.

Enlargement of the entire heart is not always caused by an enlargement of the ventricular chambers; it may be caused by enlargement of the ventricles plus atria or of the atria alone. If blood flow into the ventricle is impeded, there will be hypertrophy and enlargement of the corresponding atrium. This occurs in coronary heart disease where

30

infarction has stiffened the left ventricle, in many valvular disorders (e.g., mitral stenosis) and in primary myocardial diseases. Disorders with concentric hypertrophy such as aortic stenosis or hypertrophic cardiomyopathy may lead to substantial atrial enlargement before the left ventricle increases in size. Due to the fact that all cardiac chambers are included in the determination of the total heart volume, significant cardiac enlargement may be measurable before the echo-derived measurements of individual cardiac chambers become abnormal.

Determination of the heart volume is also useful for the early diagnosis of cardiac decompensation. On the other hand, it can be used for a quantitative assessment of the effects of cardiac volume overloading associated with atrial septal defect or aortic insufficiency. It also may be suitable for making an early diagnosis of heart failure, for example, when distinguishing between cardiac and non-cardiac edema. Finally, it is of prognostic use in heart failure, in valvular disorders, and in coronary heart disease. With 2D-echocardiography determination of cardiac volume has become an easily available quantitative measure of cardiac size.

### 3.6.2 Subtraction angiography

The principle of the subtraction technique is a photographic subtraction of two different roentgenographic images of the same body area. For example, the image of blood vessels filled with a contrast agent on one picture can be enhanced when all other structures which are identical to both images have been subtracted and are therefore made invisible.

With digital subtraction angiography (DSA) the digitized information can be manipulated to enhance, magnify, smooth-out and erase parts of the image. The subtraction technique can be adapted to many different purposes and allows for visualization of the cardiac chambers, the great arteries and veins after intravenous injection of small boluses of contrast agent. Visualization becomes more difficult as the structures get smaller and move faster. Whereas the cardiac chambers can be presented with sufficient exactness, the visualization of details inside the coronary arteries is not sufficiently sharp after intravenous contrast injection. The proximal parts of bypass grafts, on the other hand, can usually be visualized due to their larger size and limited movement.

## 3.7 Nuclear imaging techniques (see also 4.2.3)

### 3.7.1 Radionuclide ventriculography

A collimated scintillation camera placed over the heart measures the scintillation counts of radionuclide-labeled erythrocytes. With electrocardiographic triggering cumulative counting during systole and diastole can be obtained, allowing the calculation of ventricular volumes, ejection fraction, regional wall motion, and the filling and ejection rates. Cardiac output can be determined using the indicator dilution principle if the first passage of the indicator through the heart is analyzed. Forward stroke volume (SV) may be calculated from the cardiac output (CO) and heart rate (HR) where

$$SV = \frac{CO}{HR} \, .$$

A comparison of the forward stroke volume measured after bolus injection with the total stroke volume measured during steady state is a noninvasive index of the degree of valvular insufficiency or intracardiac shunting. Radionuclide ventriculography during exercise may reveal global and regional contractile abnormalities induced by ischemia (see also 4.2.3)

### 3.7.2 Thallium scintigraphy

Thallium is biologically similar to potassium. It is rapidly extracted from the blood and is avidly taken up by myocardium. An image of the myocardium can be obtained by precordial counting of radiolabeled thallium using a scintillation camera. Persistent filling defects will be seen if thallium uptake is deficient (e.g., in myocardial infarction). A temporary exercise-induced disturbance of relative coronary flow causes the phenomenon of redistribution: 1–4 h after the injection, filling defects which were seen directly after injection of thallium will no longer be found in the scintigram (see also 4.2.3).

## 3.8 Computed tomography, positron emission tomography, nuclear magnetic resonance

Computed tomography results in cross-sectional images of the internal organs similar to the ultrasound technique. For imaging of the heart a rapid scanning sequence (ultrafast CT) or electrocardiographic gating is necessary (cardiac computed tomography, CCT). Diastolic and systolic cross-sectional images of the heart allow excellent visualization of hypertrophic cardiomyopathy for example.

The metabolic activity of the myocardium can be studied with the positron emission camera. The examination requires a major financial investment, which beyond research so far does not appear justified by the clinical value of the information provided.

The application of nuclear magnetic resonance (NMR) was developed in Great Britain and is based on a revolutionary imaging principle. The nuclear spin of atomic nuclei (in this context, the most important being the hydrogen ion) is altered by strong external magnetic fields. The return of the aligned nuclei to a random order pattern of spin, induced by strong external magnetic fields, occurs with different velocities in different imaged tissues. Tissue structures can therefore be discriminated in this way. Whereas nuclear magnetic resonance imaging is indicated in studies of the central nervous system, its application for imaging of the heart is still being investigated.

# 3.9 Cardiac catheterization

In 1929, Werner Forsmann showed, for the first time, that it was possible to insert a catheter into the human heart and to measure pressures, withdraw blood samples, and visualize heart structures by injection of contrast agents. Amazingly, his first experiment was on himself and although it earned him little recognition at the time, he was awarded a Nobel Prize in 1956. Forsmann had also tried to find a therapeutic use for cardiac catheterization; e.g., he tried to augment the therapeutic effectiveness of certain medications by intracardiac administration. It was eventually another German, Andreas Gruentzig, who pioneered therapeutic cardiac catheterization when he introduced coronary balloon angioplasty in 1977.

Cardiac catheterization is the most reliable method for detecting many cardiac disorders. Figure 28 shows the approach to the right and left heart, and Figure 29 shows typical pressure curves. Intracardiac pressure measurements allow the hemodynamic consequences of valvular stenoses or shunts to be determined. The size and location of shunts can be determined by measurement of the oxygen content of blood samples obtained from different locations. Virtually all cardiac structures can be visualized using contrast agents injected into an appropriate part of the circulation and recorded on x-ray films or video. This approach is a standard one for recognizing pathologic changes of the cardiac valves and coronary arteries. Increasingly, non-invasive techniques are replacing cardiac catheterization, but so far this has not been possible for the examination of the coronary vessels. Selective coronary arteriography, first performed by Sones in 1957, is indispensable for imaging coronary anatomy. It remains the prerequisite for surgical revascularization and it is also an integral part of therapeutic coronary interventions such as angioplasty.

Complications may occur with coronary arteriography, but it has a relatively low risk (mortality rate less than 0.1%), considering how often seriously ill patients are examined.

Today, therapeutic interventions can also be performed during cardiac catheterization. Until recent years many of these interventions could be performed only during open-heart surgery and with the patient on a heart-lung machine. Coronary stenoses can be dilated with a Gruentzig balloon catheter with a good long-term result in the majority. Valvular stenoses (for example pulmonary, uncalcified aortic and mitral valve stenoses) and congenital narrowing of the great arteries may also be dilated with a balloon catheter. Finally, the cardiac catheter may be used to close congenital shunts such as patent ductus arteriosus or to create shunts for the alleviation of congenital malformations.

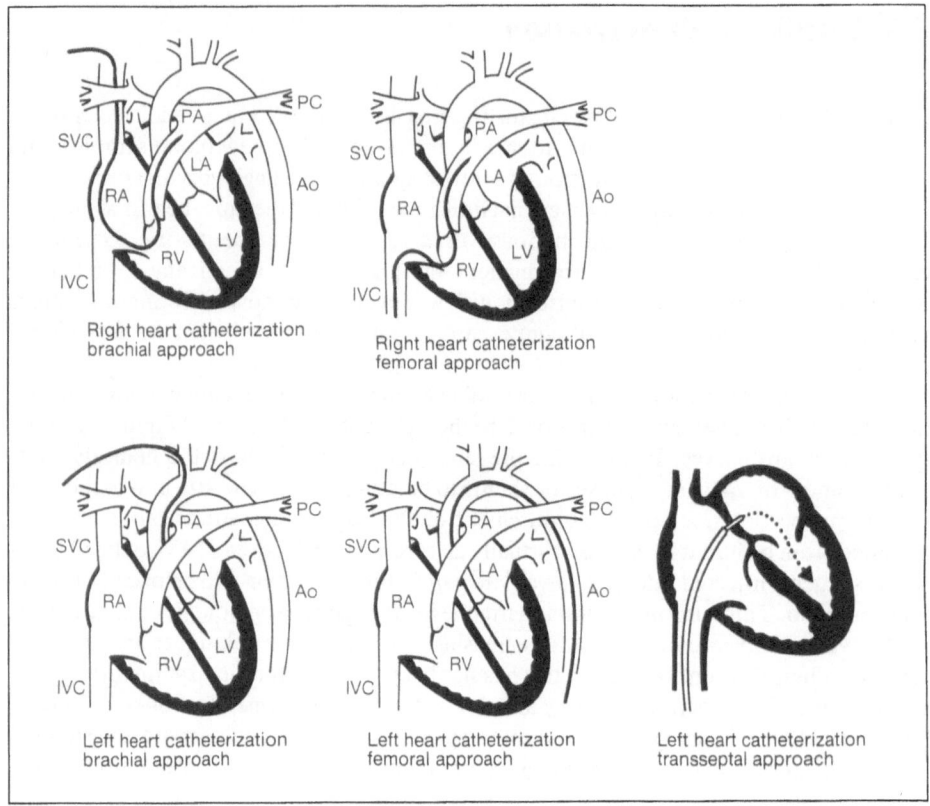

**Fig. 28.** Different approaches to right and left heart catheterization.

## 3.10 Cardiovascular measurements and their relation to body dimensions

In order to compare values obtained from individuals of different weight and size, a variety of "normalizing" methods are used. Cardiac output, the main hemodynamic parameter, is usually expressed per m² body surface area (BSA); other parameters are often given per body weight or height. For standardization purposes, a reference per normal body surface area of 1.73 m², as also widely used for renal clearance, seems attractive. A normal value referred to a body surface area of 1.73 m² is applicable to the normal adult and therefore more meaningful than a normal value referred to 1.0 m² which corresponds to a body surface area of an 8-year-old child. As far as possible, normal values are reported per normal body surface area in this book. The calculation is done with the formula:

$$\text{value/normal body surface area} = \frac{\text{value} \times 1.73}{\text{individual body surface area}}.$$

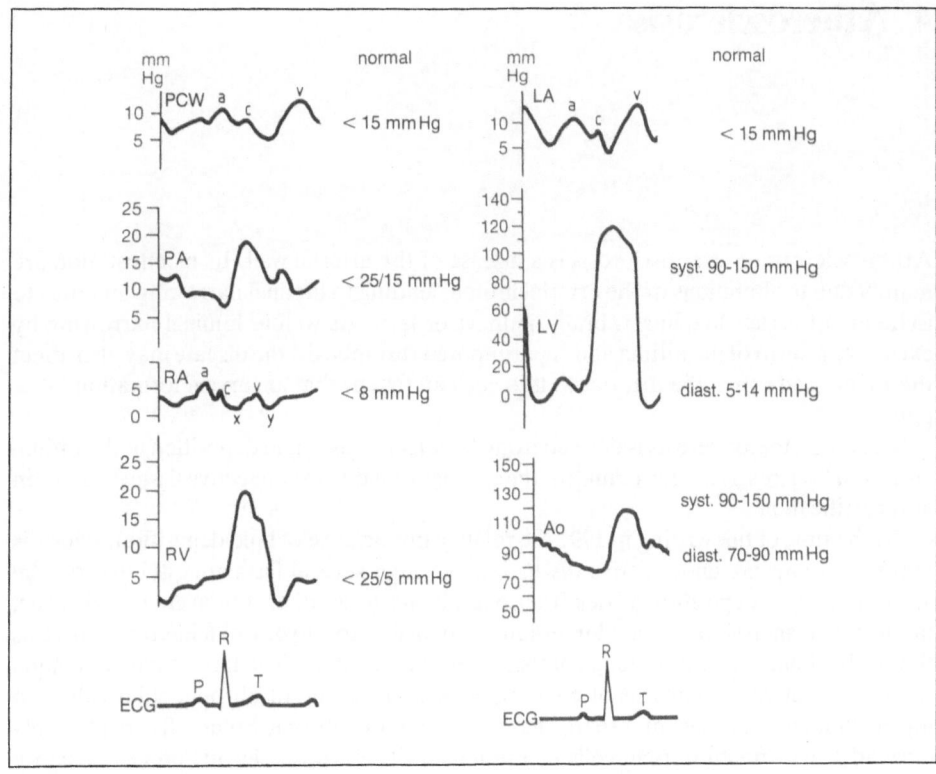

**Fig. 29.** Pressure curves and normal pressure values in the pulmonary capillary wedge (PCW), pulmonary artery (PA), right atrium (RA), right ventricle (RV), left atrium (LA), left ventricle (LV), and aorta (Ao) in relation to the ECG.

A good correlation can be made between the body surface area and the metabolically active body mass, as opposed to weight, which increases in adiposity which is of low metabolic activity. Theoretically, instead of body surface area, one might use the 4th root of the body weight raised to the third power (body weight$^{3/4}$). However this measure does not take into account differencies in height and therefore is inferior in comparing patients of identical weight but different degrees of adiposity.

Theoretical considerations, experimental findings, and practical clinical experience call for the use of anatomical and functional circulatory parameters to be referred to the average body surface area of 1.73 m$^2$. The same holds true for judging the dosage of medications. With the help of a calculator it is easy to determine the individual body surface area from the height and weight. Instead of a table or use of the more complicated formula from Dubois and Dubois, one can use a simplified version (after Mosteller, Lam):

$$\text{BSA} = \frac{\text{weight in kg} \times \text{height in cm}}{3600}.$$

35

# 4 Atherosclerosis

Atherosclerosis or arteriosclerosis is a disease of the arterial wall. Its manifestation are mainly due to alterations of the arterial intima, leading to luminal narrowing and thus to ischemia of organs like heart, brain, kidneys or legs. As well as luminal narrowing by excessive growth of the intima and superimposed thrombosis, the disease may also affect the media and soften the arterial wall to such an extent that aneurysm formation takes place.

The term atherosclerosis is derived from "atheroma" as a lipid deposition in the intima and from "sclerosis" i.e. hardening of the arterial wall due to connective tissue formation and calcification.

At the time of this writing in 1991 the relative importance of lipid deposition, sclerosis and thrombosis are under active discussion although several facts are established. The amount of lipid deposition varies from one plaque to another. On average, however, quantitative analysis performed in lesions responsible for myocardial infarction reveals that only about 5% of the tissue consists of lipid deposition. The largest part of plaque tissue – about 90% – consists of connective tissue made up of fibromuscular cells and intracellular matrix. Recent research has shown that the fibromuscular cells are probably derived from smooth muscle cells of the media. The arteriosclerotic process seen on serial histological examinations in men and animals may manifest as rapid progression or complete standstill. In the presence of increased fibromuscular cell proliferation progression occurs, while a standstill is seen if matrix is predominantly produced in such a way as seen in normal scar formation. The occurrence of restenosis after balloon angioplasty is clearly related to increased fibromuscular proliferation. Therefore an intensive search for antiproliferative drugs is now undgoing. It is also apparent that proliferation is stimulated by mechanical damage such as overstretching or excision. Many growth factors have been defined; on immunohistology their presence can be seen in the vicinity of multiplying cells.

In addition to lipid deposition and cellular proliferation the atherosclerotic process is determined by the occurrence of intraluminal thrombosis. In transmural myocardial infarction for example, formation of an occluding thrombus is responsible for the vessel obstruction causing the infarct. Thrombus formation is mostly triggered by a tear in the intima made fragile as a consequence of the arteriosclerotic process.

In modern times atherosclerosis has become the major cause of mortality and morbidity in civilized countries. It is, on the other hand, a very old disease, even recognizable in Egyptian mummies. Its predominance in modern times has been attributed to our modern lifestyle including stress and overeating. However, its emergence might also be ascribed to increased life expectancy since old age is a major risk factor for arteriosclerosis. Life expectancy has increased in the last 100 years from less than 35 years to more than 75 years of age and every year of further extension of life expectancy will produce more arteriosclerosis.

Dealing with atherosclerosis has to begin with prevention. A discontinuation of cigarette smoking is a well-documented effective measure. A healthy lifestyle with sufficient exercise, sleep, a balance between stress and relaxation, and an ideal body weight are probably beneficial as well. There is good evidence that lowering of cholesterol can be achieved by diet and drugs. Several multicenter studies are presently attempting to assess the value of this type of intervention for the evolution of the atherosclerotic process. Calcium antagonists can decrease the occurrence of atherosclerosis in animals. There is also some evidence that these drugs have an influence on human atherosclerosis. The beneficial influence of platelet aggregation inhibitors, particularly aspirin, on preventing arterial thrombosis and platelet embolism has been shown in coronary and cerebrovascular syndromes. Despite several advances, atherosclerosis remains one of the major challenges for scientific research in the nineties.

# 4.1 Coronary heart disease

## 4.1.1 Definition

Coronary heart disease or ischemic heart disease is defined as the cardiac consequences of transient or persistent coronary artery obstruction. The disease includes the symptom-free forms of myocardial ischemia, symptomatic ischemic syndromes such as angina pectoris, and heart muscle infarction caused by occlusion of coronary arteries. If a large amount of myocardium is damaged by a single large myocardial infarction or multiple smaller infarcts, coronary artery disease may lead to heart failure. The different phases of coronary artery disease may play out slowly over decades, but also very rapidly within a few hours.

## 4.1.2 Pathophysiology

The clinical manifestations depend on the degree of narrowing of the coronary arteries (Fig. 30). Physiologically, the human coronary circulation makes good provision for the myocardial oxygen requirements. Nearly all the oxygen in the coronary arterial blood is extracted by the myocardium, even at rest, so any further oxygen delivery needed during exercise must be brought by an increase in flow. The oxygen demand and coronary flow at rest corresponds approximately to one-fifth of the demand and flow at maximal exercise. Coronary insufficiency (and resultant ischemia) is defined as a mismatch between myocardial oxygen supply and demand. Such a mismatch will occur at rest only if the coronary arteries are very severely narrowed, whereas coronary insufficiency during strenuous exercise will occur with moderate narrowing.

An area stenosis of up to 50% will not result in coronary insufficiency at maximum exertion. Exercise-induced angina will usually only be clinically manifest with an area stenosis of more than 75%, and coronary insufficiency at rest only with an area stenosis of 99% (see Fig. 30). The degree of stenosis may be augmented by an increase in coronary

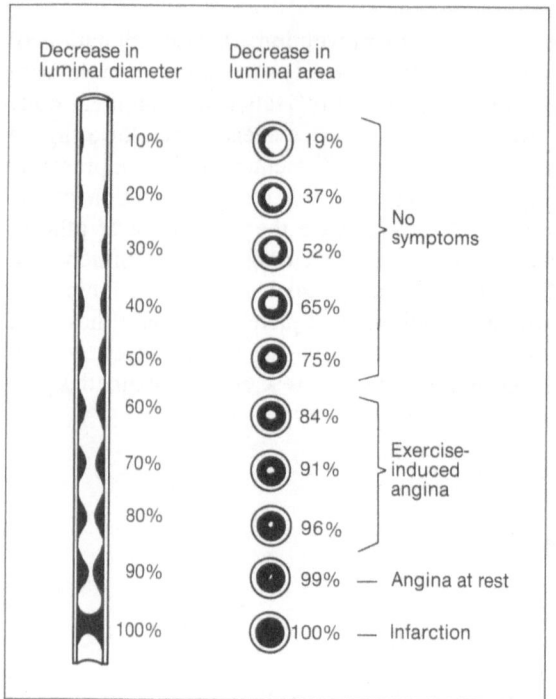

Fig. 30. Reduction in diameter caused by coronary atherosclerosis. On the left, diameter stenoses as reported from the arteriogram; on the right the resulting area stenosis. Clinical symptoms occur only with high-grade stenoses.

smooth muscle tone. Collaterals may diminish the effects of a high-grade stenosis or total occlusion in some patients.

Formerly, it was debated whether the consequences of coronary artery disease such as angina pectoris ("angina of the chest" from angeion = suffocating, seizing by the throat) and myocardial infarction were really caused by coronary artery stenoses. Heberden wrote the classical description of the symptoms of angina pectoris in 1768, and he knew that patients with this clinical manifestation were at risk of sudden death, but he did not know the cause. In one patient with typical clinical manifestations, and who had given prior permission for an autopsy, no clear cause of death could be established. It was only decades later that the location of the disease in the coronary arteries was recognized. Even up until recently there were physicians who challenged the association of coronary artery occlusion and myocardial infarction and believed that necrosis of the myocardium developed first, and that thrombotic coronary artery occlusion was only a secondary effect. However, coronary angiography during acute myocardial infarction has now shown that an occlusion, usually of thrombotic origin, occurs at the onset of nearly every transmural infarction.

Coronary atherosclerosis is, in principle, the same disease process which is found in other areas of the body. In the limbs it is known as peripheral arterial occlusive disease ("smoker's leg"), and in the cerebral arteries it causes cerebral ischemia, which manifests as transient ischemic attacks (TIAs) or as brain infarction (stroke).

### 4.1.3 Coronary arteries

The human coronary circulation is based on two major coronary arteries (Fig. 31). Typically, the left coronary artery provides blood flow for the entire anterior and lateral wall of the left ventricle and the major part of the ventricular septum, whereas the right coronary artery perfuses the right ventricle, the diaphragmatic (inferior) wall and posterior one-third of the septum. There is considerable variation in the anatomic pattern of these vessels. The most frequent pattern, seen in approximately 80% of people, has a "dominant" right coronary artery (Fig. 32) which supplies the right as well as parts of the left ventricle. The consequences of vessel occlusion depend on the anatomic pattern of the coronary arteries. Therefore, a total occlusion of the right coronary artery may be without clinical consequences in a left dominant circulation, whereas it may lead to a major inferior myocardial infarction with extension to the septum in a right dominant circulation. The right ventricle is not as vulnerable to coronary occlusion as is the left ventricle. Infarction of the right ventricle often involves multiple small necrotic areas, whereas in the left ventricle a large and fully infarcted area is usually seen.

Because the right coronary artery divides only very distally into a posterior descending branch (which supplies blood flow to the posterior septum) and a posterolateral ventricular branch, a proximal occlusion of the right coronary artery has similar hemodynamic consequences as a distal one. In contrast, the left coronary artery divides into two major branches shortly after its origin from the aorta. A total occlusion of the left main stem is therefore extremely dangerous and rarely survived.

Physiologically, the coronary arteries enlarge according to the mass of myocardium to be perfused. However, an overloaded demand (for example, induced by severe systemic hypertension or aortic stenosis) may lead to coronary insufficiency even when stenosis is absent. Diastole is the most important phase of the cardiac cycle for blood supply to the myocardium, because only in diastole is there a sufficient pressure gradient between the coronary artery and the capillary bed. A decrease in diastolic aortic pressure will therefore affect the coronary circulation in a manner similar to an increase in diastolic ventricular pressure.

The pressure in the inner layers of the ventricular myocardium is the same as the intraventricular pressure itself. The subendocardial area of the myocardium is thus most vulnerable for ischemia, because coronary arteries are epicardial and the subendocardium is the "letzte Wiese" of the blood flow ("letzte Wiese" is a German saying which means "the most remote meadow", thus the most remote area to be supplied by blood flow). In the case of severe aortic stenosis, a large subendocardial infarction may occur with normal coronary arteries. Similarly, subtotal coronary artery stenoses may lead only to subendocardial or non-transmural myocardial infarction.

### 4.1.4 Collaterals

There are vascular connections or collaterals between the right and left coronary artery. In the case of total occlusion, they may be important for sustaining a minimal perfusion. Typically, collaterals are seen in the area of the atria, the posterior wall, the septum, and

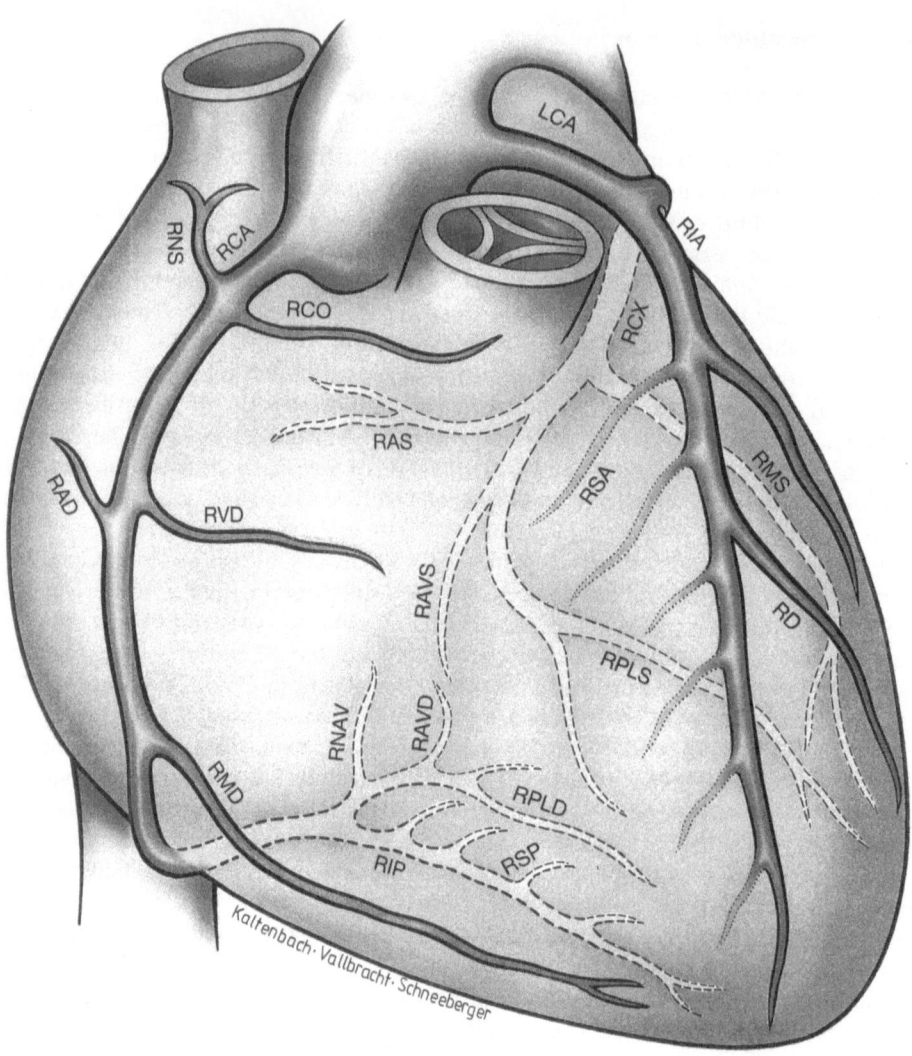

**Fig. 31.** Anatomy and classification of the coronary arteries.

<u>*RCA*</u>  Right coronary artery
(= *ACD* A. coronaria dextra)

| | |
|---|---|
| *RNS* | Ramus nodi sinuatrialis |
| *RCO* | Ramus coni arteriosi |
| *RVD* | Ramus ventricularis dexter |
| *RAD* | Ramus atrialis dexter |
| *RMD* | Ramus marginalis dexter |
| *RNAV* | Ramus nodi atrioventricularis |
| *RIP* | Ramus interventricularis posterior |
| *RAVD* | Ramus atrioventricularis dexter |
| *RPLD* | Ramus posterolateralis dexter |
| *RSP* | Ramus septalis dexter |

<u>*LCA*</u>  Left coronary artery
(= *ACS* A. coronaria sinistra)

| | |
|---|---|
| *RIA* | Ramus interventricularis anterior (often also *LAD:* left anterior descending) |
| *RCX* | Ramus circumflexus |
| *RD* | Ramus diagonalis |
| *RSA* | Ramus septalis anterior |
| *RMS* | Ramus marginalis sinister |
| *RAS* | Ramus atrialis sinister |
| *RPLS* | Ramus posterolateralis sinister |
| *RAVS* | Ramus atrioventricularis sinister |

40

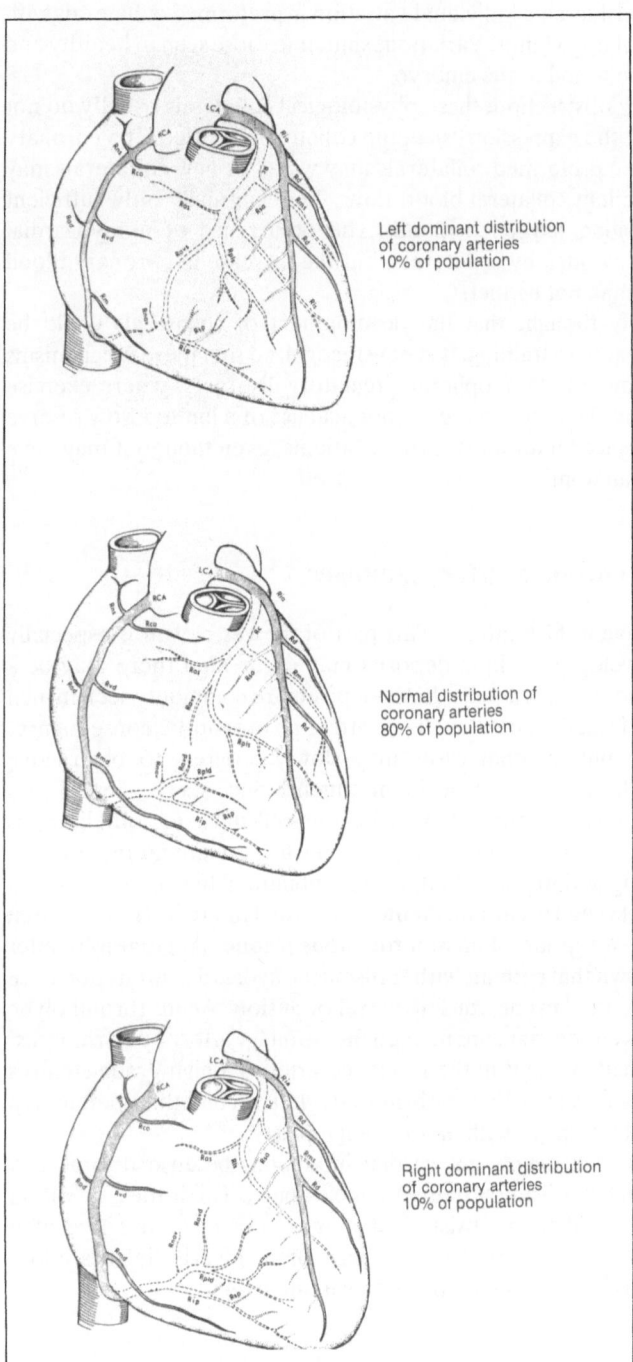

Left dominant distribution
of coronary arteries
10% of population

Normal distribution of
coronary arteries
80% of population

Right dominant distribution
of coronary arteries
10% of population

**Fig. 32.** The three typical patterns of coronary artery distribution. The normal pattern with a so-called dominant right coronary artery occurs most often (80% of cases), the extreme right or left dominant distributions make up the remainder (each about 10%). The consequences of an occlusion of the circumflex or the right coronary artery depend on the type of vessel distribution.

41

the anterior wall. There is considerable individual variation in preformed collaterals with some having a large caliber, of up to 1 mm. Variations similar to those seen in healthy and in diseased adults can also be found in the embryo.

In the absence of coronary obstruction, these physiological collaterals usually do not carry blood flow. Therefore, the expression "sleeping collaterals" is used. If a coronary occlusion occurs slowly, these preformed collaterals may widen or new collaterals may develop. But even with excellent collateral blood flow, there is usually only sufficient coronary circulation for resting oxygen demand. The occurrence of a myocardial infarction may therefore be avoided by collaterals, but the increase in coronary blood flow demanded by exercise may not be met.

Whereas it was previously thought that the development of collaterals could be induced with medication or exercise training, it is now recognized that these mechanisms have very little effect. Comparable to peripheral circulatory disorders, where exercise training of the skeletal muscles leads to a more economical use of a limited flow reserve the prescription of exercise is useful for most cardiac patients, even though it may have little effect on the coronary anatomy or coronary flow itself.

### 4.1.5 Development of coronary artery stenoses

Human coronary arteries have a thick intima. This part of the vessel wall is especially vulnerable. Edema may develop in it, lipid deposits may occur, and there may be a proliferation of fibrous or smooth muscle cells. Lipid deposits are commonly seen in men by the age of 20 to 30 years. Usually, however, these are of no prognostic consequence. Such deposits may regress, but in other cases may slowly progress to obstructive atheroma. The atheroma will then be of clinical consequence once severe stenosis has developed. The innermost layer of the intima (the one-cell-thick endothelium) is especially vulnerable. An atheroma becomes complicated when an intimal tear occurs, leading to subintimal bleeding and to platelet adhesion. Subintimal bleeding or luminal thrombosis may result in total vessel occlusion. Acute myocardial infarction is most often initiated by such a tear, i.e., a rupture of an atheromatous plaque. Angiography after thrombolytic therapy has shown that patients with transmural myocardial infarction have an occluding thrombus as the final event, causing vessel occlusion. Acute thrombolytic therapy is a therapeutic intervention that aims to open the coronary artery by fibrinolysis. This is achieved in 70% of patients, but in the reopened arteries a high-grade stenosis caused by the atheroma usually remains after fibrinolysis. In a second therapeutic step one may need to eliminate the stenosis with balloon angioplasty.

Thrombolytic therapy rarely prevents myocardial infarction, because it is usually applied after the myocardium has already sustained some damage. This is the case within 1–2 h, especially if no good collaterals exist. But a reduction in infarct size with thrombolytic therapy has been shown up to 6 h after onset of the myocardial infarction, and a beneficial effect on survival has been reported even up to 24 h.

## 4.1.6 Implications of coronary heart disease, risk factors, progression

Cigarette smoking is a well-documented risk factor. The frequency of myocardial infarction and angina pectoris correlates with the number of cigarettes smoked per day. A clear lower limit, that is an amount of cigarettes which is not dangerous, does not exist.

The risk factor of cigarette smoking is most important in young men and women, less so in persons above 60 years of age, because then age as a risk factor per se becomes of dominant importance.

The combination of cigarette smoking and hormonal contraceptives is a powerful risk combination for myocardial infarction or angina pectoris in young women. It is probably the increased tendency to form intravascular thrombi with this combination that causes both cardiac and cerebral vascular complications.

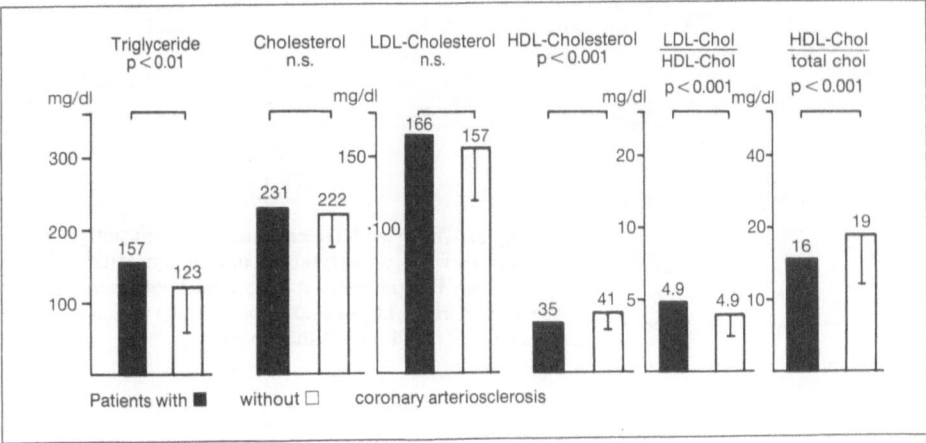

**Fig. 33.** Age and sex-adjusted comparison of patients with angiographically documented coronary artery disease with patients having normal coronary arteries. There is a small but significant correlation of disease with elevated triglycerides, with higher total and LDL cholesterol, and decreased HDL cholesterol. (Data from patients studied at Frankfurt University Hospital.)

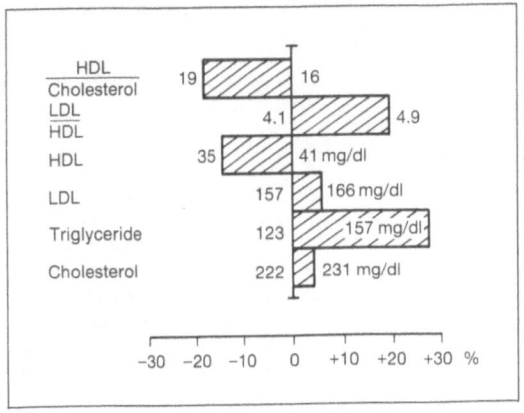

**Fig. 34.** Compared to healthy persons the average cholesterol is elevated by 4%, triglyceride by 28%, and LDL by 6% in persons with coronary artery disease, and HDL is 15% lower. The ratios change respectively.

43

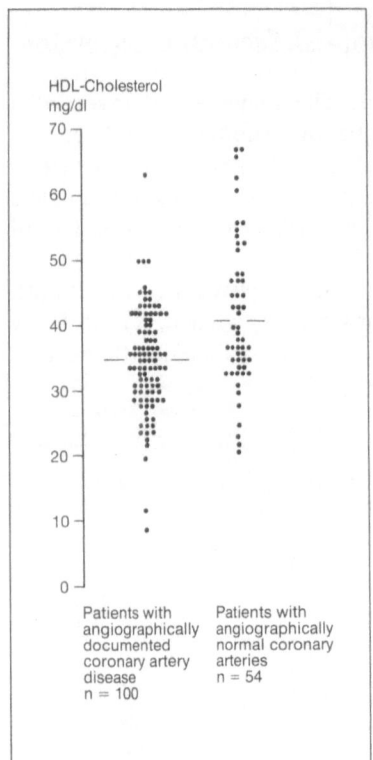

Fig. 35. The mean HDL cholesterol is significantly lower in persons with coronary artery disease compared to those without. But the levels overlap quite a lot, therefore, the level of HDL has individual prognostic value only if it is above 50 mg/dl, or less than 25 mg/dl.

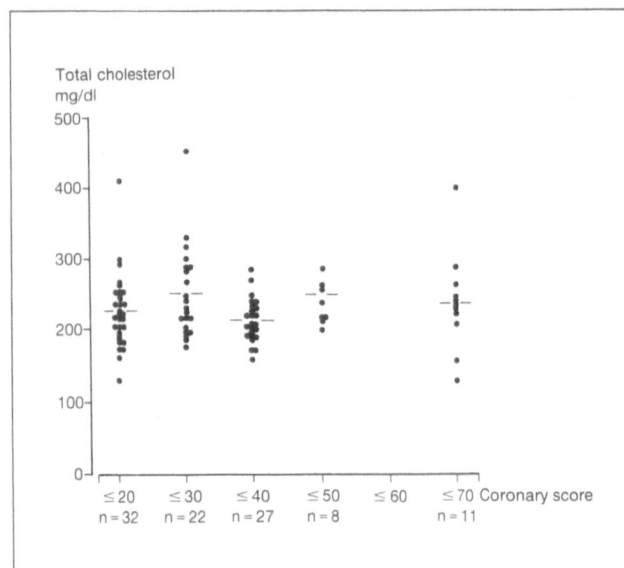

Fig. 36. No apparent relationship is seen between total cholesterol concentration and degree of angiographically documented coronary artery disease in 100 patients. A score of 20 represents mild, while 70 represents severe coronary artery disease.

Withdrawal from cigarette smoking leads, within a few years, to a reduction towards the usual base risk for progression of coronary artery disease. This consistent finding is surprising if one considers the chronicity of atherosclerosis. It is also in contrast to a continuing risk for lung cancer after quitting smoking, which mainly depends on the total quantity of cigarettes inhaled.

There is a correlation between the level of total serum cholesterol and the occurrence of myocardial infarction. A comparison of the extent of angiographically determined coronary artery stenoses with the total serum cholesterol shows less correlation (Figs. 33–36). The same applies with fractions of the lipids or ratios of the different fractions. Recent studies have shown an increase in cholesterol blood levels with age: from 200 mg at age 20, to 260 mg at age 60. If the incidence of coronary arteriosclerosis is correlated with cholesterol blood levels, this has to be taken into account.

In patients with and without angiographically visualized coronary artery disease there is significant overlap in lipid values, including HDL (see. Fig. 35). A reasonable separation of individuals with and without disease is only possible with levels greater than 50 mg/dl or less than 25 mg/dl.

In order to prevent coronary artery disease, a reduction of total serum cholesterol (by reduction of body weight and a diet low in cholesterol and fat) is recommended. Lipid-lowering drugs should only be used in lipid disorders which do not respond to diet, because their long-term benefit is doubtful in mild cases, and they may have harmful side effects. Drug therapy is indicated in familial homozygous Type IIA hyperlipidemia. Large trials completed up to 1990 have not shown a decrease in total mortality with lipid-lowering therapy; although cardiac mortality had decreased there was an increase in mortality from other causes. Even without specific disorders of lipid metabolism there seems to be a familial risk factor for early occurrence of coronary artery disease. This should be suspected if myocardial infarction or angina pectoris occurred in first degree relatives particularly before 55 years of age.

In 1990, a study was published[1] in which the influence of lipid-lowering was evaluated in a placebo-controlled double-blind design in a group of high-risk male patients (mean age 47 years) with angiographically documented coronary artery disease and a positive family history. In the follow-up arteriograms after 2.5 years, progression was shown in 23% of patients in the treatment group, as compared to 46% in the control group. Some regression was seen in 35% of treated patients as compared to only 4% of the controls. The difference in stenosis severity between placebo and treated patients was however only 3%. This is be in accordance with what can be expected from the fact that the quantitative composition of arteriosclerotic lumen narrowing is about 5% lipid deposition, while the other 95% is mainly caused by cellular proliferation.

Age and the male sex are both strong risk factors for coronary artery disease. Women, especially of younger and middle age, have a much smaller risk for coronary artery disease than men. Obesity is not an independent risk factor, but it can become a risk factor with associated disorders of lipid metabolism, diabetes or hypertension.

Systemic hypertension is of major importance in the development of stroke, but of less importance for the occurrence of coronary artery disease. Control of hypertension does not show clear benefit for prevention of coronary artery disease.

1 G Braun, JJ Albers, Ld Fisher, SM Schaefer, JT Lin, C Kaplan, XQ Zhao, BD Bisson, VF Fitzpatrick, HT Dodge (1990) Regression of Coronary Artery Disease as a Result of Intensive Lipid-Lowering Therapy in Man with High Levels of Apolipoprotein B. N Engl J Med 323:1289–1298

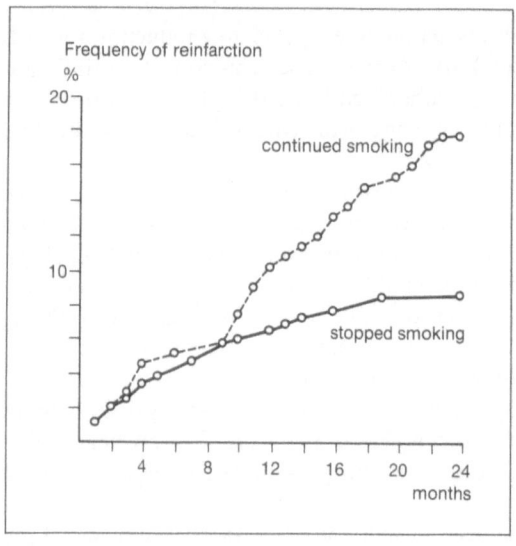

Frequency of reinfarction

%

20 —

continued smoking

10 —

stopped smoking

4    8    12    16    20    24
months

**Fig. 37.** Influence of cigarette smoking on myocardial infarction. The re-infarction rate is doubled if smoking continues.

Coronary artery disease is often linked with certain personality characteristics. The coronary patient is often seen as a tense achiever, compulsively meeting time-tables with suppressed aggression. However, scientific validation of this hypothesis is shaky and the critical physician should resist the temptation to assign coronary risk to personality traits. He should keep in mind that ischemia of the limbs or the brain is a consequence of exactly the same atherosclerotic disorder, and for these disorders, personality traits have not been implicated.

Just as in oncology, one may simplify the risk factors in cardiology by recognizing that cigarette smoking is the most important and most easily treatable risk factor. More than 25% of all tumors and myocardial infarctions could be avoided by non-smoking alone. The number of re-infarctions in patients who continue to smoke is double the rate of those who stop smoking (Fig. 37).

## 4.1.7 Prognosis

The prognosis of coronary artery disease depends on the degree of ischemia and the degree of myocardial damage.

A quantitative relationship with mortality can be established from coronary angiography: 1-, 2-, 3-vessel disease, main stem stenosis or the degree of coronary artery disease quantitated as a coronary score (Fig. 46). A similar relationship is revealed by quantification of ST-depression in the exercise ECG (Fig. 38).

The degree of impairment in left ventricular contraction, as seen in the cine angiogram, provides another important prognostic parameter. Valuable non-invasive parameters of myocardial damage may be obtained from the cardiac volume derived from x-ray or echocardiogram (Fig. 38).

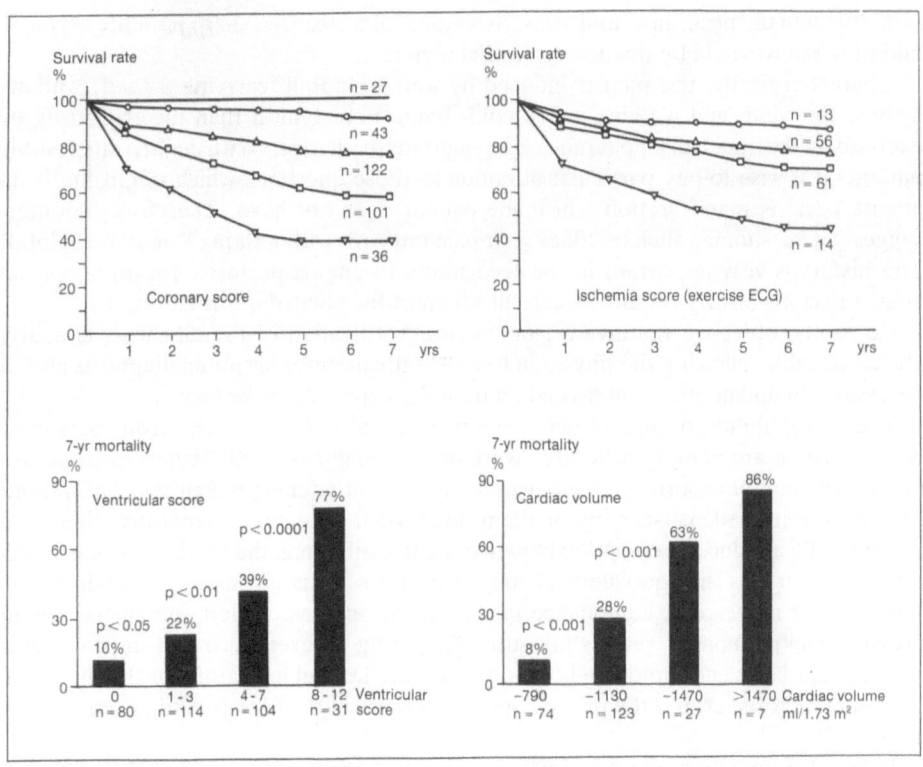

**Fig. 38.** Prognosis for the patient with coronary artery disease depends on the degree of angiographically documented coronary artery disease (coronary score see also Fig. 46). The degree of ischemia seen in the exercise ECG (ischemia score) is of equal prognostic importance (above left and right). Prognosis is also determined by the degree of myocardial damage. This can be evaluated from the angiogram of the left ventricle (ventricular score) or from the cardiac volume which are determined noninvasively (below left and right).

## 4.2 Diagnosis

### 4.2.1 History and physical examination

Coronary artery disease should be diagnosed as early as possible. The diagnosis is often first made when symptoms of ischemia occur with exercise. Symptom-free coronary artery disease, in contrast, is difficult to detect clinically. The diagnosis of an acute myocardial infarction is usually not difficult, but often it comes too late. About half of patients do not survive their first myocardial infarction.

Angina pectoris is the major clinical manifestation of myocardial ischemia. Angina pectoris refers to a sensation of tightness in the chest, and is a term which is used today only for myocardial ischemia. Chest pain due to other causes is not labeled with this term. The typical pain of angina pectoris is a tight dull heaviness behind the sternum, often radiating into the neck, jaw, and arms. Symptoms of a localized sharp pain are atypical, and only rarely would be due to myocardial ischemia.

Characteristically, the pain is induced by walking uphill, carrying a load, walking against the wind, and walking in the cold. Even more typical than the triggering by exercise is the rapid disappearance of symptoms with rest. With highly suggestible patients it is wise to pay particular attention to those questions which might imply an angina pectoris manifestation which the patient does not have. Therefore, counter-suggestive questioning such as "does your pain improve with walking?" may be helpful. The history is very important in the recognition of angina pectoris. Taking a correct angina pectoris history requires a careful sifting of the elicited information.

Currently, objective noninvasive or invasive verification of the diagnosis is nearly always possible, allowing the physician to constantly monitor his initial diagnosis and, if necessary, to update the diagnosis taken from the original case history.

The susceptibility to anginal pain from myocardial ischemia varies from person to person. There are patients who are aware of even slight ischemia, whereas there are others who do not experience pain even during life-threatening ischemia or infarction. This is known as silent ischemia or silent myocardial infarction. Generally, these are patients with a reduced perception of pain or neuropathy (e.g. diabetics). Some persons report dyspnea as an equivalent of angina pectoris. This is caused by an ischemic reduction of myocardial compliance leading to an increase in left ventricular filling pressure and pulmonary venous pressure. Triggering by exercise, rapid improvement after nitroglycerin and rapid amelioration at rest are helpful indicators for the diagnosis of angina pectoris, even if the pain component is more in the background or not present at all.

Physical examination may give further clues to a diagnosis of coronary artery disease. Absence of peripheral pulses or murmurs auscultated over the great arteries are highly suggestive of generalized arterial atherosclerotic disease. Ratschow's test and Doppler pressure measurements help in evaluation. The presence of systemic hypertension and elevated blood lipids lower the threshold for diagnosis.

If the ECG at rest does not show any significant change, it is advisable to obtain an exercise ECG for further evaluation. Myocardial ischemia is recognized on the ECG by changes in the ST-segment. Characteristically, ST-segment depression is seen, although rarely there is ST-segment elevation. The ECG changes are seen only with a certain individual level of ischemia. Therefore, exercise has to be sustained over several minutes at an exercise workload which induces insufficient myocardial blood flow. Usually, the patient will report typical angina pectoris symptoms or its equivalent, such as increasing dyspnea. Monitoring (observation and questioning) the patient during exercise testing is therefore necessary; this is especially important since there is some risk of complications with exercise during ischemia.

## 4.2.2 Exercise ECG

Exercise testing for myocardial ischemia should be performed with a defined workload and reproducible forms of testing. Exercise tests that use a bicycle, a step test or treadmill are suitable in clinical practice (Fig. 39). Each form of testing has its own specific advantages and disadvantages. Stress tests with a bicycle ergometer are often stopped

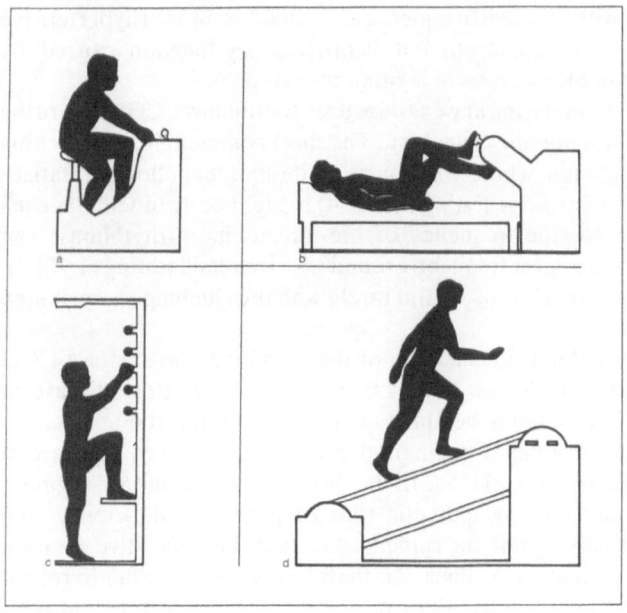

**Fig. 39.** Four types of exercise tests: **a** bicycle in sitting position, **b** bicycle in recumbent position, **c** step test, **d** treadmill.

prematurely before the cardiac reserve is exhausted, due to fatigue of the lower leg muscles. This holds true especially for patients who experience angina pectoris only with strenuous exertion. In such cases bicycle ergometry in the recumbent position may induce ischemia earlier, because myocardial ischemia occurs at a 25% lower workload when recumbent versus sitting. The augmented caval blood flow from the lower parts of the body during recumbency causes a higher filling pressure. This provokes earlier myocardial ischemia because the higher filling pressure during recumbency impairs diastolic coronary blood flow. Exercise testing in the recumbent position therefore leads more easily to dyspnea, and in some circumstances, even to pulmonary edema.

During exercise testing while sitting or standing upright, the increase in filling pressure is not as rapid. The work capacity of the coronary patient is therefore higher. During the climbing step test there is no premature leg muscle fatigue, because the arms and the back muscles are used in addition to the leg muscles. Milder impairment of coronary blood flow may therefore be more easily detected or excluded with this type of exercise testing.

Maximal exercise testing can also be achieved quite well with treadmill testing. However, the elderly may develop anxiety or insecurity with the moving walkway. Possibly, this is one explanation for the higher rate of ventricular fibrillation during treadmill versus step testing, as there is a correlation between mental stress and the occurrence of cardiac arrthythmias.

The heart rate is recorded from the ECG during the exercise test. The workload-dependent increase in heart rate is excessive in the hyperkinetic heart syndrome, whereas in disturbed sinus node function the increase in rate is reduced (Fig. 40). Systemic blood-pressure measurement during exercise is of limited accuracy. Whereas the systolic blood-pressure may be recorded reliably, the diastolic pressure can be measured less accurately. However, accurate measurements can always be performed immediately after the

49

exercise. There are patients with an excessive increase in blood pressure (hypertensive regulatory disorder), whereas during acute left ventricular dysfunction caused by myocardial ischemia, a drop in blood pressure is often observed.

Because arrhythmias may occur during any exercise test, continuous ECG monitoring and the availability of a defibrillator are obligatory. The most common life-threatening arrhythmia is ventricular fibrillation, which will require defibrillation. Following statistical analysis of different forms of exercise testing (Table 4) it might be assumed that each form of testing has its own specific frequency of life-threatening arrhythmias. For example, ventricular fibrillation is most frequently found with treadmill testing (1:2000), less often during bicycle ergometry (1:14000), and rarely with the climbing exercise step test (1:40000).

With careful performance and individualization of the workload, the exercise ECG provides valuable information on whether or not there is coronary artery disease as determined by signs of acute coronary ischemia (Fig. 41). If doubtful, the test can be repeated with a higher workload; if the ST-segment depression is caused by myocardial ischemia it will increase with a higher workload. In the case of non-ischemic ST-segment depression – for example, increased sympathetic tone or potassium deficiency, the amount of depression will usually remain the same or decrease. False-positive exercise ECGs may be obtained from patients on digitalis; it is therefore advisable either to repeat the test after a 2–4 week digitalis-free interval, or perform alternative testing that does not use an electrical end-point (e.g., thallium perfusion scan).

While the specificity of the exercise ECG is 90% for men, it is less in women (70%). The diagnostic value of the exercise ECG increases considerably if, through careful history-taking, a pre-test likelihood of coronary artery disease can be categorized as probable, doubtful or improbable. The occurrence of angina pectoris during exercise testing further sharpens the accuracy of the test.

**Table 4.** Life-threatening complications from exercise testing of 2 million patients

|  | Bicycle in recumbent position | Bicycle in sitting position | Step test | Treadmill |
|---|---|---|---|---|
| Ventricular fibrillation | 1:18000 | 1:10000 | 1:43000 | 1:2100* |
| Pulmonary edema | 1:29000 | 1:257000 | Ø | 1:170000 |
| Infarction | 1:33000 | 1:51000 | 1:43000 | 1:2800 |
| Mortality | 1:59000 | 1:103000 | 1:128000 | 1:20000 |

After: 1) Irving JB, Bruce RA (1977) Am J Cardiol 39:849; 2) Kaltenbach M, Scherer D, Dowinski S (1982) Eur Heart J 3:199; 3) Rochmis P, Blackburn H (1971) JAMA 217:1061; 4) Stuart RJ, Ellestad MH (1980) CHEST 77:94; 5) Wendt Th, Scherer, D, Kaltenbach M (1984) Dtsch med Wschr 109:123

* Mean values from 1) frequency of ventricular fibrillation (1:2140) and 4) frequency of ventricular fibrillation or severe arrhythmia which required intravenous medication (1:2092).

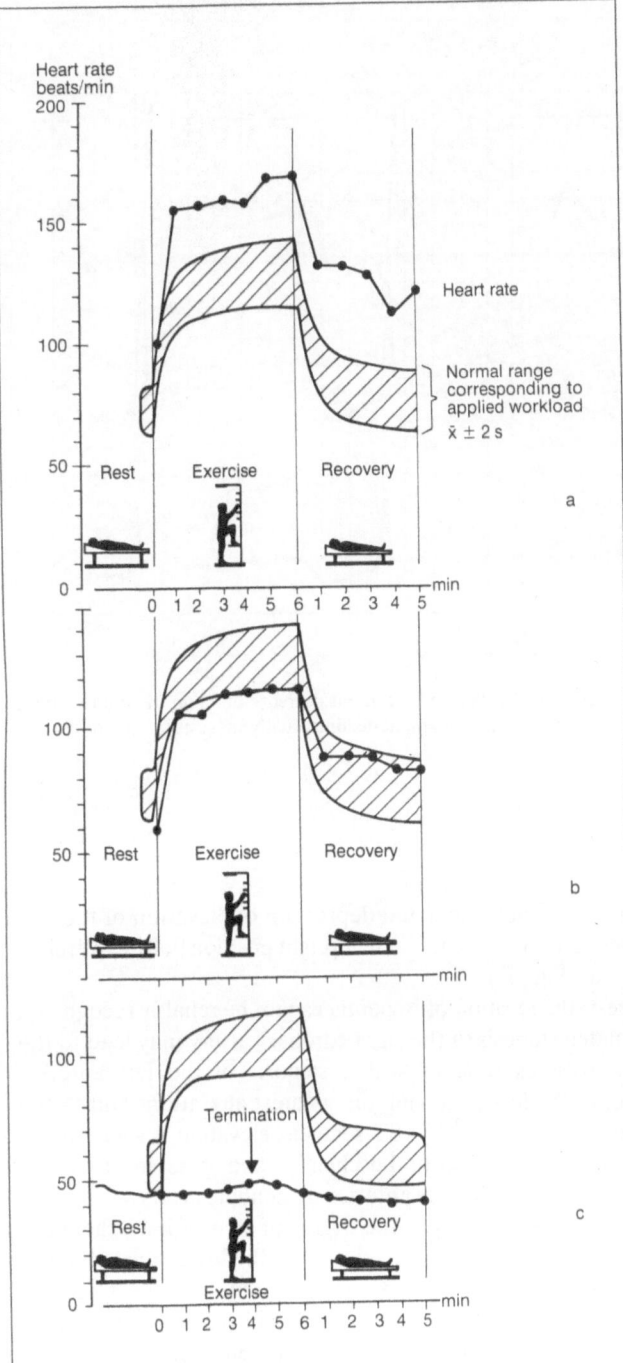

**Fig. 40.** Actual heart rate in comparison to the normal range (cross-hatched area); the normal range was determined for different workloads – separately for men and women. The workload is related to the standard body surface area to account for differences in body size and constitution. **a** Excessive heart rate in hyperkinetic disorder; **b** heart rate of an athlete who has been under endurance training; **c** lack of increase in heart rate with complete heart block.

51

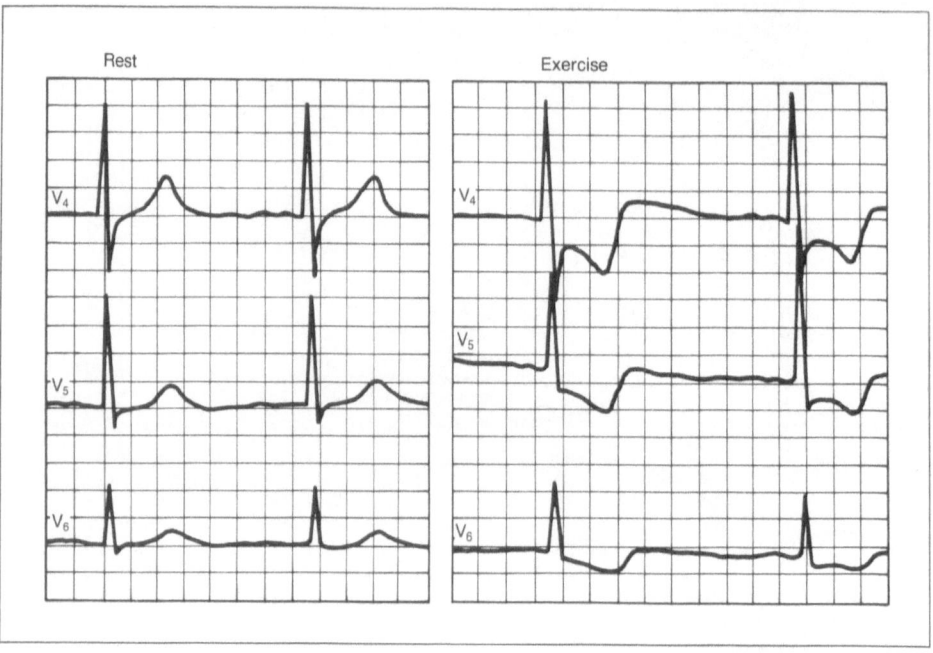

**Fig. 41.** Signs of ischemia in the exercise ECG with an ST-segment decrease of 5 mm in a patient with triple-vessel coronary disease. Such a pronounced ST-segment decline usually suggests left main stenosis or triple-vessel disease.

Isolated T-wave changes (i.e., without associated depression or elevation of the ST-segment) or ST-segment depression which occurs in the upright position before exercise, do not have any diagnostic value (Fig. 42).

In contrast to the ECG at rest, the location of ischemia cannot be reliably recognized with an exercise ECG. An isolated stenosis of the right coronary artery may lead to the same ST-segment depression with exercise as will a stenosis of the left anterior descending artery with respect to the leads showing the greatest alterations and to the amount of ST-segment depression. Occasionally, ST-segment elevation is seen on the exercise ECG. It is a sign of severe transmural ischemia, and it seems to occur preferentially with high-grade stenosis of the left anterior descending artery.

A quantitative evaluation is possible in so far as the degree of myocardial ischemia is greater with a more pronounced ST-segment depression, and the lower the tolerated workload is. From the degree of ST-segment depression in mm, and the tolerated workload in watts a ratio can be calculated ("ischemia score") which correlates with the degree of coronary disease and prognosis (Fig. 43, see also Figs. 38, 46).

Nuclear imaging techniques may complement the exercise ECG. These techniques are especially useful in those cases in which the exercise ECG does not show any ST-segment changes, although there is a typical history of angina pectoris, or in which a positive exercise ECG is recorded, but the history is negative.

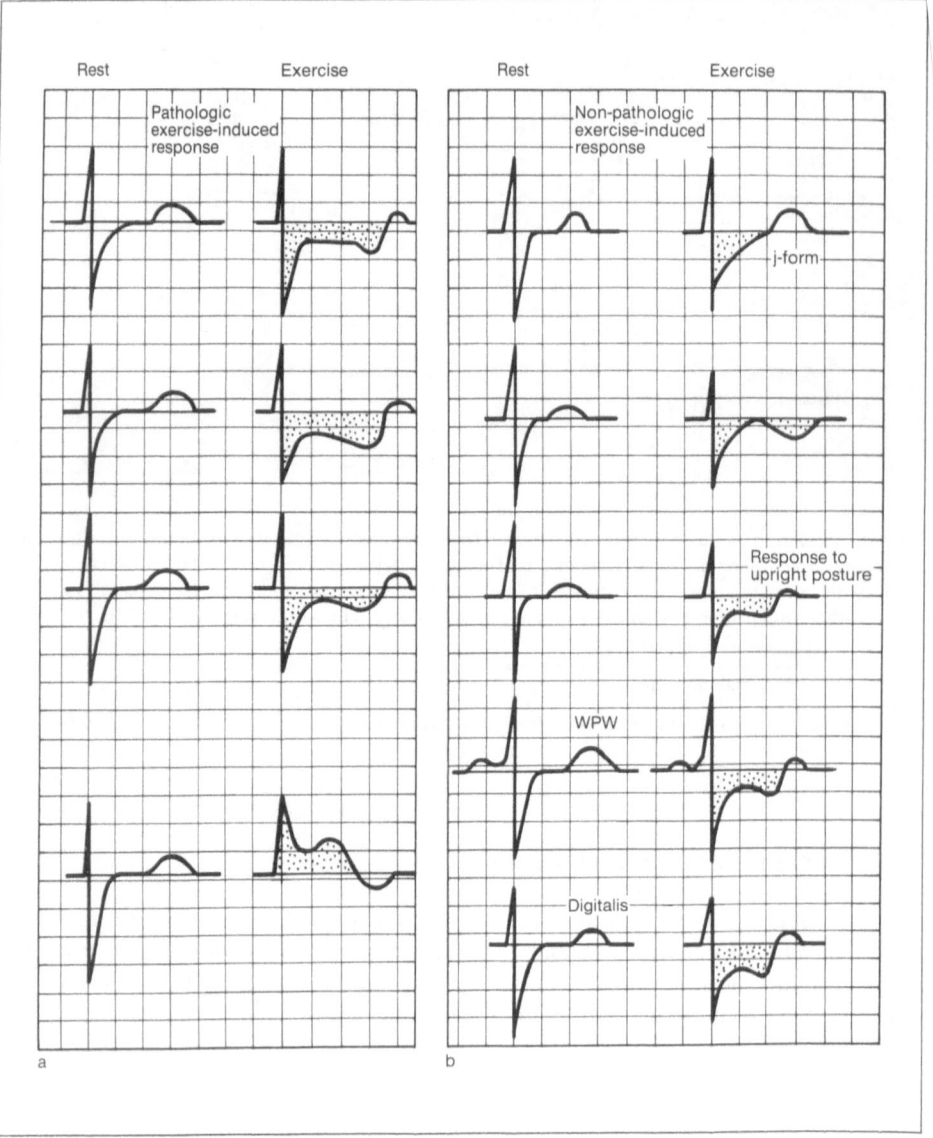

**Fig. 42.** Typical ischemic response with ST-segment depression or ST-segment elevation (**a**) and non-pathologic exercise-induced changes (**b**).

**a** An abnormal ischemic response is defined as a horizontal or down-sloping ST-segment depression of more than 0.1 mV (1 mm) in the precordial leads. In rare cases, ST-segment elevation occurs during exercise testing. This expecially severe form of ischemia may be judged as a sign of ischemia only in ECG recordings showing no residual signs of myocardial infarction. This alteration is usually associated with a peaking of the T-wave.

**b** Up-sloping J-point depression (J-form) is not pathologic, however, occasionally it may be the first sign of ischemia. In cases of doubt the exercise testing should be repeated with a higher workload. Isolated positive or negative T-wave changes are not pathologic. ST-segment depression as a result of the upright posture (before the exercise) is caused by increased sympathetic tone and is not indicative of ischemia. In the WPW syndrome and other intraventricular conduction disturbances there is often non-ischemic ST-segment depression during and after exercise testing. Patients on digitalis with ST-segment depression found in the exercise ECG may not be interpreted as definitely ischemic, even if the ECG at rest does not show signs of digitalis therapy (i.e. sagging ST-segment depression).

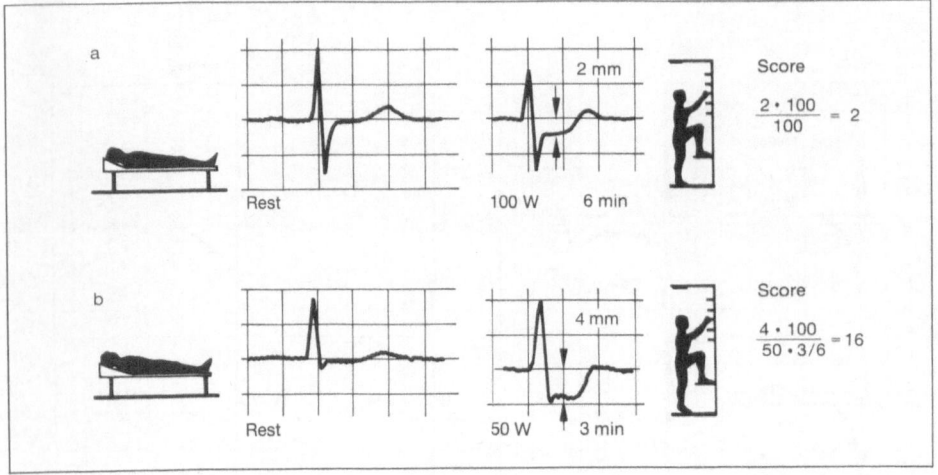

**Fig. 43.** Calculation of the ischemia score from ST-segment depression, workload, and duration. The score correlates with the degree of ischemia. **a** ST- segment depression of 2 mm at 100 watts at 6 min in a patient with coronary single-vessel disease. **b** ST-segment depression of 4 mm with 50 watts at 3 min in a patient with severe main stem stenosis of the left coronary artery. The score is calculated with the formula:

$$\frac{\text{ST segment depression (mm)}}{\text{watt} \times \text{time}} \times 100 \,,$$

where the time, that is, the duration of exercise at the same workload is calculated in 1/6 up to 6/6; 1/6 corresponds to an exercise duration of 1 min, 6/6 to 6 min.

## 4.2.3 Nuclear imaging techniques

In radionuclide ventriculography scintillation counts over the ventricles are recorded using radiolabeled erythrocytes and a gamma camera. ECG-triggering is used to cumulate counts during sequential intervals of the cardiac cycle. The test is performed with the patient recumbent. The left ventricular ejection fraction can be estimated as

$$\frac{\text{end-diastolic counts minus end-systolic counts}}{\text{end-diastolic counts}} \,.$$

Whereas this fraction will normally increase by 1–5% with exercise, it decreases during myocardial ischemia. It is important to evaluate regional wall motion in addition to the global ejection fraction by comparing the scintillation counts at rest and during exercise above the respective ventricular areas, because coronary disease usually affects some segments more than others. Finally, the sequence of contraction can be timed; ischemia induces a retardation of contraction in diseased areas (Fig. 44).

Thallium scintigraphy may also reveal myocardial ischemia during exercise. The diagnostic accuracy depends on the amount of ischemia present at the very moment when thallium is injected intravenously and myocardial uptake occurs. Therefore, the patient is exercised until ischemic signs appear, then thallium is injected and the exercise continued for some time. Similar to potassium uptake, there is rapid uptake of thallium

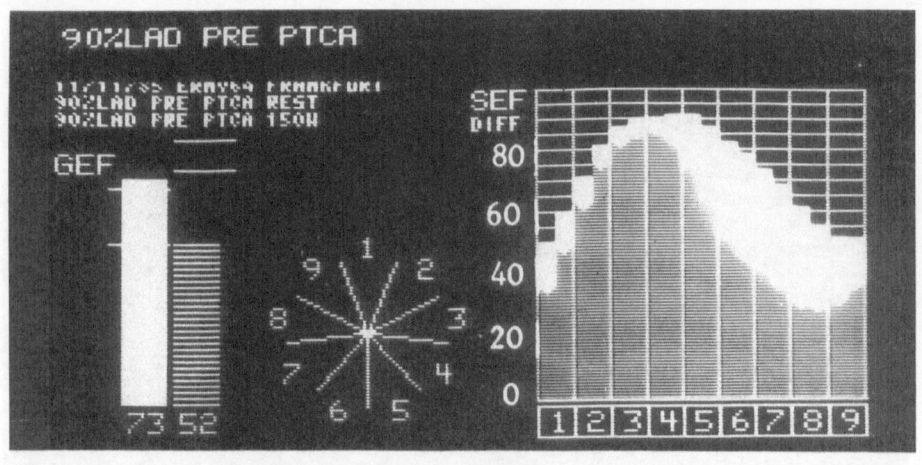

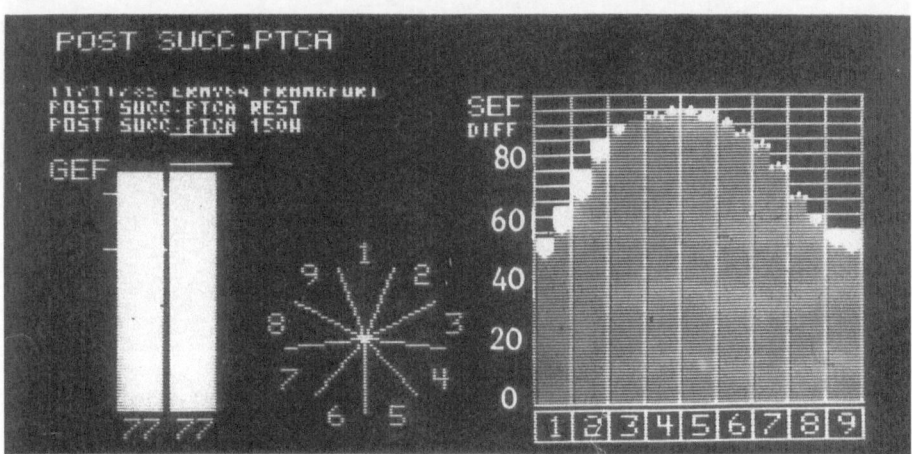

**Fig. 44.** Radionuclide ventriculogram in a patient with effort angina. Global ejection fraction (GEF) was normal at rest (**a**). During exercise (150 watt, 6 min) it fell. The computerized regional evaluation showed a reduction in sectional ejection fraction (SEF), occuring predominantly in segments 1 and 4–9. It is indicated by the white arrows pointing downwards (**b**). After successful angioplasty resting global EF is unchanged. After exercise no decrease is seen (**c**), (**d**). (Fig. 44 and 45 from the Department for Radionuclear Medicine, Frankfurt, Prof. Dr. G. Hör.)

into the myocardial and skeletal muscle cells. Ischemic regions show diminished thallium uptake (filling defect). The scintigraphic measurement is repeated some hours later and any filling-in of the defect (redistribution) is recorded (Fig. 45). This redistribution phenomenon is typical of transient exercise-induced ischemia. In the case of myocardial scars, a filling defect will persist; redistribution does not occur.

Nuclear imaging techniques are used in the diagnosis of coronary artery disease if history and other techniques are inconclusive. The techniques are not useful for

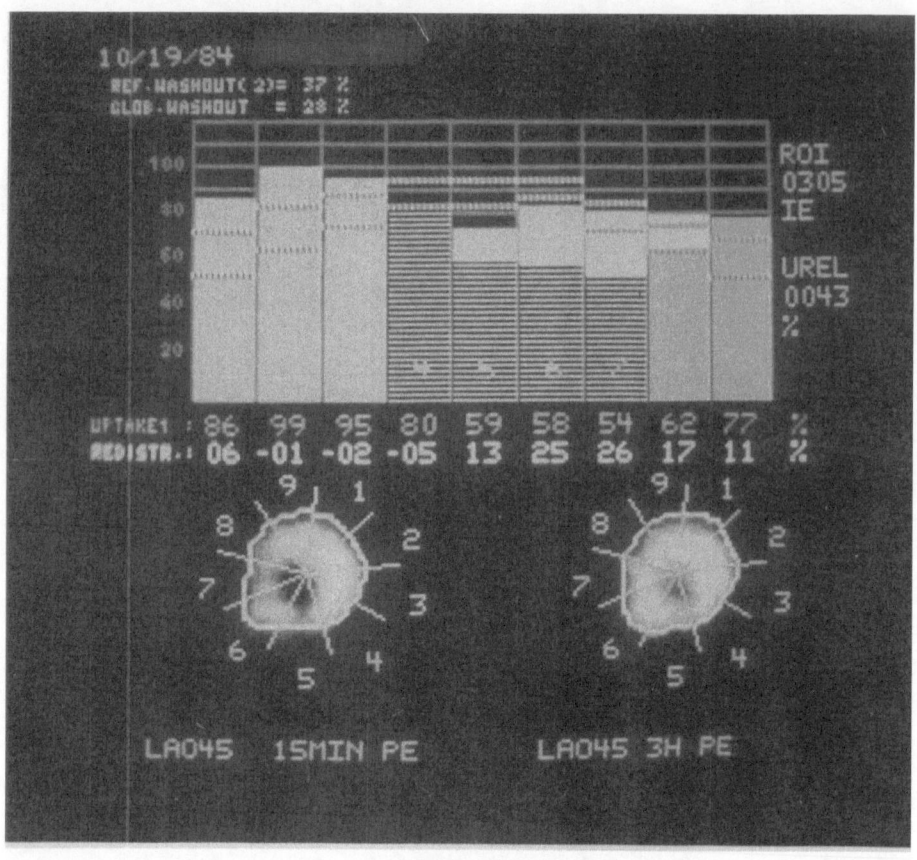

**Fig. 45 a.** A large thallium defect is seen in the anterior wall during exercise in segment 4–7, but thallium has "redistributed" into this area 1 h later indicating an exercise-induced perfusion deficit.

screening, because they are associated with a certain amount of radiation exposure and are also costly (specially trained personnel and expensive materials). These techniques have a limited sensitivity and specificity, just as do all other noninvasive techniques for the diagnosis of coronary disease. Their diagnostic accuracy is only good if they are used in conjunction with careful history taking. If applied in a hazard way for screening, they have little value. Bayes theorem states that for the evaluation of the diagnostic correctness of a test, the prevalence of the disease in the examined group is of importance. False-positive results increase when there is a low prevalence; false-negative results increase when the prevalence is high.

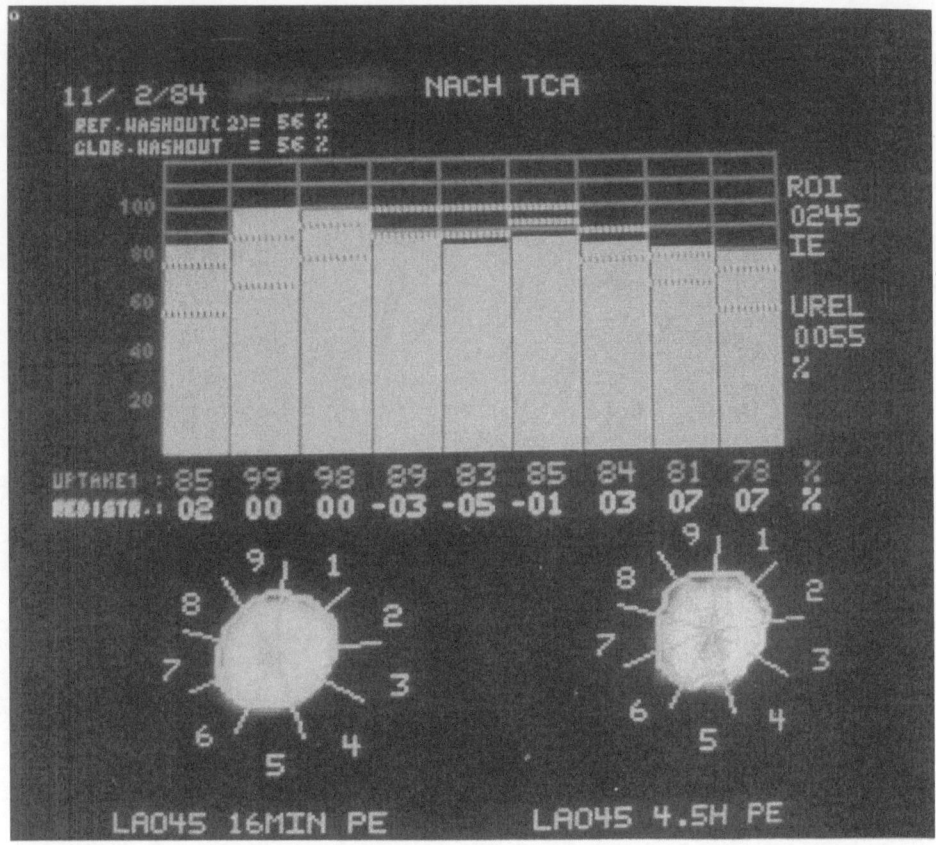

**Fig. 45b.** After successful angioplasty the test is repeated. Thallium uptake is now normal in all segments.

## 4.2.4 Coronary arteriography

When myocardial ischemia is suspected, from the patient's history and from noninvasive testing, coronary arteriography is frequently performed for further clarification. The technique was pioneered by Mason Sones at the Cleveland Clinic, Ohio, USA, during the late 1950s and early 1960s. It was later modified by Judkins, Amplatz, Schoonmaker, and others.

Coronary arteriography has the aim of verifying the diagnosis and also documenting the localization and degree of coronary artery stenoses. These x-ray studies of the coronary arteries are performed after selective catheterization of the coronary arteries, using a special catheter introduced via the femoral or the brachial approach. The arteries are visualized by injecting 2–8 mls of contrast agent. Because coronary arteries show considerable individual variation and different branches often overlap in the same view, it is necessary to use different projections, including the hemiaxial, craniocaudal, and caudocranial directions of the x-ray beam. Clear visualization of the vessels is possible

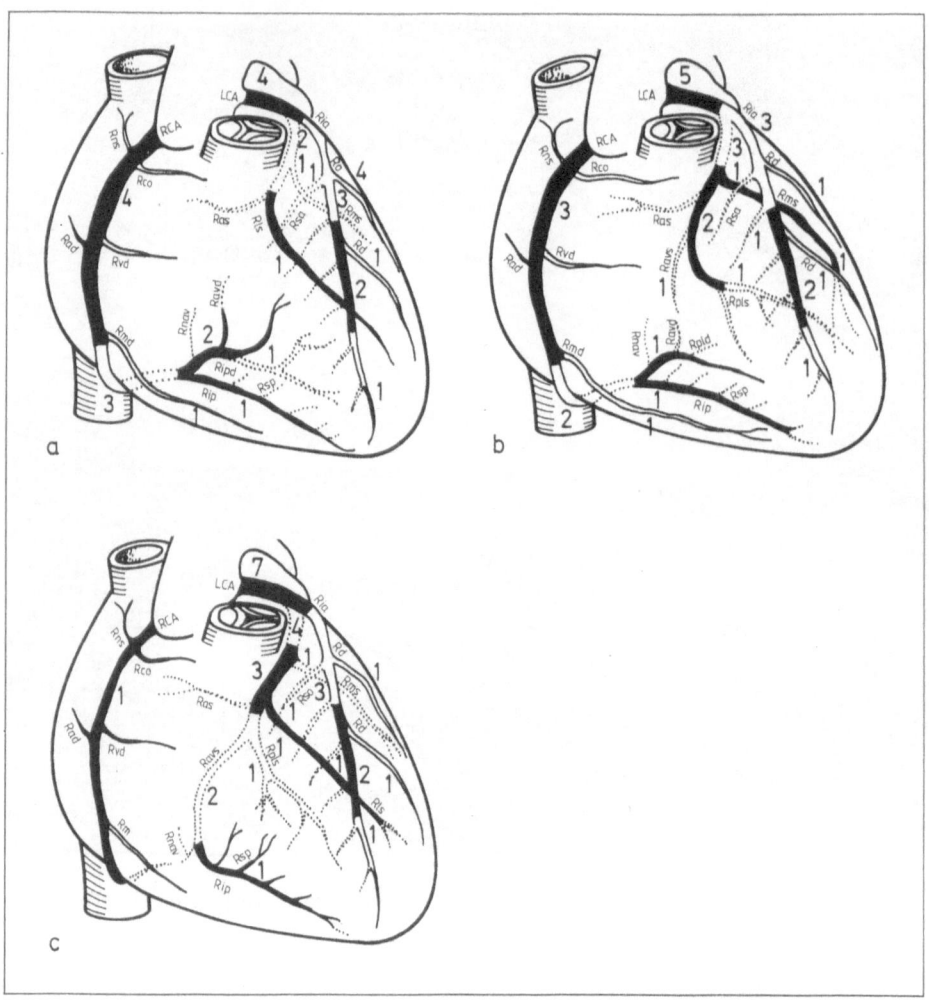

**Fig. 46.** Calculation of the coronary score for quantifying the degree of coronary artery disease. For each coronary segment a score is calculated from a weighting for location, multiplied by a factor representing the severity of stenosis. The patient's score is the sum of all the segment scores. If in a coronary segment there are multiple stenoses, only the most marked stenosis is used for measurement. The location weighting factor can be seen in the diagram. The factor for the severity of stenosis is:

| Stenosis % | 1–39 | 40–59 | 60–79 | 80–99 | 100 |
|---|---|---|---|---|---|
| Factor | 1 | 2 | 3 | 4 | 5 |

An isolated 75% proximal LAD stenosis in a normal vessel perfusion pattern (**b**) has a score of $3 \times 3 = 9$; an occlusion of the proximal right coronary artery in a right predominant vessel type (**a**) has a score of $4 \times 5 = 20$.

with powerful x-ray equipment. Arteries with a luminal diameter as small as 0.3 mm may be recorded with the help of magnification techniques.

Coronary arteriography is done under local anesthesia from the groin or the elbow. It is usually not associated with pain; additional use of analgesics or sedatives is therefore not necessary. However, the procedure carries some risk. Fatal complications occur in 0.05% of cases. This rate is very low if one considers that patients are often severely ill and already at risk of myocardial infarction or left ventricular failure. Coronary arteriography may be easily repeated, for example, following angioplasty or coronary surgery if the clinical course of the disease warrents it. However, the enthusiasm for doing arteriography must also be balanced by the radiation exposure and the costs involved.

When there is typical angina pectoris and a pathologic exercise ECG, coronary arteriography will reveal a severe coronary artery stenosis or occlusion in more than 90% of the patients. In many patients, atheromata are localized, in others, changes are diffuse with long stenoses or occlusions in several branches.

The follow-up of patients who have had coronary arteriography has shown that prognosis depends mostly on the severity of coronary artery disease and ventricular function. The degree of coronary artery disease may be quantified as a coronary score. In a method shown in Fig. 46, this is computed as the sum of an individual weighting appropriate for each coronary segment, multiplied by a factor for the degree of the stenosis in that segment.

The severity of coronary artery disease is of major importance when considering the indications for coronary surgery. Single-, double- and triple-vessel disease is defined as greater than or equal to 50% narrowing of the lumen diameter in one, two or three vessels. Surgery is usually indicated only for left main coronary stenosis or two to three diseased main branches. In single-vessel disease the stenosis can usually be dilated with angioplasty, thereby avoiding surgery. Increasingly double- and triple-vessel cases are also treated less invasively by angioplasty if stenoses amenable to balloon dilatation are present.

## 4.3 Clinical course of angina pectoris

### 4.3.1 Stable angina pectoris

Stable angina pectoris is characterized as a disorder where the exercise-induced symptoms of angina have not changed significantly over a long period of time (more than 3 months).

### 4.3.2 Unstable angina

Unstable angina is a clinical manifestation where the angina pectoris threshold has significantly decreased. Often, there is a change in symptoms, such that anginal pain occurs with a much lower workload than usual. Such a change in symptoms should be regarded as serious, and it usually necessitates referral for hospital care. This course often reflects an increase in coronary stenosis, triggered by subintimal bleeding or intraluminal thrombosis.

The syndrome of unstable angina includes many different manifestations. There may be frequent changes in the anginal pattern. Sudden severe anginal attacks may occur one day, whereas on other days there are no reports of attacks, or only of angina induced by strenuous exercise. These patients have a higher risk for myocardial infarction. Arteriography and intracoronary angioscopy during surgery in such patients have shown that thrombotic deposits often occur on already existing atheromata and it can be assumed that it is their changing size which causes the change in symptoms. A decrease in symptoms is explained by intermittent resolution of thrombi by endogenous fibrinolysis. Measures to prevent thrombosis, such as the administration of platelet aggregation inhibitors, heparin, and fibrinolytic agents, are therefore of specific therapeutic importance.

### 4.3.3 Angina pectoris at rest

Exercise-induced angina or unstable angina may change into angina at rest, if coronary blood flow decreases below the value needed even at rest. This will only occur with subtotal vessel stenosis or occlusion, as coronary arteries are wide enough to provide a reserve of blood flow at least five times the necessary rest flow (see Fig. 30, page 38).

Sometimes angina at rest is induced by intermittent coronary narrowing; for example, so-called Prinzmetal angina is characterized by anginal attacks suffered exclusively at rest. The diagnosis is based on the symptoms and on signs of severe ischemia on an ECG obtained during a myocardial ischemic episode. Characteristically, the ECG shows transient focal ST-segment elevation similar to that seen in acute myocardial infarction. Patients often tolerate a good workload and are free of symptoms during the interval between attacks. In the absence of associated severe fixed coronary artery disease, the exercise ECG may be normal. Prinzmetal angina can be attributed to coronary artery spasm, which may occur in vessel segments that have only mild underlying stenosis. Therefore, between attacks myocardial blood flow is maintained even with strenuous exercise due to sufficient coronary reserve. Anginal attacks will only occur if the tone of the smooth muscle of the coronary artery is increased. This rarely occurs with an increase of catecholamine secretion, but more often occurs at rest, and occasionally in association with strong vagal stimulation. Therapy includes the use of vasodilating agents, especially nitroglycerin and calcium channel blockers. A diagnostic evaluation with coronary arteriography is usually necessary. If there is diagnostic uncertainty, provocation of spasm may be performed with ergonovine, by cold stimulus or by hyperventilation to produce respiratory alkalosis (Fig. 47).

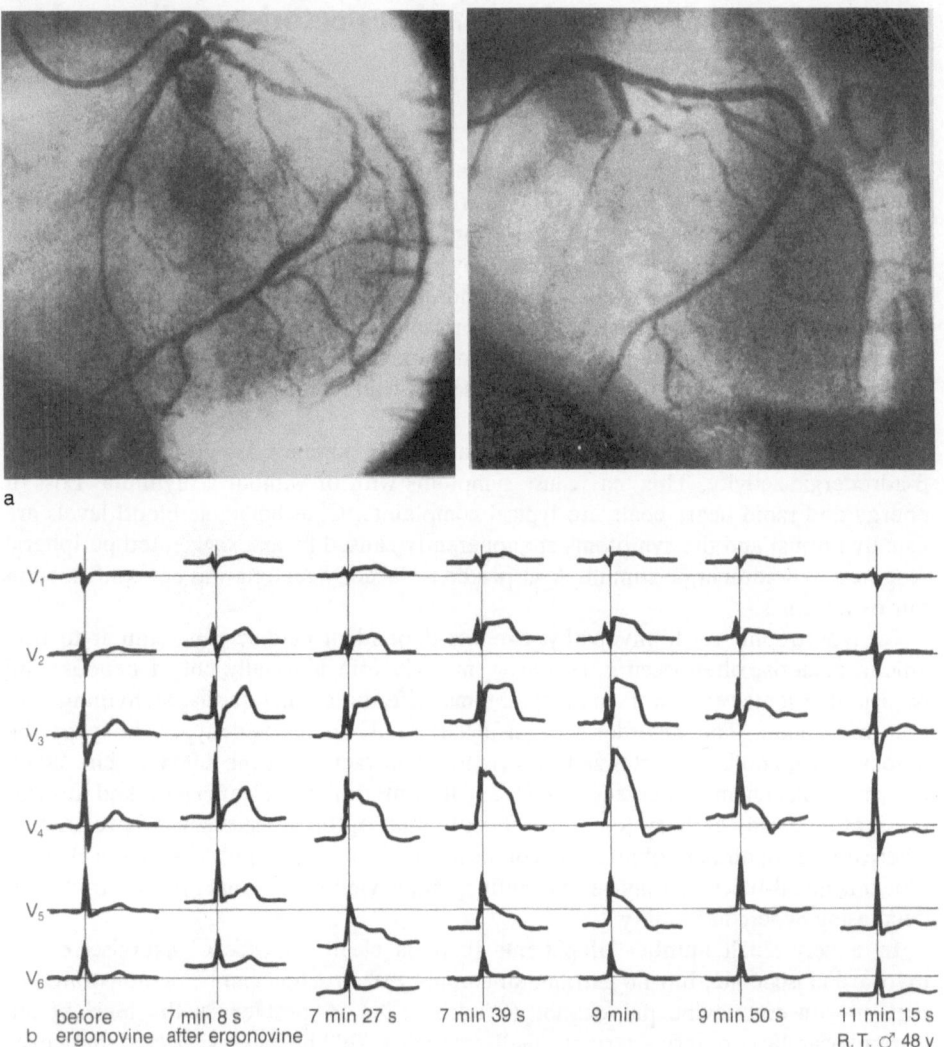

**Fig. 47.** Ergonovine-induced coronary artery spasm as cause of myocardial ischemia: **a** intermittent occlusion of the LAD in the coronary angiogram (right); **b** significant ST-segment elevation on the ECG (from [6]).

61

## 4.4 Differential diagnosis of angina pectoris, cardiac and non-cardiac chest pain

Whereas true angina pectoris indicates myocardial ischemia, pain or sensations in the cardiac area may also be linked to other cardiac disorders, such as pericarditis, cardiac arrhythmias, and mitral valve prolapse. More frequently, however, non-ischemic chest symptoms are caused by other organs. It may be chest or intercostal muscle pain or pain caused by the pleura, esophagus, costochondral junction or the skin and subcutaneous tissue. Pain may also be caused by nerve or radicular irritation. Cardiac arrhythmias, especially extrasystoles, may be experienced as cardiac pain. Finally, there are chest or cardiac complaints without any organic cause, for example those arising from anxiety or cardiac neurosis.

In the hyperkinetic heart syndrome (see also 11.1), patients demonstrate augmented β-adrenergic activity. This may cause symptoms with or without arrhythmia. Loss of energy and rapid heart beats are typical complaints. Catecholamine blood levels are usually normal and the symptoms are apparently caused by an exaggerated peripheral response to β-adrenergic stimuli. A suspected reduced vagal tone was not confirmed in our own studies.

In hypertrophic cardiomyopathy, exercise-dependent cardiac pain, similar to true angina pectoris, often occurs. However, nitroglycerin is usually not of benefit, and occasionally it may even worsen the symptoms. Life-threatening cardiac arrhythmias are not uncommon. The disorder (see also 9.3) leads to marked hypertrophy of the myocardium, and is characterized by increased contractility of the left ventricle. When the ventricular chamber decreases in size and the anterior mitral leaflet is sucked towards the septum during early systole, the left ventricular outflow is subsequently restricted. There is also impairment of relaxation of the myocardium. Therapy with calcium channel blockers and β-blockers may be of benefit by improving relaxation of the ventricle and decreasing hypercontractility.

In a very small number of patients there is clear evidence of exercise-related myocardial ischemia, but no extramural coronary obstruction can be demonstrated at rest or with ergonovine provocation (Syndrome X). A problem at the level of the intramyocardial coronary arteries ("small-vessel disease") has been suspected, but never conclusively proven. Mitral valve prolapse is associated with a wide range of chest pains and arrhythmias. The degree of subjective complaint is entirely independent of whether there is hemodynamically significant mitral insufficiency or not. Most often, mitral valve prolapse is seen in thin young women. The prognosis is usually excellent and only occasionally is mitral valve prolapse associated with severe mitral insufficiency, life-threatening arrhythmias or endocarditis.

Retrosternal pain may be caused by esophageal dysfunction. There may not be any relationship of the pain to food intake. The symptoms may even occur with exertion and therefore are very similar to angina pectoris. A simple radiologic examination of the esophagus will provide a positive result only in cases with marked abnormality such as achalasia. The disordered sequence and vigor of contractility of the lower esophagus, which is often the cause of the complaint, will not be recognized. Abnormal pressure changes can be recorded with esophageal manometry. Drug therapy with nitroglycerin and calcium channel blockers is sometimes effective under these conditions, as well as for esophagitis or diaphragmatic hernia. Antacids, $H_2$-receptor blockers, and surgery may also be indicated.

Thoracic pain, caused by increased local muscular tone, does not occur retrosternally, but in the area of the pectoral or intercostal muscles. Pain can be severe and may persist for weeks and months. In some cases, symptoms will be reported as appearing suddenly. Thorough history-taking will reveal common causes, such as unusual stress during snow-shoveling. The diagnosis is confirmed by physical examination. One will palpate contraction and spasm of affected muscular areas, and palpation will induce pain. Therapy consists primarily of physiotherapy based on muscle stretching and relaxation exercises. Deep muscular massage and application of heat may also be effective.

Pain along the sternal border may occur in the area of the costochondral junction (Tietze's syndrome). The pain and tenderness to touch may be treated by infiltrating with local anesthetics. It may also subside spontaneously with or without the associated use of mild oral analgesics.

Pain originating from subcutaneous tissue may be detected by palpation or when the skin is gently pinched. With palpation, firm, thickened areas are discovered which cannot be as easily moved about as can healthy areas. These disorders are part of a clinical spectrum that includes panniculitis and cellulitis.

Severe precordial pain may be caused by herpes zoster, even before the typical vesicles appear.

Cardiac neurosis may appear without any cardiological causes, but may be associated with other functional symptoms. Cardiac neurosis is usually seen in connection with traumatizing personal events. The clinical history may reveal factors that are linked to the symptoms and chronologically linked to their onset, thus suggesting possibilities for therapy.

The differential diagnosis of cardiac and non-cardiac chest pain is of major practical importance. A false diagnosis may have far-reaching consequences. The patient's history is fundamental for the diagnostic evaluation because a further intervention is only helpful if it is used with a clear aim. Furthermore, the entire personality of the patient has to be taken into account, in order to prudently apply further diagnostic measures. The best physician is not the one who makes most use of all diagnostic procedures available, but is the one who establishes a complete diagnosis with the least technical effort and the least harm to the patient.

# 4.5 Therapy of angina pectoris

The therapy of myocardial ischemia is based on an accurate diagnosis. The diagnostic steps of history, ECG, noninvasive tests, and coronary angiography are modified according to the possible therapeutic consequences. The therapy of angina pectoris includes three steps:
1) general measures;
2) drug therapy;
3) revascularization.

### 4.5.1 General measures

The patient's active participation is needed for adjusting lifestyle and controlling possible risk factors. This participation can only be obtained if the physician informs the patient thoroughly about the importance and consequences of his disease. The physician makes a "therapeutic deal" with the patient.

Adjusting the lifestyle includes consistent nonsmoking, sufficient exercise, normal body weight, diet and, if needed, specific behavior modification. It is important not to overburden the patient in his zeal for additional tasks. For example, rather than exercising daily for 30 min on an "exercycle" or jogging 5 kilometers, it may be more suitable to walk to work instead of using the car. In this way, the patient gains time for emotional regeneration, even if it is a less strenuous physical performance. If hypertension or diabetes coexist, it is appropriate to strive for optimum control.

### 4.5.2 Antianginal drug therapy, thrombosis prophylaxis

Drug therapy begins with the prescription of sublingual nitroglycerin. Nitroglycerin has been used for angina pectoris therapy for more than a century. It is not only effective in relieving attacks of angina, but it can also be used prophylactically. After administration of nitroglycerin, exercise can be better tolerated and the patient may not reach the anginal threshold. The response to nitroglycerin during an attack is prompt, an observation that can be helpful in confirming the diagnosis of the chest pain. In true angina, nitroglycerin is effective within 5 min of sublingual application. If this is not the case, the diagnosis is in doubt.

Isosorbide dinitrate and 5-isosorbide mononitrate (still experimental in the United States) may be used orally, and they have a sustained effect over 4 h, whereas sublingual nitroglycerin is only active for 20–30 min. The chronic effect of different oral nitrates is partially based on the appearance of effective metabolites after having passed through the liver (first-pass metabolism).

Oral therapy may be started with isosorbide dinitrate or 5-isosorbide mononitrate. Both agents act via 5-isosorbide mononitrate. After sublingual aaministration isosorbide dinitrate is active, therefore, it may also be used this way for a more prompt effect. Transdermal therapy with nitrate patches is of dubious clinical value, because of the development of tolerance. It appears that tolerance develops if constant plasma levels of nitrates are sustained over several hours. This is the case with nitrate patches, intravenous nitrate infusions and the two or three times daily application of long lasting preparations.

Usually, non-sustained-release 20–40 mg dinitrate or 5-mononitrate is used three times daily. Some authors recommend a single daily dose of approximately 100 mg of the agent in its slow-release formulation. Nitrates may cause vascular headaches. Often they diminish within several of continued application. However, in 5% of patients nitrates have to be stopped because of these headaches. A temporary dose decrease, change of the formulation, or the use of a nitrate analogue such as molsidomine (experimental in the United States) is often helpful.

A second group of antianginal agents is the calcium channel blockers. Agents of the verapamil or diltiazem type are especially useful. Nifedipine is suitable, especially in combination with nitrates in patients with bradycardia, but less so with a normal heart rate because it may induce an adverse increase in heart rate. The usual daily dose for verapamil is 80–120 mg three times daily, for diltiazem 30–60 mg three times daily, and for nifedipine 10–20 mg three times daily. Each of these is now also available in a slow-release formulation.

β-receptor blocking agents form a third group. These agents exert effective antianginal activity, especially in combination with nitrates. However, their bronchoconstrictive and coronary constrictive activity has to be kept in mind. β-receptor blockers and calcium antagonists may slow the sinus node rate and atrioventricular conduction.

### 4.5.3 Pharmacodynamics of antianginal agents

A reduction in filling pressure of the left ventricle is important, because ischemia is enhanced by an increase in the filling pressure which impairs blood flow to the inner layers of the myocardium. Most coronary blood flow occurs during diastole and it is significantly improved by a reduction in filling pressure. Nitrates are the most potent agents for reducing the filling pressure (Fig. 48).

Reducing the left ventricular afterload lessens myocardial oxygen needs and this may be achieved by nitrates, calcium channel blockers and β-receptor blocking agents.

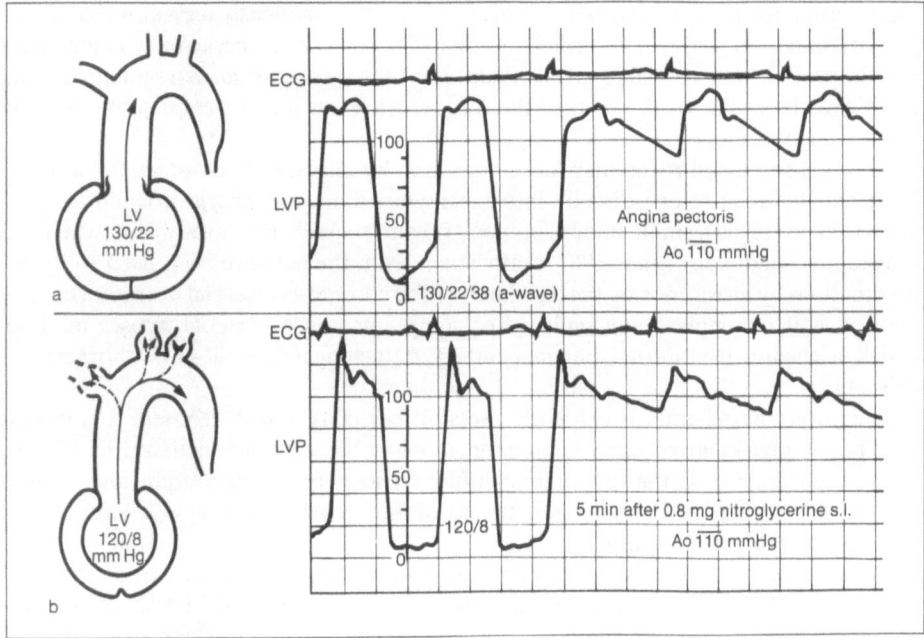

**Fig. 48.** Pressure curve of the left ventricle and of the aorta **a** during a sudden anginal attack and **b** after interruption of the attack by nitroglycerin. Use of nitrates reduced the elevated left-ventricular filling pressure during the attack. The aortic pressure curve shows a decrease in pressure amplitude and a change in form due to a fall in the elastic resistance (decrease in tone of the great arteries) after nitroglycerin.

Dilation of dynamic coronary vessel stenoses may occur with nitrates and calcium antagonists; β-blockers, however, may lead to further constriction. These changes are not as important in stable angina as in angina at rest, where there may be a predominant vasoactive component to the coronary narrowing.

Agents which predominantly affect the coronary arteriolar resistant vessels are no longer used for the therapy of angina, because they may aggravate the problem via a "steal" phenomenon. This is true for agents like dipyridamole and also calcium channel blockers with a coronary arteriolar dilating effect. In individual cases, these drugs may lead to a paradoxical increase in symptoms.

The antianginal efficacy of β-blockers is based on their reduction of myocardial oxygen consumption due to a decrease in heart rate and contractility. This effect is especially relevant under conditions of sympathetically mediated increases in heart rate and contractility such as during anxiety or exercise.

### 4.5.4 Surgical and angioplasty revascularization

Efforts to restore cardiac blood flow are the logical consequence of the knowledge that myocardial ischemia is caused by limitation of blood flow. A coronary arteriogram of high image quality is a prerequisite for coronary revascularization. On the cineangiogram it should be possible to resolve three pairs of lines per millimeter in order to correctly recognize stenoses in coronary vessels of less than 1-mm diameter. Generally speaking, intervention for revascularization is indicated if there is medically unresponsive angina pectoris and/or objective myocardial ischemia. The coronary artery to be revascularized should provide flow to viable myocardium, not to a scar. Such an assessment is made from examining the contraction of the left ventricle on the cineangiogram, or from radionuclide studies.

The first successful revascularization was done by implanting the internal mammary (internal thoracic) artery directly into the myocardium (Vineberg procedure). This approach produced a small amount of blood flow to the ischemic myocardium via newly developing collaterals. Since 1967, grafts taken from the leg have been used to bypass obstructions by anastomosing the distal part of the coronary vessel and to the aorta. This method is increasingly being replaced or complemented by arterial bypass methods which use mainly the internal mammary artery, detaching it from the inner thoracic wall (Fig. 49).

If myocardial ischemia is caused by isolated coronary vessel stenoses, it is usually possible to revascularize using balloon angioplasty, an approach initiated in 1977 by Gruentzig (Fig. 50). In the case of long diffuse stenoses or coronary occlusions, bypass graft surgery is preferred. High-grade stenosis of the left main coronary artery represents an indication for prompt surgery.

Because angioplasty is not as invasive as bypass surgery, it is preferred whenever possible (Figs. 51, 52). Using current state-of-the-art angioplasty technique, balloon angioplasty can be done in about 50% of patients who need revascularization. Its use does mandate the availability of immediate bypass surgery in case of complications. However, the rate of complications is low and mortality is about 1%. The mortality rate of bypass surgery is in the range of 1–3%, depending on the severity of the patient's disease and the skill of the surgical team.

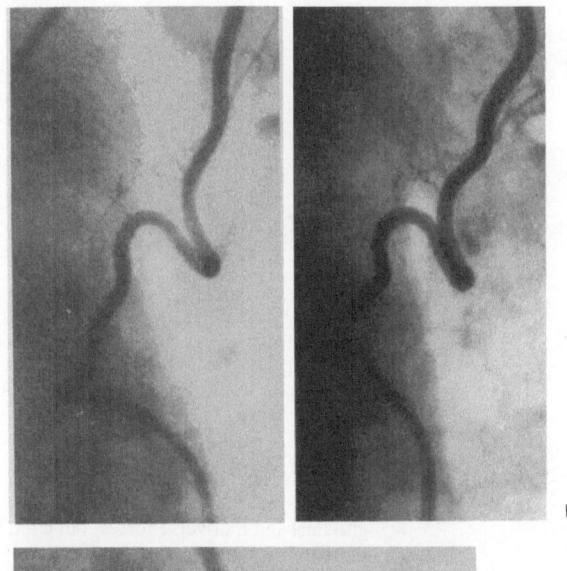

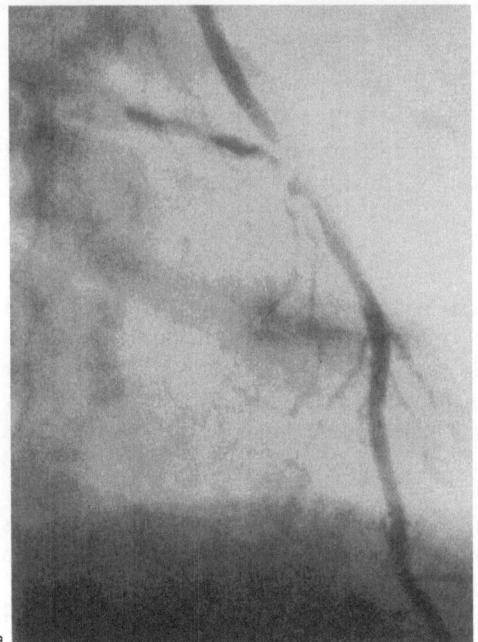

**Fig. 49.** Aortocoronary arterial bypass with anastomosis from the internal mammary artery (A. thoracica interna) to the LAD (R. interventricularis anterior). The arteriogram after operation (**a**) shows a smaller diameter of the artery than the second arteriogram performed two years later (**b**). This increase in diameter of the mammary artery occurs in order to match the blood demand of the myocardium. It is regularly seen if serial arteriograms are performed.

A variety of other catheter technologies is being developed to complement the balloon angioplasty approach. These include methods that remove plaque (atherectomy), melt it or grind it away (laser, rotablation), or mechanically hold the vessel open (stents). Each of these approaches is finding a small but useful role alongside the balloon method. Low speed rotational angioplasty is used to reopen total occlusions.

Antithrombotic drugs are of major importance as therapy after surgery or dilatation, because platelet deposition and thrombi may produce acute occlusion and progressive

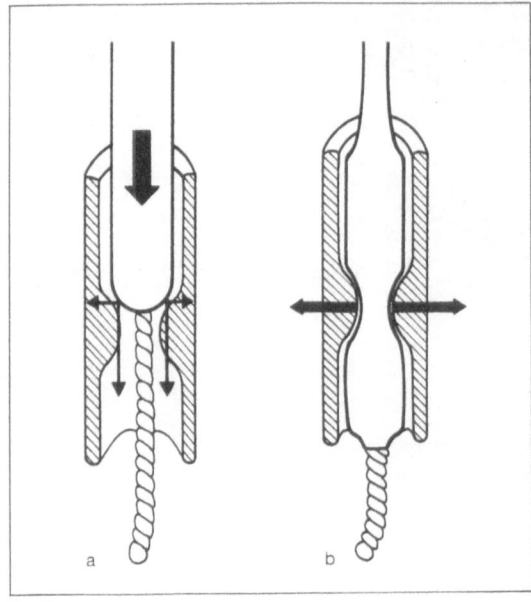

**Fig. 50. a** The older Bougie-method of dilating stenoses is based both on longitudinal and transverse forces, but **b** the more gentle balloon angioplasty relies only on transverse force.

graft narrowing. Agents that inhibit platelet aggregation, especially salicylates (0.1–0.9 grams per day), have been beneficial. Anticoagulants are sometimes also used in problem cases.

### Long-term results

The initial or primary success rate for balloon angioplasty is about 90%. After successful dilatation, recurrences occur in 20–40% of patients. These can usually be treated with a second dilatation (Fig. 53). Including redilatations the medium-term success rate for balloon angioplasty is around 80%. It can be expected that coronary artery stenosis may be dilated successfully in 80 of 100 patients. The long-term prognosis of these patients is very good and superior to patients with similar degrees of heart disease but unsuccessful angioplasty (Fig. 54).

Angiographic follow-ups of up to 8 years have shown that restenosis usually occurs during the first 3 months, predominantly 2 months after the procedure (Fig. 55). Often the dilated stenosis can hardly be seen any more on a follow-up angiogram (Fig. 56). Recurrent angina after a longer time period is usually due to new stenoses at other locations. These can often be treated by additional balloon dilatation (Figs. 52, 53).

Occlusions or stenoses of large or middle-sized coronary arteries can be bypassed surgically. One year after saphenous vein aortocoronary bypass surgery, approximately 80% of grafts remain open. Due to degeneration of the transplanted vein, there is a further yearly occlusion rate of about 2–3%. Ten years after surgery only 50% of vein grafts remain open and an additional percentage are stenosed. Subsequent surgical interventions are possible, but are more difficult in comparison to the initial procedure. If instead of a venous bypass, the internal mammary artery is used, long-term patency results are better. For this reason, most graft surgery procedures now incorporate at least

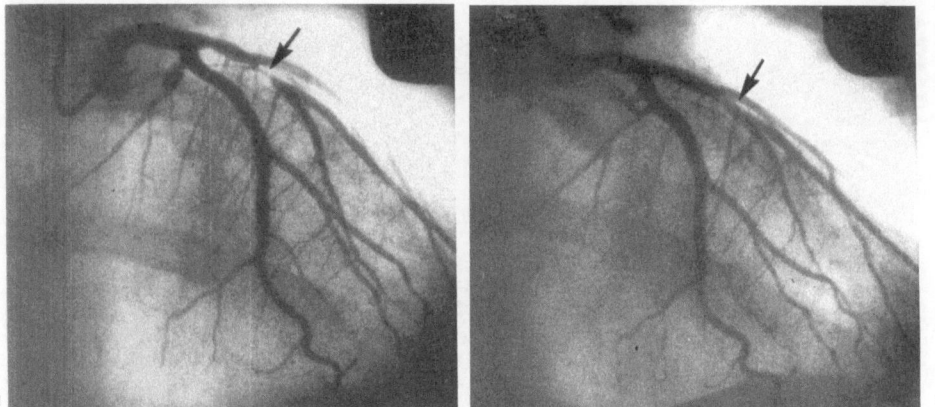

a                                                      b

**Fig. 51. a** Isolated stenosis of the left anterior descending artery; **b** widening of the stenosis by balloon angioplasty. The stenosis is no longer seen at follow-up angiography. Angina pectoris and ST-segment depression during exercise ECG were relieved.

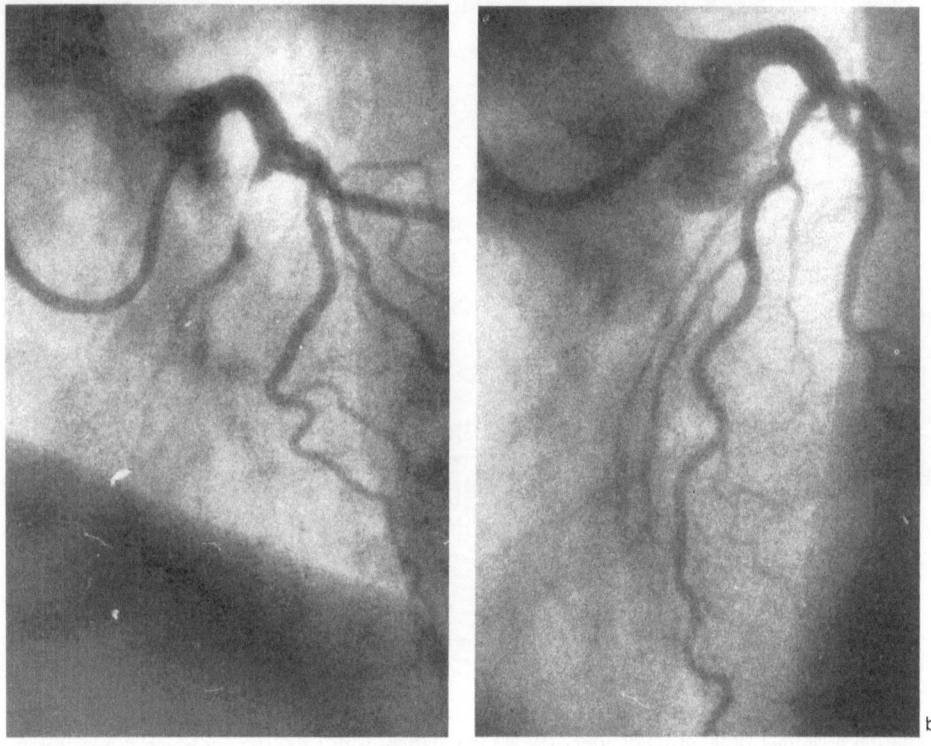

a                                                      b

**Fig. 52. a** Subtotal "99%" stenosis of the left anterior descending artery with limited and slow contrast filling of the distal vessel in a patient with severe angina pectoris and ischemia during exercise ECG. **b** After balloon angioplasty the stenosis is hardly recognizable and the distal vessel shows excellent filling. There were no pathologic changes in the other coronary vessels and the patient became completely asymptomatic. After 3 years, angina recurred, but it was due to disease of the right coronary artery (see Fig. 53).

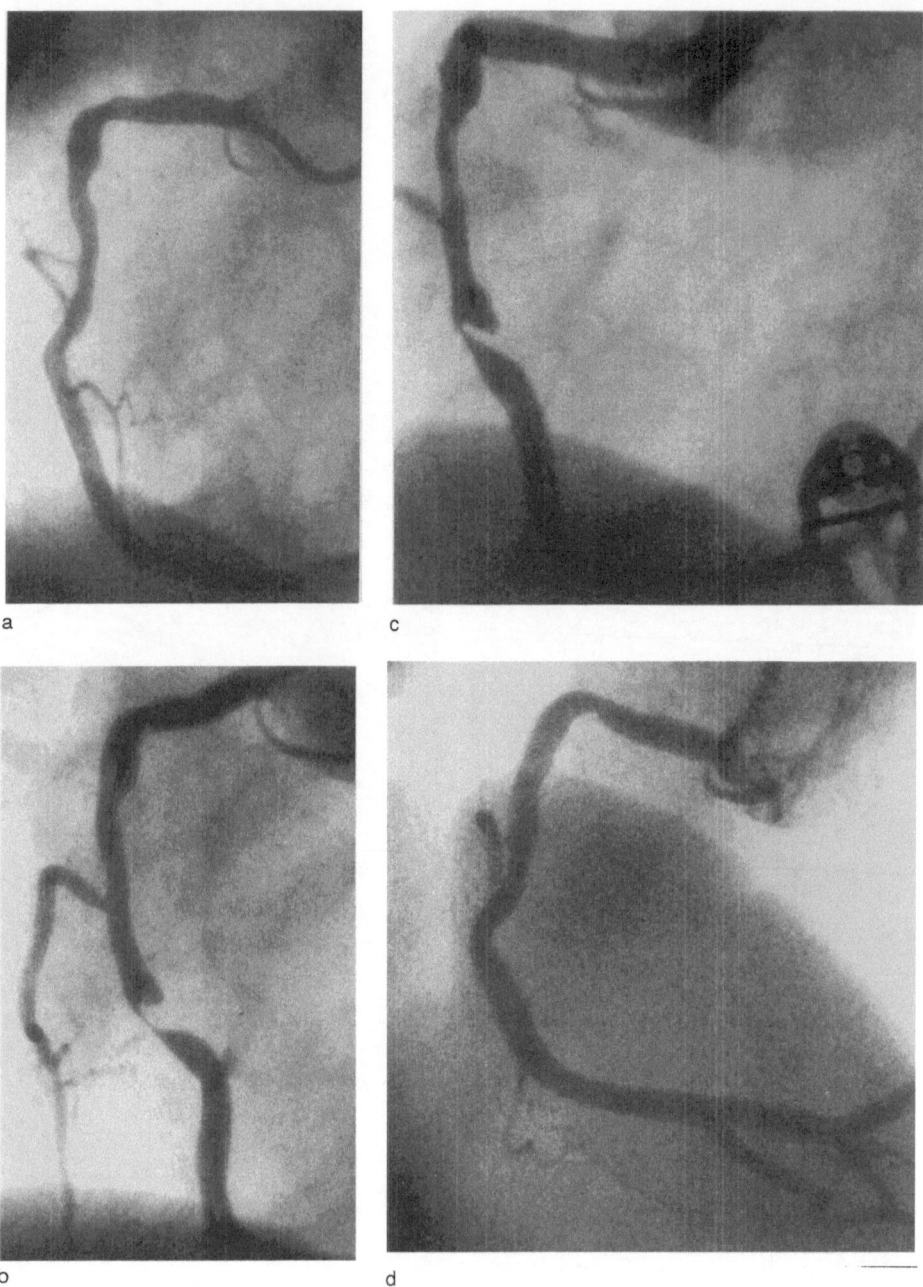

a

c

b

d

**Fig. 53. a** Normal right coronary artery (RCA) in a patient with LAD stenosis which was successful treated by PTCA (see Fig. 52); **b** Three years later the patient had renewed angina which was now due to a stenosis in the RCA. The stenosis appears subtotal and very eccentric; **c** After successful PTCA of the RCA stenosis recurrence of angina occurred 2 months later; in the angiogram a restenosis is seen which is very similar to the original stenosis but somewhat shorter; **d** After redilatation a good long-term result is angiographically documented 4 months after redilatation.

70

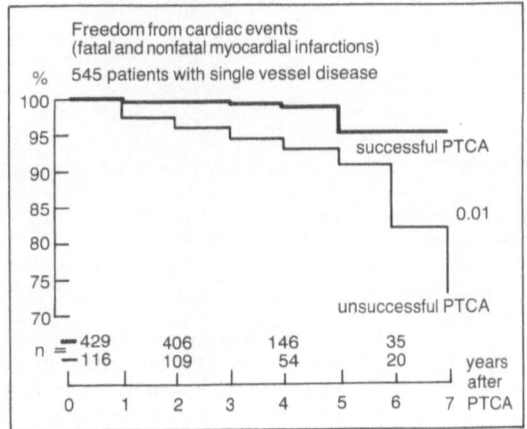

Freedom from cardiac events
(fatal and nonfatal myocardial infarctions)
545 patients with single vessel disease

successful PTCA

0.01

unsuccessful PTCA

**Fig. 54.** Long-term outcome after angioplasty shows a very good prognosis after successful PTCA. In patients in whom angioplasty was not successful, the long-term results are less favourable. The severity of coronary artery disease was identical in both groups as was the amount of left ventricular impairment.

The procedures were performed in 1977–1984. During this time PTCA was unsuccessful in 30% of patients due to technical difficulties. Today this percentage has decreased to 5%. Therefore most patients with unsuccessful PTCA than would be successfully treated today; thus, this retrospective comparison may give an reasonable idea of the benefit of PTCA.

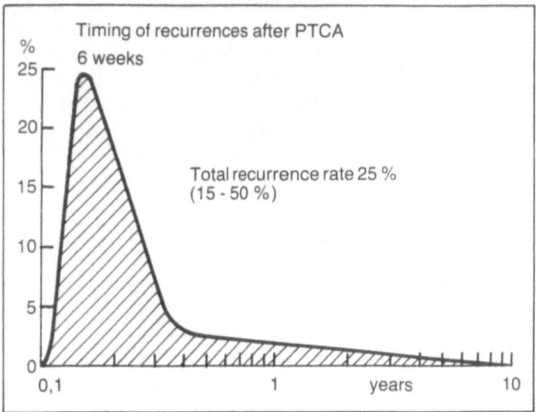

Timing of recurrences after PTCA
6 weeks

Total recurrence rate 25 %
(15 - 50 %)

**Fig. 55.** After successful angioplasty recurrences occur essentially within 3 months after the procedure. There is a peak at about 6 weeks after angioplasty.

D. L., 58 yrs ♂

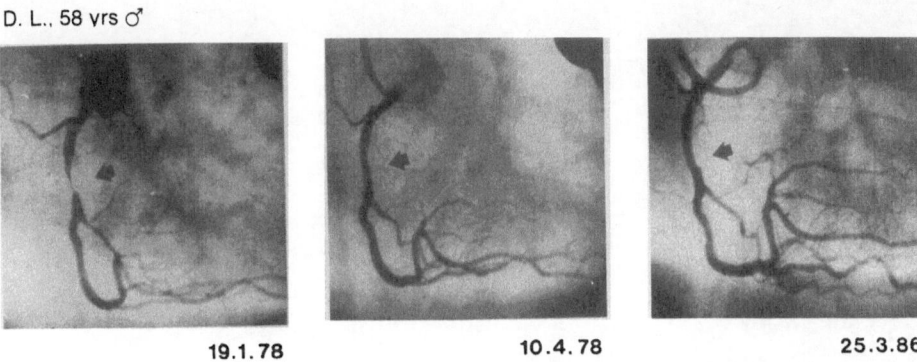

19.1.78        10.4.78        25.3.86

**Fig. 56.** Right coronary artery of a 58-year-old man with typical angina pectoris during exercise. The high-grade stenosis was successfully treated with angioplasty. A follow-up angiogram performed 3 months after PTCA showed a good medium-term result. Another follow-up angiogram performed 8 years later confirms a very good long-term result. In more than 90% of patients who have good angiographic results 4 months after angioplasty a good long-term result can be anticipated.

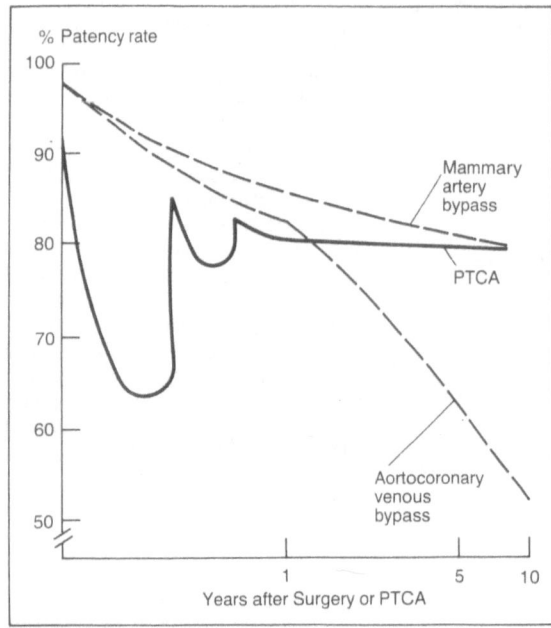

**Fig. 57.** Patency rate of coronary artery vessels after revascularization using internal mammary artery bypass (IMA), aortocoronary vein bypass (ACVB), and percutaneous transluminal coronary angioplasty (PTCA). In the case of angioplasty the curve shows changes during the first months due to restenosis and additional second or third angioplasties. Long-term results of IMA and PTCA are very similar.

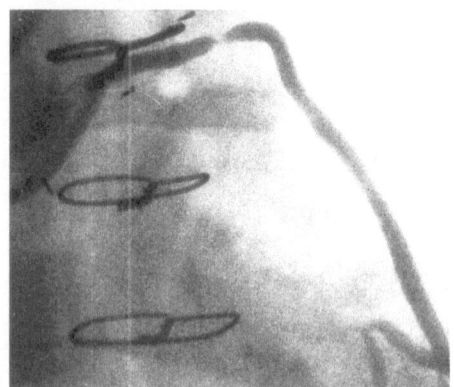

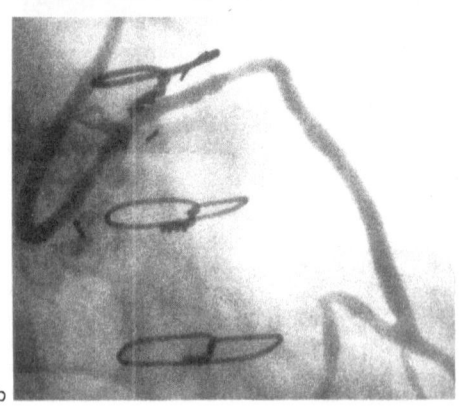

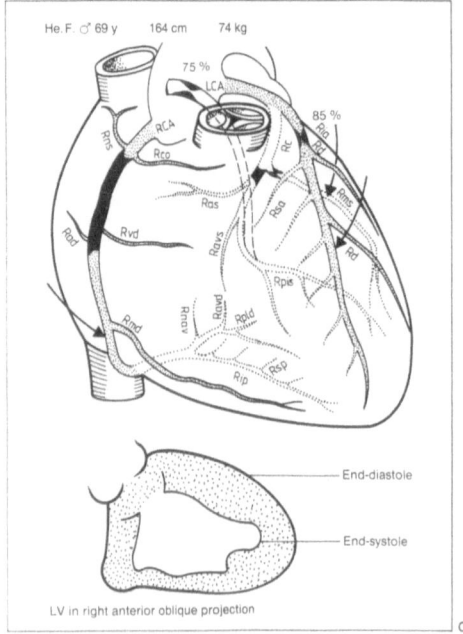

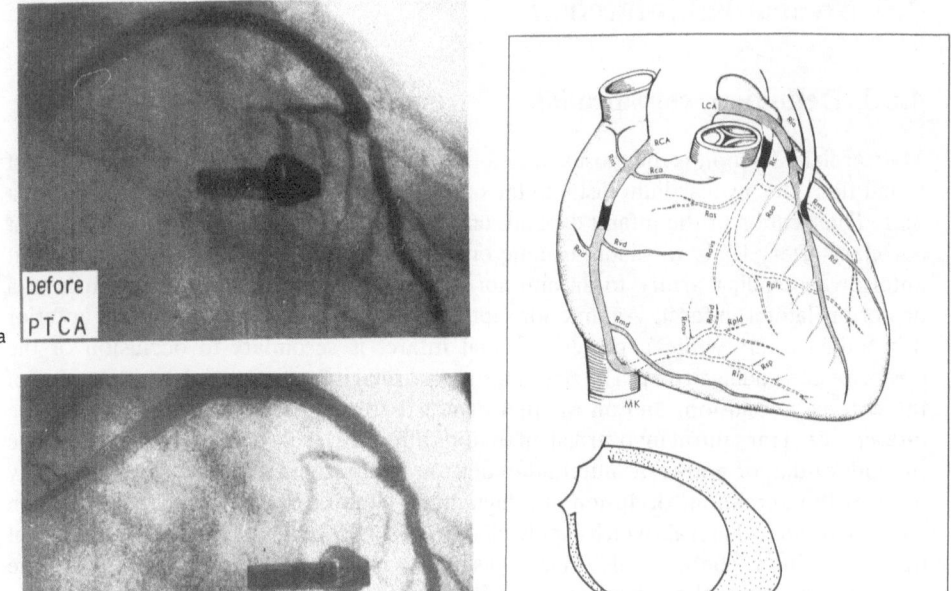

**Fig. 59.** This 46-year-old patient also had two of three venous grafts occluded. The open LAD-bypass had a 80% stenosis at the distal anastomosis (**a**). One year after PTCA a good result of PTCA was documented (**b**). Despite occlusion of RCA and RCX symptoms improved and reoperation was not necessary. The ventriculogram shows akinesia due to an infarct scar in the perfusion area of RCA and RCX (**c**).

one internal mammary graft. In Fig. 57 long-term patency rates are compared using the three different forms of revascularisation.

Angioplasty and coronary surgery are revascularization techniques which complement each other. Balloon angioplasty will be used if anatomically possible, but it necessitates surgical stand-by. In 5% of patients, where angioplasty seems possible, surgical intervention is nevertheless necessary, because the procedure – usually due to anatomic difficulties – is not feasible. In 4% of angioplasty cases a vessel occlusion occurs which necessitates emergency bypass surgery in about 0.5%.

Vice versa, balloon angioplasty may be used as a second intervention in 10% of primary surgical patients in order to avoid further surgical interventions. Balloon angioplasty as a second procedure may be useful in patients with bypass graft stenosis or graft occlusion (Figs. 58, 59).

◀ **Fig. 58.** Bypass operation and balloon dilatation as complementary procedures: In a 69-year-old patient with triple vessel obstruction two of three bypasses were occluded. The only open bypass had a high-grade proximal stenosis (**a**). After balloon dilatation this bypass remained open (**b**). Schematic representation (**c**).

73

# 4.6 Myocardial infarction

## 4.6.1 Definition, classification

Myocardial infarction is the most severe form of coronary insufficiency. Due to a loss of blood flow, the myocardium distal to the occlusion dies, becomes necrotic and forms a scar. The location of the infarct depends on the vessel occluded. Occlusion of the right coronary artery leads to diaphragmatic or inferior myocardial infarction, of the left anterior descending artery to an anterior infarct and of the circumflex branch to a posterior (lateral) infarct. An anterior septal infarct is associated with the left anterior descending artery while a posterior septal infarct is secondary to occlusion of the posterior descending artery. The size of the myocardial infarction depends on location of the coronary occlusion, and on whether or not there are preformed collaterals to the infarct area. Transmural myocardial infarctions affect all layers of the myocardium while subendocardial or non-transmural infarctions are of partial thickness. The latter may occur with intermittent occlusion of a high-grade stenosis or with persistent occlusion combined with collaterals which supply blood flow to the less susceptible outer layers of the myocardium. There are also infarctions, which in their central area affect the entire wall, but affect only the subendocardium in marginal areas.

## 4.6.2 Development of myocardial infarction

A transmural infarction is usually the consequence of an intra-arterial thrombus, which develops at the site of an atheroma. The initiating event is usually a tear of the intima or rupture of the plaque which leads to platelet deposition and thrombus formation. Often, it is an atheroma which has been present for many years, but suddenly ruptures and produces occlusion. In the case of a total coronary occlusion a myocardial infarction occurs; if there is only a partial luminal decrease, prolonged or crescendo angina may occur. The change from an uncomplicated to a complicated atheroma is independent

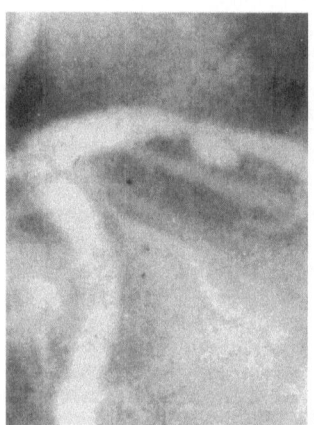 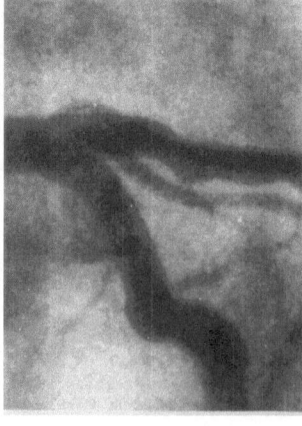

a      b

**Fig. 60. a** High-grade stenosis and a deep ulcer due to dissection of the intima in a 45-year-old man with angina pectoris. The high-grade stenosis of the left anterior descending was treated by angioplasty. **b** The ulcer healed after the procedure, and the patient became asymptomatic.

from the pre-existing luminal narrowing. In the case of a flat atheroma, the infarction may occur without premonitory symptoms. In the case of an atheroma that has previously caused high-grade stenosis, anginal attacks will usually have been present before the infarction. The often stepwise course of coronary artery disease is brought about by multiple tears with subintimal bleeding and/or thrombosis occurring in the same plaque. Figure 60 shows the angiogram of a chronic atheromatous ulcer (consequence of plaque rupture) distal to a coronary stenosis which was dilated by angioplasty.

### 4.6.3 Pathologic, angiographic and angioscopic findings

Necrosis of cardiac muscle cells occurs in areas without blood flow. Initially, leukocyte infiltration can be seen and, in the course of the following weeks, a fibrous scar forms. Usually, at autopsy, thrombi can be seen in the appropriate coronary artery supplying the infarct area, but not always. For a long time, there was uncertainty as to whether coronary artery thrombosis was of primary importance or whether it was simply a secondary event. Coronary arteriography during the development of acute myocardial infarction has shown that coronary thrombosis virtually always exists in transmural infarctions. The occluding thrombus is often resolved by drug therapy or intrinsic thrombolysis. Although the infarction can rarely be fully prevented, it can be diminished in size by early fibrinolysis. Usually myocardial necrosis occurres within 30 min to 2 h of persisting vessel occlusion.

### 4.6.4 Clinical manifestations

The typical myocardial infarction is a dramatic, life-threatening event. The patient experiences pain and a feeling of tightness behind the sternum, which is often associated with a feeling of immediate danger to life. The patient turns pale and sweaty, and often develops nausea, collapse, and impaired consciousness. Sudden cardiac death may occur with circulatory arrest due to ventricular fibrillation or asystole, or secondary to cardiogenic shock or severe left ventricular failure. Mortality is as high as 50%.

The arterial blood pressure is normal, elevated or depressed. On auscultation heart sounds may be soft; a third heart sound or a mitral insufficiency murmur may be heard. Extrasystoles nearly always occur and pulmonary congestion may develop early.

In other patients the clinical manifestations are not as dramatic. Atypical symptoms lead to infarction not being recognized and to a false diagnosis of rheumatic musculo-skeletal or gastrointestinal disorder. Because of radiation of the pain into the lower jaw, a patient with an acute myocardial infarction may see a dentist. In a diaphragmatic or inferior infarction, the symptoms may be perceived as epigastric pain, again confusing the diagnosis. In 30% of all infarctions, no pain at all is reported ("silent infarction"). This usually is seen in a patient group who, similar to those with "silent angina", are relatively insensitive to pain.

The hemodynamic consequences of an infarction are strongly correlated with the infarct size. A subendocardial infarction usually has the least hemodynamic consequence. A localized diaphragmatic or inferior infarction usually does not lead to pump failure unless bradycardia is marked or there has been prior anterior infarct. In contrast, a large anterior wall infarct with septal involvement may cause profound left ventricular failure, or cardiogenic shock.

The initial phase of a myocardial infarction is the most dangerous for the patient. The infarcted myocardium is at first soft and bulges outwards in systole like an aneurysm. Increase in pump function of the healthy myocardium may not compensate the loss. When the diseased myocardium is infiltrated by leukocytes, it changes in stiffness and compliance. The filling pressure will increase and the pump function improves. Coronary blood flow is, however, further impaired by an increased diastolic pressure.

In certain situations, even a small infarction may become life-threatening. This occurs if a papillary muscle becomes ischemic or necrotic, and severe mitral insufficiency results, or if in septal infarction a perforation of the septum occurs with left-to-right shunting. A rupture of the free ventricular wall will generally only occur with extensive infarction. Life-threatening arrhythmias are more frequent in larger infarctions, but ventricular fibrillation does also occur even with a small infarction. The physician should be motivated by the following motto when first confronted with a patient with ventricular fibrillation: "A heart in ventricular fibrillation is too good to die."

### 4.6.5 Diagnosis

The diagnosis is simple in typical cases and may be suggested by the patient himself or by his relatives. The ECG shows ST-elevation and T-wave peaking. There are four consecutive phases of ECG changes which vary in duration from hours to days (Fig. 61). At first, only the ST-segment is changed on the ECG. T-wave elevation occurs ("T-wave peaking"), thereafter ST-elevation is seen. These changes are largely reversible. But changes in the QRS complex, such as loss of R-wave or development of Q-waves, indicate irreversible necrosis. During the ensuing course a negative T-wave develops. Later, only Q-waves will remain as a sign of a previous infarction.

Characteristic ECG changes can be found in different recordings depending on the site of the infarction (Fig. 62). Inferior myocardial infarction is seen in Leads II, III and aVF; anterior myocardial infarction in standard Leads I and aVL, and chest leads V2–V6; posterior myocardial infarction in the anterior chest leads V1–V3, where there are reciprocal changes – instead of the typical ST-elevation, ST-depression is seen and, instead of R-wave loss, R-wave elevation and S-loss occurs. The cineangiogram of the left ventricle shows in the infarcted area a decreased contraction (Fig. 63).

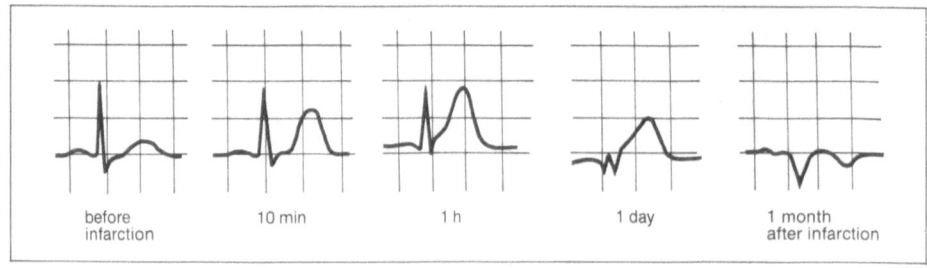

|  |  |  |  |  |
|---|---|---|---|---|
| before infarction | 10 min | 1 h | 1 day | 1 month after infarction |

**Fig. 61.** Sequence of ECG changes in myocardial infarction. In some cases the chronological order may vary substantially from these average values.

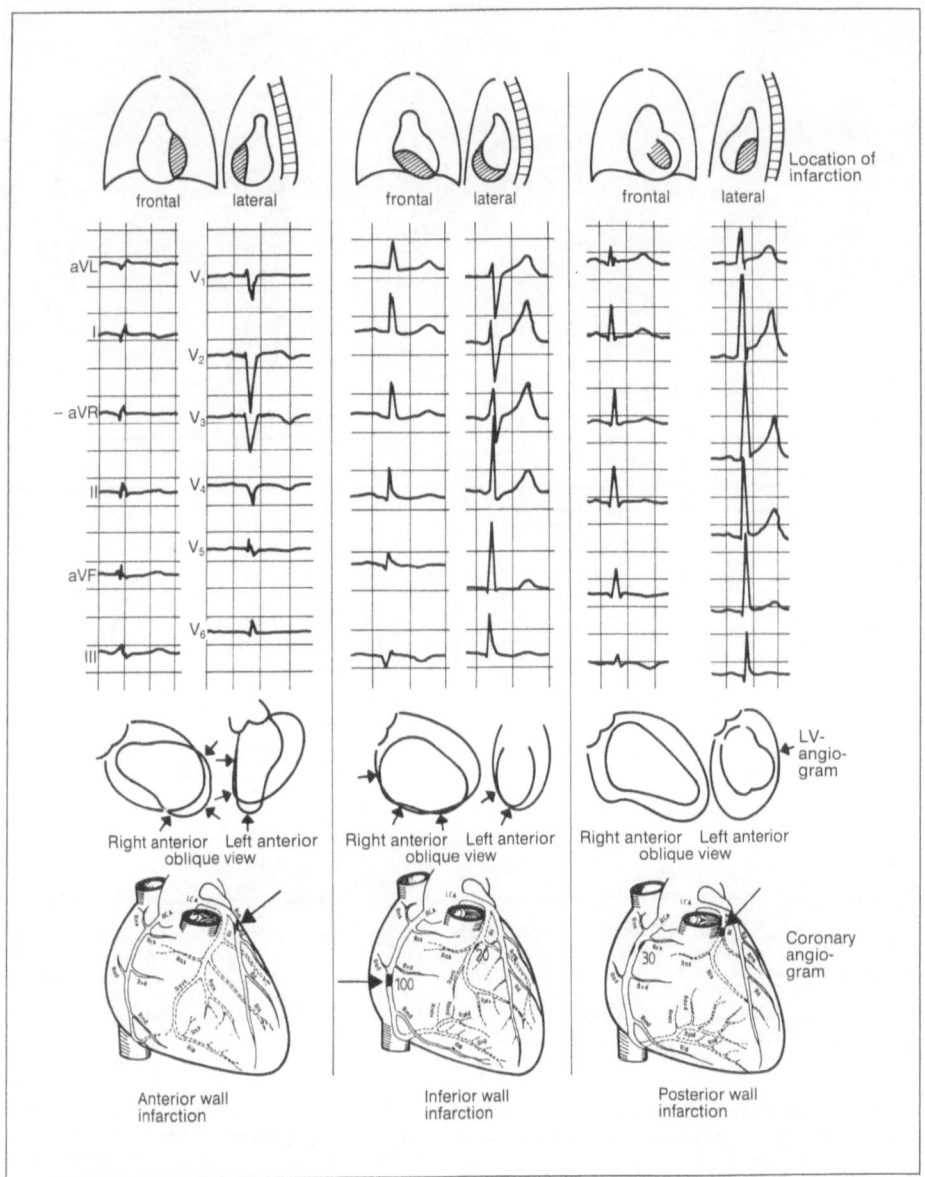

**Fig. 62.** Synopsis of location of infarction, ECG, ventriculogram, and coronary arteriogram in anterior, diaphragmatic (inferior), and posterior myocardial infarctions. From top down, the location of the infarct, the ECG, the ventriculogram (in right anterior and left anterior oblique projections), and the coronary arteriogram is shown. The systolic and diastolic contours of the ventricle are shown on the left ventriculogram with the contractile defect indicated with arrows. The location of the occlusion, as seen on the arteriogram, is also indicated with an arrow.

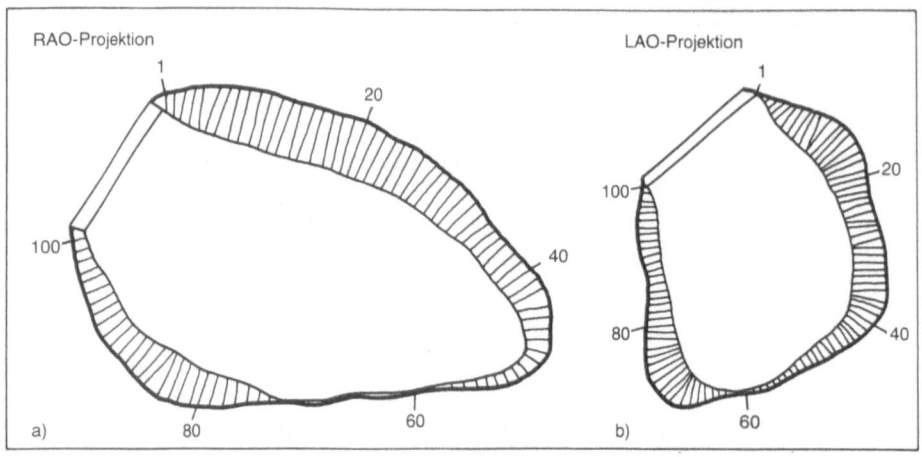

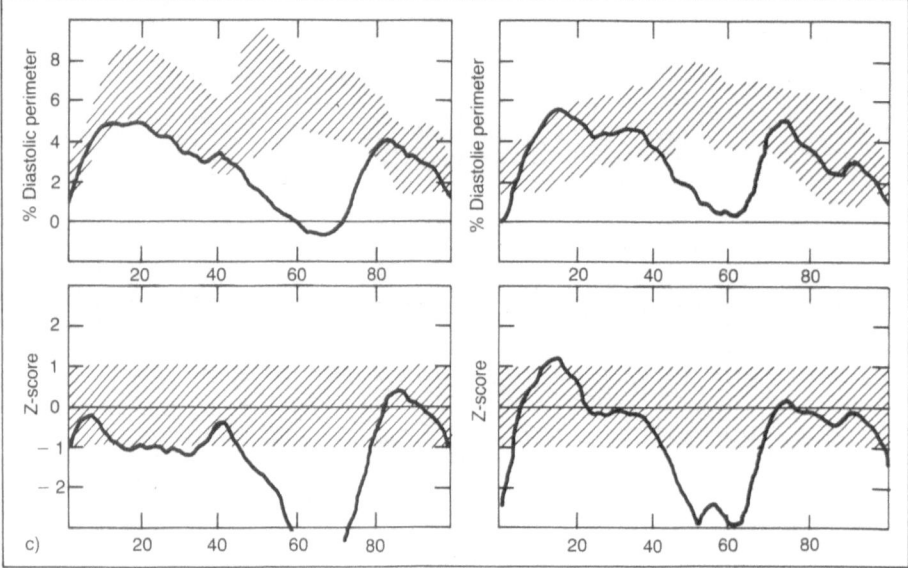

**Fig. 63.** Cineangiogram of the left ventricle in a patient with diaphragmatic (inferior) infarction. **a** The diastolic and systolic contours show akinesia in the inferior wall. Regional analysis of contraction demonstrates hypo- or akinesia in segments 40–80. **b** The dotted area represents the normal range ($\times \pm \sigma$) in % of diastolic perimeter. In **c** the same pattern is displayed with the normal range as a horizontal band comprising the average value of contraction as zero line plus/minus one sigma.

Myocardial necrosis induces a typical elevation of enzymes in the peripheral blood, which begins 4–6 h after the infarction and persists for several days (Fig. 64). Usually the ECG will show changes before the enzymes increase. Whereas elevation of creatinine phosphokinase (CPK) may result from necrosis of many types of cells, and can therefore also be caused by intramuscular injections, elevation of the cardiac muscle isoenzyme

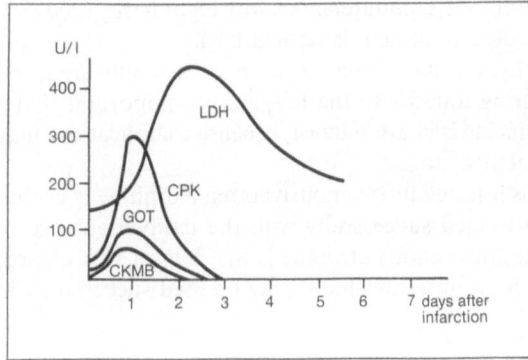

**Fig. 64.** Time-course of enzyme release after acute myocardial infarction.

(CPK-MB) is quite specific for myocardial necrosis. If the MB isoenzyme level is more than 5–10% of the total CPK (depending on the specific laboratory), then myocardial infarction is highly likely. The amount of increase in CPK and CPK-MB reflects the size of the infarction. Fever, leukocytosis, and hyperglycemia also occur.

### 4.6.6 Therapeutic interventions and diagnostic procedures in acute myocardial infarction

The fate of a patient with myocardial infarction is mostly determined within the first minutes or hours. Almost half of the patients die before the physician or the ambulance arrives. Since sudden cardiac death in acute myocardial infarction is usually due to arrhythmias, which by themselves are not lethal, there have been many attempts to decrease the high primary mortality rate with cardiopulmonary resuscitation by laypersons. It seems to be beneficial that the public in general knows about cardiopulmonary resuscitation. The probability for success is higher if earlier and more specific interventions (in particular, cardiac defibrillation) are performed, irrespective of who applies them.

During resuscitation of someone found unconscious, the *ABCD-rule* should be remembered:

$A$ = *a*irways clear
$B$ = *b*reathing (in respiratory arrest)
$C$ = *c*ompression of the chest (in circulatory arrest)
$D$ = *d*efibrillation, *d*iagnosis, and use of *d*rugs

This sequence applies to patients with an unwitnessed circulatory arrest. In a witnessed sudden circulatory arrest (usually due to ventricular fibrillation or asystole) therapy begins with a precordial thump. This may lead to spontaneous contraction in the case of asystole. Ventricular fibrillation will only rarely be interrupted by mechanical stimulation alone. If this intervention fails, the patient is placed on a hard surface and closed-chest massage is performed. Correct application without using any other intervention will usually lead to spontaneous breathing and restoration of consciousness; exceptions are mostly seen in patients with a circulatory arrest lasting several minutes. Ventricular fibrillation is corrected by nonsynchronized DC countershock with high energy (200–360 joules), in Table 5 the emergency medical treatment is summarized.

For a documented or suspected myocardial infarction, even if uncomplicated, the patient is promptly hospitalized. During transfer to the hospital it is important that a physician or emergency medical technician is in attendance, because complications may require urgent intervention at a moment's notice.

If pain is prominent, an analgesic is injected intravenously; often morphine is useful. Ventricular arrhythmias are usually treated successfully with the intravenous use of lidocaine. In the case of bradycardia, intravenous atropine is the drug of first choice. Nitroglycerin – formerly thought to be contraindicated – may be used successfully in

**Table 5.** Medical treatment in acute myocardial infarction.

| | | |
|---|---|---|
| *1) General* | | |
| Nitroglycerin | 1–3 mg/h i. v.<br>0.4–0.8 mg s. l. | except in patients with systolic<br>BP < 90 mmHg |
| Heparin i. v. | 1000 U/h | |
| Aspirin p. o. | 100–300 mg/d | |
| *2) Thrombolysis in patients with infarcts < 6 h* | | |
| Streptokinase | 1.5 million U i. v. within 1 h | avoid repeat application<br>(allergy) |
| Urokinase | 1.5 million U i. v. within 15 min | |
| rt-PA | 100 mg in 4 h | |
| APSAC | 30 mg in 5 min | avoid repeat application<br>(allergy) |
| *3) Heart failure, pulmonary edema* | | |
| Nitroglycerin | 10–50 µg/min (0.6–3 mg/h)<br>0.8 mg s. l. | |
| Captopril | 6.25 mg p. o. | |
| Furosemide | 20–40 mg i. v. | |
| *4) Arrhythmias* | | |
| Bradycardia  Atropine | 0.5–1 mg i. v. | |
| Ventricular  Lidocaine<br>arrhythmias | 80–130 mg i. v.<br>2–4 mg/min i. v. | |
| *5) Shock* | | |
| Dobutamine | 5–20 µg/kg/min i. v. | |
| Dopamine | 3–15 µg/kg/min i. v. | |
| Nitroglycerin | 10–50 µg/min i. v. | |
| Intraaortic balloon pump | | |
| Emergency coronary angiography | | |

acute myocardial infarction, especially if the filling pressure is elevated. This can be clinically documented by dyspnea with basilar rales caused by pulmonary congestion. In any case, it is advisable to initially use only a small dose of nitroglycerin (e.g., 0.4 mg sublingually, or 1 mg/h i. v. infusion) and to monitor the response. If there is inadequate improvement after 5 min and no adverse effect, then higher doses can be used. Nitroglycerin is especially effective as a first-line intervention in pulmonary edema.

In cardiogenic shock due to severe pump failure the therapeutic possibilities are restricted. In addition to drug therapy, for example dobutamine and nitroglycerin infusion, the use of other methods may be tried. The most promising intervention is immediate use of an intra-aortic balloon pump and restoration of blood flow by passing a guide wire through the coronary thrombus, and subsequent balloon angioplasty.

Patients hospitalized without cardiogenic shock have a relatively good prognosis. With intensive care, the hospital mortality rate is less than 10%. A very important intervention is ECG monitoring. Life-threatening arrhythmias can be successfully controlled in a coronary care unit environment. Other interventions aim at reducing the amount of infarction. The left ventricular filling pressure can be measured using Swan-Ganz right heart catheterization, but it can also be estimated from clinical manifestations such as basilar rales or visible pulmonary congestion on the x-ray. Therapy with nitrates is a good first step. Nitroglycerin may be used sublingually or infused intravenously. Oral administration of isosorbide dinitrate or isosorbide 5-mononitrate also improves ventricular function and may lower the mortality rate.

Following pioneering work by Chazov in Moscow and Rentrop in Germany, thrombolytic drug therapy has now been established as a first-line procedure. A variety of agents (see Table 5) are effective in reopening about two-thirds of acutely occluded coronary arteries. The most important limitation of this procedure is that the infarct has often reached its final size when the patient is hospitalized. Exceptions are with those patients where the myocardial infarction occurred less than 6 h prior to treatment, or where the infarction has developed only slowly due to good collaterals. Systemic thrombolysis with streptokinase, urokinase, rt-PA, or APSAC may be used. There is currently no clear clinical advantage of one over another. If the diagnosis is clear, intravenous thrombolysis may be initiated outside of the hospital.

Intracoronary thrombolysis benefits from the fact that higher local concentrations can be achieved and lower total dosages are needed. It may be combined with or replaced by mechanical recanalization, achieved most easily with balloon angioplasty. However, such an invasive therapeutic intervention needs a properly-equipped cardiac laboratory and 24-h stand-by. The therapeutic gain justifies the large effort only in special situations, such as in shock or severe LV failure. This approach may also be an optimal one when acute infarction develops within the hospital setting or close by.

Prophylaxis against rethrombosis is achieved with aspirin and with heparin infusion (see Table 5) the therapy being commenced simultaneously with thrombolytic therapy.

Thromboembolic complications usually occur in the subacute phase, i.e., several days after the myocardial infarction. Prophylaxis is accomplished with platelet inhibitors, heparin, and, in some patients, oral anticoagulants. This step is especially important in patients with left ventricular mural thrombus recognized by echocardiography. In patients with or without lysis complete coronary occlusions can persist. If the myocardium distal to the occlusion is still viable angioplasty reopening may be attempted (Figs. 65, 66).

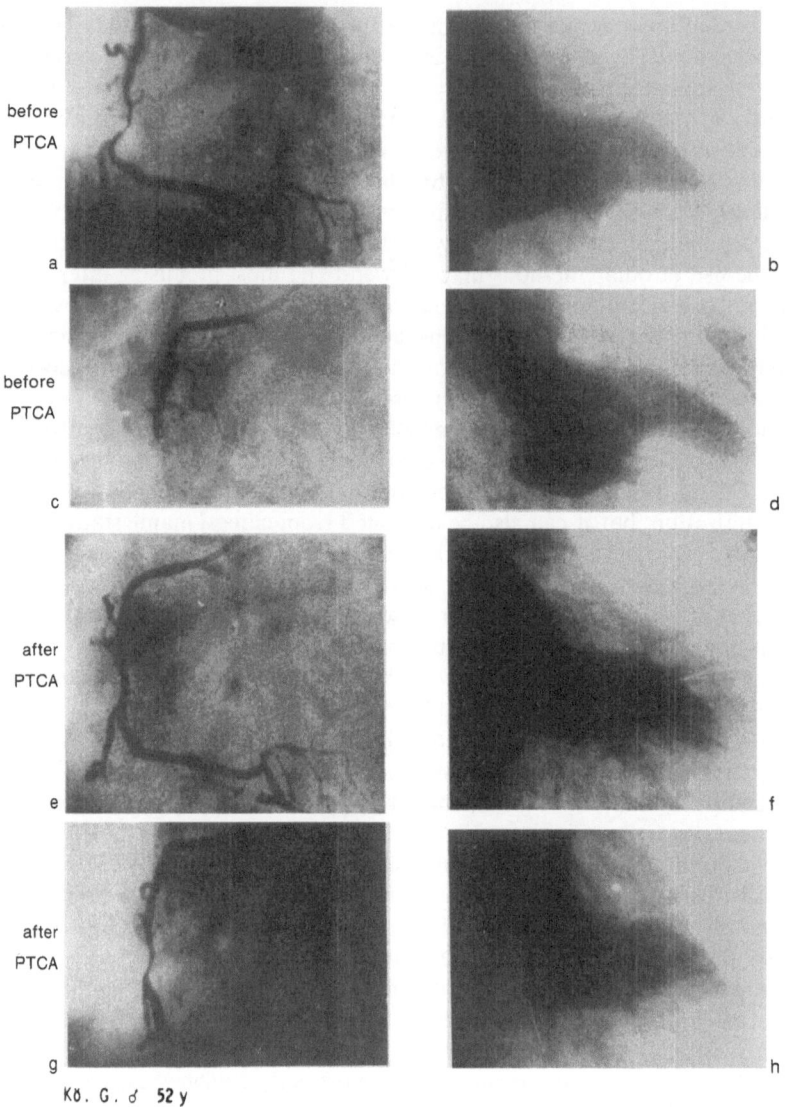

before
PTCA

a

b

before
PTCA

c

d

after
PTCA

e

f

after
PTCA

g

h

KÖ. G. ♂ 52 y

**Fig. 65.** Right coronary artery of a 52-year-old man with severe angina pectoris. At the diagnostic angiography a high-grade stenosis of the RCA (**a**) is seen. The systolic contour of the left ventricle shows normal contraction (**b**).

Two months later when the patient was scheduled for coronary angioplasty, the right coronary artery was totally occluded (**c**) and the left ventricle showed an akinetic area in the diaphragmatic wall (**d**).

After successful reopening (**e**) the right coronary artery looked normal and left ventricular function also returned to normal (**f**).

Two months later angina reappeared and the follow-up angiogram showed a restenosis (**g**) which is not as narrow and has smoother contours than in (**a**).

The left ventricle is still normal (**h**). In this particular patient, who was treated in 1978, bypass surgery was performed. Today a reangioplasty would be performed.

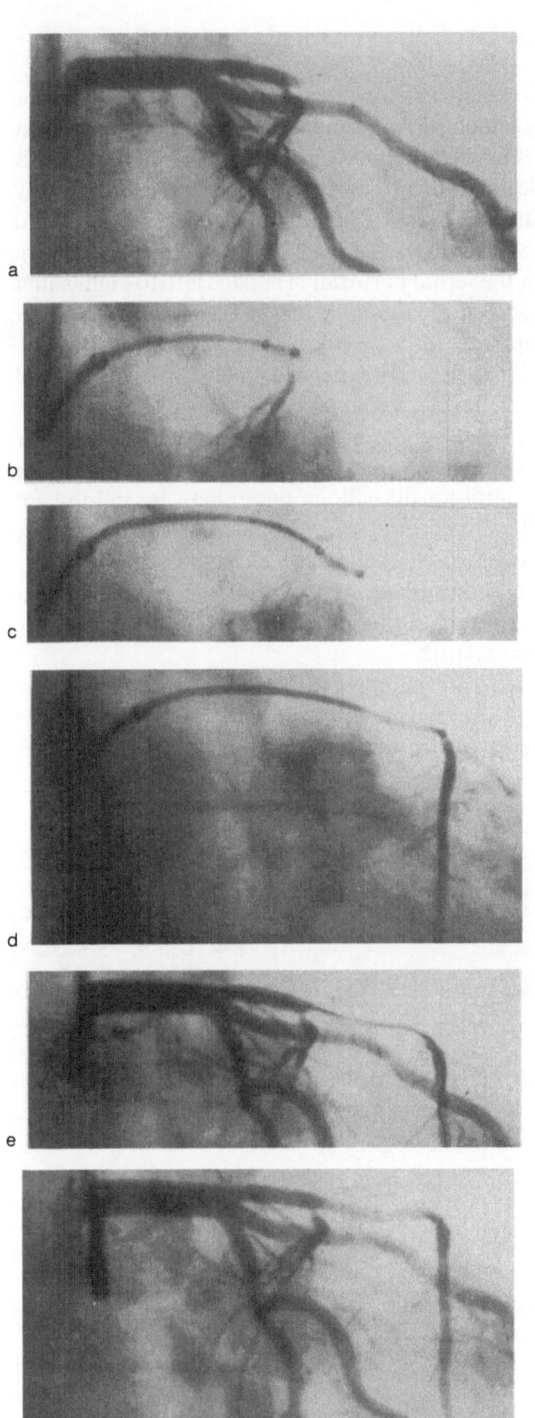

a

b

c

d

e

f

**Fig. 66. a** Chronic occlusion of the LAD in a 30-year-old man with a well preserved left ventricle and typical angina. The total occlusion was already demonstrated at an angiogram performed 3½ months earlier. The distal LAD is faintly filled by "bridging" collaterals. Reopening was not possible with a conventional guide wire technique. **b** Therefore, a slowly rotating flexible steel catheter with a rounded tip (Rotacs) was introduced and advanced in the obstruction during slow rotation at 200 rpm. **c** One can see how the flexible catheter had to find its way upward in the obstruction. **d** After several centimeters the olive of the rotating catheter points downwards. Repeated contrast injection through the Rotacs now shows superselective filling of the distal LAD. **e** An exchange wire is introduced through the central lumen of the Rotacs and the Rotacs is removed. Contrast injection through the guiding catheter shows re-established antegrade filling and the channel created by the Rotacs catheter. **f** After additional balloon angioplasty the obstructed part of the LAD is efficiently widened. The patient became symptom free.

83

### 4.6.7 Complicated myocardial infarction, ventricular aneurysm

In cardiogenic shock due to pump failure in the first few hours of myocardial infarction, immediate restoration of blood flow by catheter intervention (balloon dilatation) is most promising. In some cases, only surgical intervention may save the patient's life. This is especially true when there are mechanical complications such as septal rupture. This may occur either in anterior or inferior infarction. Clinically, the complication is recognized by the sudden appearance of a loud systolic murmur at the left sternal edge in the third intercostal space. On echocardiography the septal perforation and the left-to-right shunt are often visible. The oxygen saturation in the pulmonary artery is significantly higher than in the right atrium when blood samples are obtained through a Swan-Ganz catheter.

If the infarction involves the anterior or posterior papillary muscle, severe mitral insufficiency may result. Pump failure occurs due to volume overloading of the ventricle. Drug therapy with nitroglycerin often leads to hemodynamic improvement. If the hemodynamics cannot be stabilized, emergency surgery with valvular replacement or repair is necessary. In some cases an intra-aortic balloon pump may be helpful for temporary stabilization until surgery. This intervention lowers the cardiac workload by means of an ECG-triggered, diastolic expansion of a balloon which has been placed in the aorta via a catheter. The additional diastolic pumping action of the balloon assists forward blood flow, supports coronary perfusion, and lowers end-diastolic aortic pressure in readiness for the next cardiac systole.

Small cardiac aneurysms, i.e., localized wall segments with systolic outward bulging, may have little hemodynamic consequence. However, large aneurysms cause heart failure. In cases where the non-infarcted myocardium contracts well, aneurysm ectomy

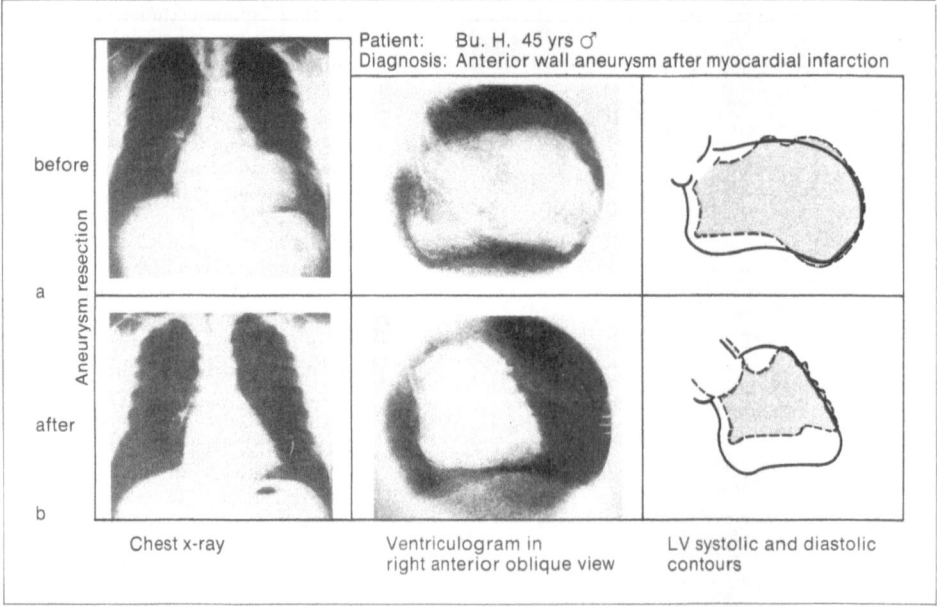

Patient: Bu. H. 45 yrs ♂
Diagnosis: Anterior wall aneurysm after myocardial infarction

Aneurysm resection

before
a
after
b

Chest x-ray | Ventriculogram in right anterior oblique view | LV systolic and diastolic contours

**Fig. 67.** Surgical resection with reduction in size of the ventricle in a patient with severe left heart failure due to ventricular aneurysm. The operation led to sustained clinical improvement.

may achieve excellent results by reducing the ventricular volume, decreasing the wall tension, and eliminating relative blood stasis (Fig. 67). Extensive akinesis without a clearly defined aneurysm is not an indication for surgery.

Arrhythmias occur with nearly every acute myocardial infarction and they are often life-threatening. In the later post-infarct course, they are less frequent, but still are the main cause for sudden cardiac death. There is a direct correlation between the frequency of arrhythmias and the severity of ventricular dysfunction. In individual cases, however, even small scars may, due to a change in conduction velocity and by promoting reentry, be the cause of recurrent ventricular tachycardia or recurrent ventricular fibrillation. If it is possible to locate the responsible segment (with intraoperative ECG recordings), surgical excision of the scar or an encircling ventriculotomy may abolish the arrhythmia. In some circumstances, implantation of an automatic defibrillator is necessary.

## 4.6.8 Cardiac rehabilitation, diagnostic procedures after infarction

Mobilization of the infarct patient should be instituted as early as possible (Fig. 68). In the case of an uncomplicated infarction without significant hemodynamic consequences, the patient should start to be mobilized the next day. The patient is helped to the toilet; hemodynamic measurements have shown that defecation while sitting is much less demanding than it is in the recumbent position. "Easy-chairs" should be available within the first days.

Late in the first week or early into the second week, the patient is usually fully mobilized. A modified (less stress than usual) exercise ECG should be done before discharge. If the ECG shows no pathologic changes at a reasonable workload, the patient may be discharged. If there is ischemia or anginal pain during the exercise, coronary arteriography will be necessary.

In order to estimate the myocardial reserve it is useful to get an idea of the size of the myocardial infarction. An estimation can be obtained from the determination of the cardiac volume by x-ray or, more usually, by echocardiography. Except for patients in whom, due to pulmonary emphysema, a good quality ultrasound cannot be achieved, two-dimensional (2D) echocardiography is especially helpful for locating and quantifying the myocardial infarction. Radionuclide ventriculography (ECG-triggered cardiac radionuclide imaging) allows estimation of the end-diastolic and end-systolic volume of the ventricle with determination of global and regional ejection fractions. The patient's prognosis is directly correlated with the size of the infarct. The less extensive the scar appears on echocardiography, the less the ejection fraction is reduced, and the better the prognosis.

Surgical aneurysmectomy has good results in the case of large, well-defined, ventricular aneurysms. On the other hand, severe diffuse damage has an unfavorable outlook. These patients often develop progressive cardiac failure which can be a challenge for therapy. Drug therapy includes digitalis, diuretics, vasodilators, and ACE inhibitors. If heart failure is refractory, cardiac transplantation should be considered if patients are younger than 60 years and meet specific physical and emotional criteria.

In addition to the contractile state of the myocardium, the condition of the coronary arteries is important in prognosis. If there are no signs of ischemia on an exercise ECG

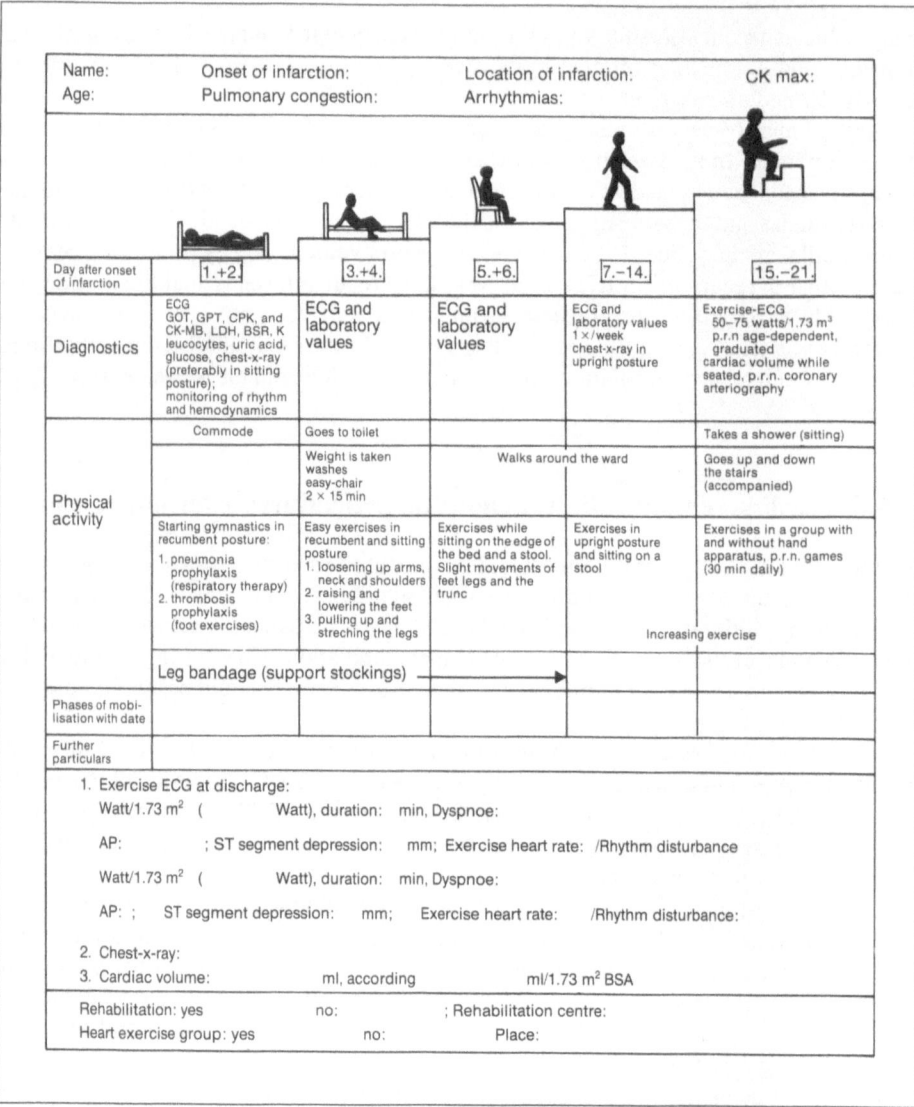

| Name:<br>Age: | Onset of infarction:<br>Pulmonary congestion: | Location of infarction:<br>Arrhythmias: | | CK max: |
|---|---|---|---|---|
| **Day after onset of infarction** | 1.+2. | 3.+4. | 5.+6. | 7.-14. | 15.-21. |
| **Diagnostics** | ECG<br>GOT, GPT, CPK, and CK-MB, LDH, BSR, K leucocytes, uric acid, glucose, chest-x-ray (preferably in sitting posture); monitoring of rhythm and hemodynamics | ECG and laboratory values | ECG and laboratory values | ECG and laboratory values 1 ×/week chest-x-ray in upright posture | Exercise-ECG 50–75 watts/1.73 m³ p.r.n age-dependent, graduated cardiac volume while seated, p.r.n. coronary arteriography |
| **Physical activity** | Commode | Goes to toilet | | | Takes a shower (sitting) |
| | | Weight is taken washes easy-chair 2 × 15 min | Walks around the ward | | Goes up and down the stairs (accompanied) |
| | Starting gymnastics in recumbent posture:<br>1. pneumonia prophylaxis (respiratory therapy)<br>2. thrombosis prophylaxis (foot exercises) | Easy exercises in recumbent and sitting posture<br>1. loosening up arms, neck and shoulders<br>2. raising and lowering the feet<br>3. pulling up and streching the legs | Exercises while sitting on the edge of the bed and a stool. Slight movements of feet legs and the trunc | Exercises in upright posture and sitting on a stool | Exercises in a group with and without hand apparatus, p.r.n. games (30 min daily) |
| | | | | | Increasing exercise |
| | Leg bandage (support stockings) ——————————→ | | | | |
| **Phases of mobilisation with date** | | | | | |
| **Further particulars** | | | | | |

1. Exercise ECG at discharge:

    Watt/1.73 m² (     Watt), duration:  min, Dyspnoe:

    AP:     ; ST segment depression:   mm; Exercise heart rate: /Rhythm disturbance

    Watt/1.73 m² (     Watt), duration:  min, Dyspnoe:

    AP: ; ST segment depression:   mm; Exercise heart rate:  /Rhythm disturbance:

2. Chest-x-ray:
3. Cardiac volume:     ml, according     ml/1.73 m² BSA

Rehabilitation: yes     no:      ; Rehabilitation centre:

Heart exercise group: yes     no:     Place:

**Fig. 68.** Rehabilitation schema after acute myocardial infarction. The chronological order of the mobilization measures is adapted to the specific situation and the clinical course.

with an adequate workload and no complaints of angina pectoris or increased dyspnea, one may predict that there is reasonable coronary reserve. This is usually the case with single-vessel coronary disease; otherwise, coronary arteriography is indicated. If there are critical stenoses or occlusions in vessels perfusing noninfarcted myocardium, bypass surgery or balloon angioplasty should be considered.

### 4.6.9 Non-transmural myocardial infarction

Non-transmural infarction is a clinical myocardial infarction with increase of the enzymes, but without the development of Q-waves or loss of R-waves on the ECG. ST-segment changes such as peaked and inverted T-waves may persist or regress slowly. During follow-up, patients may be asymptomatic or suffer anginal attacks. The exercise ECG will indicate whether myocardial ischemia occurs with exercise. Coronary arteriography is usually indicated, because patients with non-transmural infarction are prone to suffer further, transmural infarctions. Often high-grade proximal coronary artery stenosis easily accessible for angioplasty is seen. It is quite likely that non-transmural infarction is caused by a complete thrombotic occlusion of a high-grade stenosed coronary artery which is quickly reopened by natural or administered fibrinolysis.

### 4.6.10 Cardiac rehabilitation

Rehabilitation of the coronary patient should begin in the intensive or coronary care unit. The impressions and understanding that the patient receives during the acute phase of myocardial infarction may be important for the long-term. Early rehabilitation, i.e., mobilization of the patient as soon as possible and as much as possible, is generally accepted today. Concerns as to whether the infarction might extend, and aneurysm or ventricular rupture may occur, have not been substantiated. Early mobilization has also proven to be the most effective protection against thromboembolic complications. It also undoubtedly contributes to the emotional and physical rehabilitation of the patient. If mobilization is instituted in time, it is usually possible to perform an exercise ECG with an adequate workload (from 75 to 150 watts for 6 min, depending on age and sex) within the first to third post-infarction week. The results will show whether or not coronary arteriography is necessary.

After hospitalization, further progressive rehabilitation at home or in a rehabilitation center continues over several weeks. In addition, special attention is given to motivation to live a healthy life, to stop smoking, and to correct other risk factors. If diagnostic procedures have not been done in the acute setting, they are further considered at outpatient follow-up 2–4 weeks after hospital dismissal.

Ambulatory sports groups have proven to be very useful, not only for many patients following myocardial infarction, but also for patients after surgery or angioplasty. There are several thousand groups in Germany in which psychologic support is offered in addition to exercise therapy with gymnastics and games. Group dynamics, if wisely monitored, may be helpful. The physician involved has to find the proper balance between controlling anxiety and fear, giving encouragement, and softening the overzealousness which sometimes "infects" members of a group.

Pure self-help groups are not recommended because some patients will not overcome their fear of reinfarction, and others with excessive zeal may tend to dominate and put other group members under pressure.

### 4.6.11 Psychologic support of post-infarct patients

To what extent the modern lifestyle contributes to myocardial infarction has frequently been discussed. Myocardial infarction has been classified as a "manager-disorder", since it may occur more frequently in certain stress situations or with inadequate stress relief. However, there are arguments against all these hypotheses. It must be borne in mind that the epidemiologic data linking infarction with stress should be interpreted cautiously, as it is observational and does not provide a test of causality. Perhaps one should also not talk any longer of "manager-disease", because the predominance of managers among infarct patients has disappeared with changing smoking habits. Infarcts are more common today in lower-income classes, where cigarette smoking is most common. On the other hand, some investigations do indicate that people with a hostile, driving, time-conscious behavior are prone to myocardial infarction. It is appropriate for those patients to develop opportunities for relaxation and stress reduction, although a clear causal connection between a specific pattern of behavior and the occurrence of myocardial infarction has not yet been proven. Measures for rehabilitation, including the psychologic aspects, must always be applied with care and attention to the individual personality of the patient.

Premature retirement does not improve the prognosis, and it may rather induce depression or neurotic disturbances. It may actually shorten life expectancy ("retirement death").

### 4.6.12 General lifestyle, chronic drug therapy

Sufficient exercise and normal body weight are important. Giving up smoking is a must for every infarct or coronary patient, just as for any other patient with atherosclerosis. Only a physician who is a non-smoker has a chance of being listened to on this issue. It is advisable to keep to a low fat diet. Plant lipids with a high percentage of unsaturated fatty acids should be used for cooking. Therapy with lipid-lowering drugs should be restricted to patients with severe disturbances of lipid metabolism.

Prevention of recurrent coronary artery thrombosis is important after myocardial infarction. This is especially true for patients with multivessel disease, where ulceration of new atheromas may occur at any time. The best documented antithrombotic intervention is chronic aspirin therapy and it should always be introduced if no contraindication (recurring gastric ulcer, gastritis, aspirin allergy) exists. The daily dose is between 0.1 and 0.5 g. Beneficial results have been achieved with both high and low doses. Daily administration of 0.1 g may be sufficient.

Some studies have found a beneficial effect of β-receptor blockers on late mortality and reinfarction. Other studies have not confirmed such an effect, and they were even terminated prematurely because of the drugs' unfavorable effects. Most of the studies with a negative result used β-blockers with concomitant β-receptor-stimulating effects. Whether these characteristics are responsible for the lack of mortality effect has not yet been verified. Therapy with calcium antagonists is indicated in patients with unstable angina, and after non-transmural infarction. Recently, a benefical effect has also been reported after transmural infarction.

# 5 Inflammatory cardiac disorders

## 5.1 Endocarditis

Bacterial endocarditis is to be distinguished from rheumatic endocarditis. It encompasses acute, and also subacute and chronic courses. This serious disease is found in all age groups, as opposed to rheumatic endocarditis, which occurs predominantly in children or juveniles. Although rheumatic fever is the result of a bacterial infection, contrary to bacterial endocarditis it is not caused through direct bacterial involvement of the heart, but through an inflammatory-allergic reaction of the endocardium to bacterial toxins produced by streptococcal infection in the nasopharynx.

### 5.1.1 Bacterial endocarditis

Bacterial or infectious endocarditis is a serious disease which, before institution of antibiotic therapy, was almost uniformly fatal. Today, the success rate is excellent for the majority of patients, but even so, the fatality rate is 10–20%. The endocardium of the cardiac valves is a tissue with little blood flow, despite the fact that the valves "swim in blood". Therefore, the endocardium of the cardiac valves is especially receptive to infection (predominantly the mitral and the aortic valves). In the drug addict, endocarditis will also affect right heart valves. The endocardium in the area of previously damaged valves or of congenital disorders is especially susceptible for infections, for example, in former rheumatic valvular lesions, congenital aortic stenosis, mitral valve prolapse, patent ductus arteriosus or ventricular septal defect.

Acute septic endocarditis usually occurs after bacterial sepsis. Causative agents are staphylococci, streptococci, and E. coli bacteria with staphylococcal sepsis seen more often in recent years. Bacterial endocarditis is often seen in association with a bacterial infection such as abscess, peritonitis, infection in the biliary or urinary tract, or pneumonia. It may also be induced by medical procedures such as endoscopy, infusions or surgery.

Cardiac valve disorders due to bacterial endocarditis include ulcers, bacterial vegetations, and thromboses. Beyond destruction of the valves, these may lead to septic emboli to the cerebral arteries, kidneys, spleen, and extremities. Clinically, with acute septic endocarditis, there is fever with temperatures up to 40°C and intermittent chills. The spleen is often enlarged and the digits show small red spots (infarcts) resulting from bleeding after microembolism. Usually, a murmur can be auscultated over the heart. The murmur may develop or change during the course of the disease. A change in the character of the murmur often indicates progressive disease of the cardiac valves. A typical consequence of valvular endocarditis is mitral insufficiency. This can be especially dramatic when caused by ruptured chordae tendineae. Septic endocarditis may lead to perforation of the aortic valve and, consequently, to acute aortic insufficiency with severe hemodynamic consequences.

Subacute endocarditis differs from the acute form in that it is characterized by a relatively silent and slowly progressive course. Bacterial colonization of the cardiac valves is caused by bacteremia, often associated with nasopharyngeal infection or after dental procedures, yet without general sepsis. Bacterial vegetations occur with the same frequency on both the mitral and aortic valve; in 15–20% of the patients both valves are affected. The most common causative agents are streptococci (streptococcus viridans 50%) and enterococci (15%). Bacteria cannot be found in the blood of approximately 10% of the patients, especially if blood cultures are obtained after some antibiotics have been administered.

Symptoms such as fatigue and weakness occur for weeks or months, and often the patient will consult a physician long after symptoms have started. A "dusky" paleness of the skin is characteristic; the patient has transient fevers; the spleen is enlarged, and fingers and toes show signs of petechial bleeding. Further symptoms are cardiac murmur, anemia, and a markedly elevated erythrocyte sedimentation rate, often with concomitant focal nephritis.

It is not too difficult to diagnose this disease, as long as the physician bears it in mind. It may be rapidly confirmed by blood culture, but blood cultures are only reliable if they have been obtained prior to antibiotic therapy.

### Treatment

Antibiotic therapy is most effective and has the least adverse effects if it is aimed at the causative agent found in the blood culture. Group D streptococcal endocarditis is usually treated with high-dose intravenous infusions of penicillin (e.g., 4 mega penicillin G daily), sometimes combined with an aminoglycoside, for 4 to 6 weeks. Cure is achieved in more than 80% of patients. Even higher cure rates are seen with shorter (2-week) courses of penicillin in patients who have streptococcus viridans endocarditis.

Staphylococcal endocarditis associated with sepsis is a very severe disorder with a mortality rate above 50%. Successful treatment depends on the diagnosis being made in a timely fashion, and on the virulence and sensitivity of the micro-organism. It is especially difficult to treat hospital-acquired infections as well as patients with an impaired immune response (drug addicts, patients with chronic illness). Besides penicillin, penicillinase resistant agents (for example oxacillin), cephalosporins, and vancomycin have their place in therapy.

Infected thrombi or septic valvular vegetations may often be directly visible with echocardiography. Septic foci, or abscesses which do not respond to antibiotics, can often be treated surgically. Also, if destruction of the valves, rupture of chordae, or valvular perforation cause refractory heart failure, surgical intervention with valvular replacement may demand urgent consideration. Surgical success rates are remarkably high even during the most severe phases of the disease.

Many cases of bacterial endocarditis follow bacteremia induced by dental, genitourinary or gastrointestinal manipulation. Therefore, appropriate antibiotic prophylaxis is recommended when patients with valvular heart disease undergo these procedures (Tables 6, 7). Special care is also necessary with intravenous infusion lines; bacterial contamination may occur if the infusion set remains in place for several days.

90

**Table 6.** Prophylaxis for infective endocarditis in adults, recommended by the German Cardiac Society.

| Procedure | Regime |
|---|---|
| Dental treatment: (e.g., tooth extraction, gum treatment, scaling) | Oral penicillin: 1 million units Penicillin V (= 2 × 0.6 G) 1 h prior to and 6 h after the procedure |
| Instrumentation of the upper respiratory tract: (e.g., bronchoscopy) | ditto |
| Instrumentation of the urogenital or gastrointestinal tract: | Amoxicillin: 1 G orally 1 h prior to and 6 h after the procedure |

**Table 7.** Bacterial endocarditis prophylaxis, recommendations of the American Heart Association*.

*A) Dental and upper respiratory tract procedures*

1. Amoxicillin 3 G p.o. 1 h prior, followed by
   1.5 G p.o. 6 h later
2. For patients unable to take oral medications:
   Ampicillin 2 G i.v. 30 min prior, followed by
   1 G i.v. 6 h later
3. For penicillin-allergic patients:
   Erythromycin ethylsuccinate 800 mg p.o. 2 h prior, followed by
   400 mg p.o. 6 h later

*B) Gastrointestinal and genitourinary tract procedures*

1. Ampicillin 2 G i.v. or i.m. plus,
   Gentamicin 1.5 mg/kg (max 80 mg) i.v. or i.m. 30 min prior, followed by
   Amoxicillin 1.5 G p.o. 6 h later
2. For low risk patients:
   Amoxicillin 3 G p.o. 1 h prior, followed by
   1.5 G p.o. 6 h later
3) For penicillin-allergic patients:
   Vancomycin 1 G i.v. over 1 h, plus
   Gentamicin 1.5 mg/kg (max 80 mg) i.v. or i.m. 1 h prior, and repeated 8 h later

* For further recommendations see JAMA 264:2919, 1990; note also that doses for children are lower

## 5.1.2 Rheumatic endocarditis

Endocarditis associated with rheumatic fever is an inflammation which predominantly affects the endocardium of the mitral valve, the aortic valve, and the left atrium. Wart-like (verrucal) deposits occur where thrombi might develop. The inflammation often leads to fusion of the mitral commissures and the chordae tendineae. Interestingly, the hemodynamic effects seen during the acute phase are often those of mild mitral insufficiency, whereas the most common later manifestation is mitral valve stenosis, manifesting as late as 20 years after acute endocarditis. The myocardium is affected by perivascular foci of inflammation. Some of the late sequelae after rheumatic fever are probably caused by inflammatory myocardial damage.

Rheumatic pericarditis, in contrast, rarely leads to late complications, with the exception of occasional pericardial calcification.

Rheumatic fever occurs in children and juveniles between the ages of 5 and 15 years; it rarely occurs after the 21st year, and it is preceded by an infection with Group A β-hemolytic streptococci. In some patients – probably those with a genetic or environmentally determined susceptibility – the bacterial inflammation leads to an immune reaction which induces a response in the large joints and occasionally in the skin and subcutaneous tissue. If this same process extends to the brain, a characteristic movement disorder (chorea minor) develops.

The interval between the streptococcal infection, manifested as acute tonsillitis, and the appearance of rheumatic fever ranges from 2–3 weeks. Endocarditis occurs in subsequent weeks, whereas chorea minor only manifests after several months. Polyarthritis usually occurs in connection with the endocarditis.

Besides fever and a general feeling of malaise, joint complaints are prominent. Involvement of the cardiac valves is recognized by a newly developed murmur, typically one of mitral insufficiency. Mitral stenosis usually occurs only several years later.

It is not difficult to establish a diagnosis if a clear history can be obtained. A high erythrocyte sedimentation rate and an elevated antistreptolysin (ASO) titer are almost invariable during the acute phase. Treatment of acute disease is accomplished with anti-inflammatory analgesics, such as high doses of aspirin and occasionally steroids. Chronic therapy involves prophylaxis against further attacks. It is best achieved with penicillin given either as an intramuscular injection of benzathine penicillin 1.2 million units every 4 weeks or oral penicillin 250 mg b. i. d.

Penicillin therapy of streptococcal pharyngeal infections is recommended as a way of preventing rheumatic fever. If streptococcal infection is documented with a smear, then penicillin therapy is indicated.

## 5.1.3 Rare manifestations of endocarditis

Loeffler's endocarditis is a rare disease in which there is an excessive peripheral blood and myocardial accumulation of eosinophilic leukocytes. Cardiac involvement leads to thickening of the endocardium, and often there is superimposed thrombus formation.

Cardiac involvement may occur in ankylosing spondylitis, with aortic valve endocarditis and subsequent aortic insufficiency. Clinical endocarditis in lupus erythematosus is uncommon, even though verrucal lesions are often found at autopsy. Similarly, pathology findings of a thrombotic endocarditis are relatively common in patients who have died of metastatic cancer (marantic endocarditis), even though this process rarely causes clinical symptoms or sequelae.

# 5.2 Myocarditis, pericarditis

Myocarditis is an inflammatory disease of the myocardium characterized by cellular necrosis and leukocytic infiltration. Formerly, this disorder was diagnosed relatively often, with clinical manifestations such as tachycardia, hypotension, and arrhythmias. After the introduction of myocardial biopsy, it was often found that the clinically suspected diagnosis could not be confirmed histologically. In many cases, however, even the histologic findings are ambiguous.

Pathologic examinations show that inflammatory cell infiltration of the myocardium is not uncommonly a concomitant of systemic inflammatory disorders. Myocarditis occurs in association with typhus, malaria, and diphtheria. In acquired immune deficiency syndrome (AIDS), involvement of the heart occurs in 30–50% of patients. An inflammatory reaction of the myocardium may also occur in systemic disorders such as lupus erythematosus, lymphogranulomatosis, sarcoidosis, and Whipple's disease.

Myocarditis, as an independent disease, was found in only about one in 1000 autopsies (Table 8) among a total of 2507 cases examined at Frankfurt University Hospital.

There is no combination of clinical manifestation that makes the diagnosis easy and certain. General inflammatory manifestations such as fever, leukocytosis, and tachycardia may not be present. Arrhythmias and ECG changes often occur, but are nonspecific (Fig. 69). Possibly in the future, noninvasive diagnostic imaging may be facilitated by the use of radiolabeled myocardial monoclonal antibodies. Myocardial biopsy from the right or left ventricle is indicated where there is clinical suspicion and where definite confirmation will alter the clinical approach.

**Table 8.** In only two of 2507 autopsies was myocarditis seen as a separate disease and as being of major influence on the clinical course, without any other basic disease.

| Autopsies | 2507 | 100 |
|---|---|---|
| | n | % |
| Mononuclear cell infiltration | 84 | 3.3 |
| – with general sepsis | 20 | 0.8 |
| – with other associated diseases | 61 | 2.4 |
| – sarcoidosis | 1 | 0.04 |
| Myocarditis | | |
| – as primary cardiac disease with major influence on the patients' outcome | 2 | 0.01 |

Pericarditis may manifest as a dry fibrinous reaction or as an exudative process with effusion. If the epicardial pericardium is significantly affected, the inflammation may extend into the outer layers of the myocardium ("myopericarditis").

With fibrinous pericarditis, a systolic and diastolic friction rub is heard on auscultation. Exudative pericarditis leads to an increase in the area of cardiac dullness on percussion, and an enlargement and smoothing-out of the cardiac shadow (Fig. 70a, b). It also leads to an echo-free zone around the heart on the echocardiogram. Intracardiac pressure recordings show equally elevated diastolic pressures in both ventricles in severe cases; the pressure curve shows a "dip-plateau" phenomenon (Fig. 70c, d).

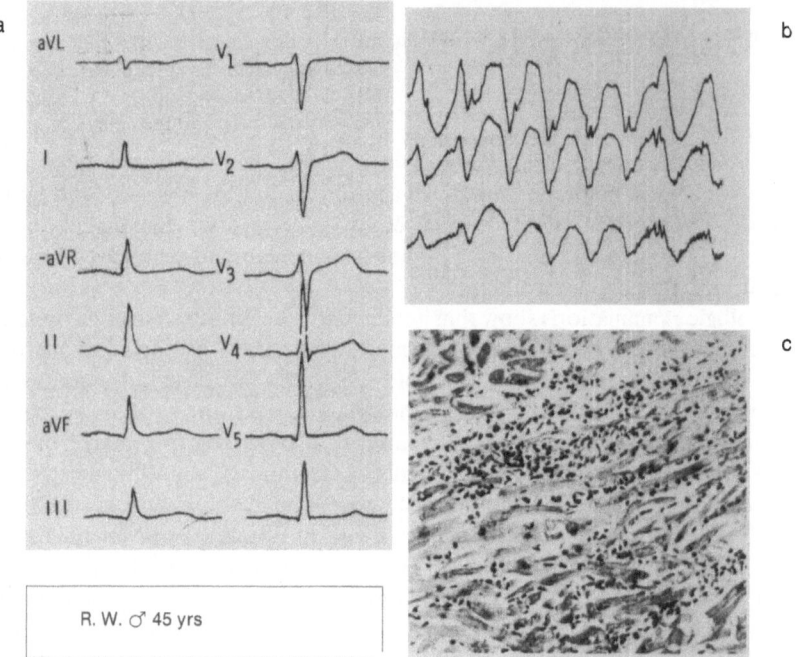

R. W. ♂ 45 yrs

**Fig. 69.** Acute myocarditis in a 45-year-old man, who was hospitalized because of syncopal attacks.
**a** normal ECG, **b** ventricular fibrillation during exercise testing, which was treated by defibrillation;
thereafter, the patient was asymptomatic. Two weeks later spontaneous ventricular fibrillation occurred,
which was refractory to therapy. At autopsy **c** diffuse inflammatory infiltration of the myocardium was
seen.

Severe hemodynamic consequences may result from inflammatory, and also from non-inflammatory or bloody pericardial effusions. These latter effusions are often more severe, develop faster, and may cause cardiac tamponade. The possibility of tamponade has to be borne in mind in cases of chest trauma, medical interventions such as application of central i.v. catheters, cardiac catheterization, transseptal puncture, and temporary pacemaker implantation when a sudden loss in blood pressure occurs, associated with decreasing volume of the heart sounds, and symptoms and signs of shock. Immediate pericardial aspiration may be life-saving; this is most easily performed by needle-puncture from the apical or subxiphoid approach, using echocardiographic guidance.

Pericarditis is not a rare disease. It may occur by itself, but it usually occurs in association with infectious, systemic or malignant disorders. Most often, pericarditis is seen with infections caused by Coxsackie Group B viruses. Some are "idiopathic". Repeated pericardial exsudation is not uncommon. It can be treated by antiphlogistic and antiproliferative medications but sometimes requires surgical pericardectomy.

Constrictive pericarditis may be a late sequel of any form of pericarditis. This clinical manifestation is especially typical for tuberculous pericarditis, but may develop even after Coxsackie pericarditis. Pericardial calcification is typical, but frequently not present. Surgical resection of the thickened and relatively rigid epicardial and pericardial scarring is the treatment method of choice.

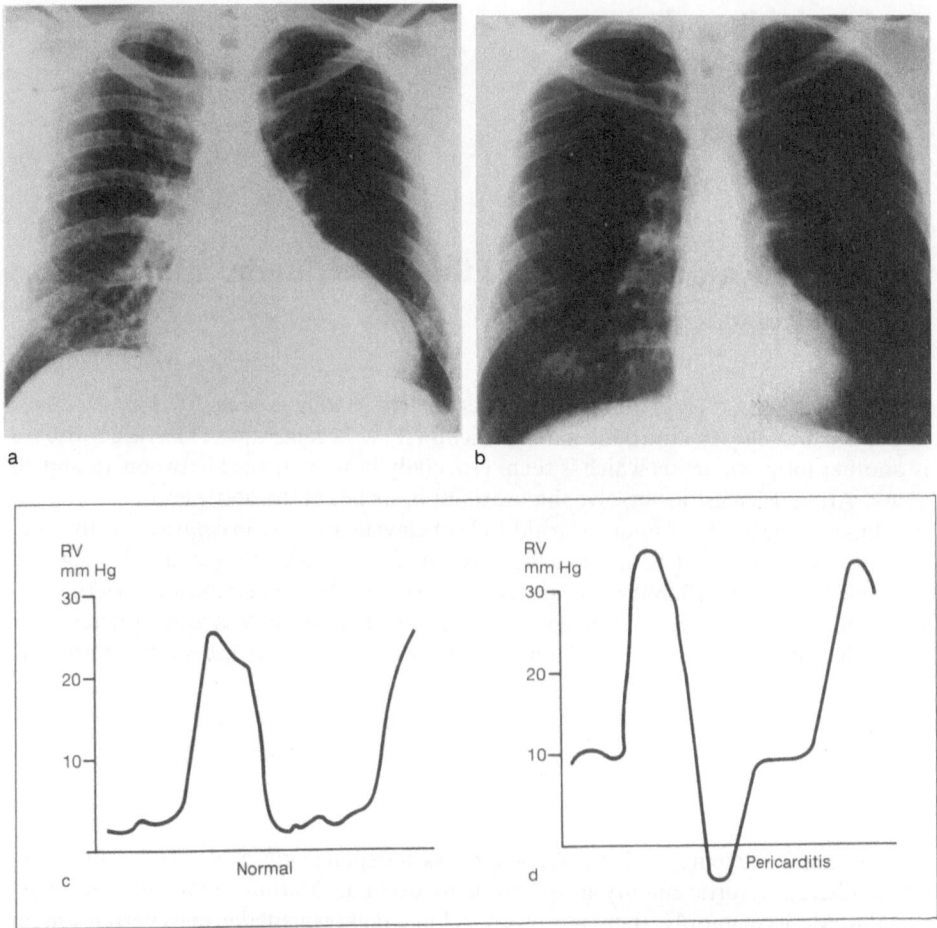

**Fig. 70. a** X-ray cardiac enlargement due to pericardial effusion, **b** after drainage of 1200 ml exudate, the cardiac contours are normal. **c, d** In constrictive pericarditis the diastolic filling pressure is elevated due to a restriction of diastolic ventricular expansion; the diastolic pressure equalizes in all cardiac chambers.

# 6  Aortic disorders

## 6.1  Inflammatory diseases of the aorta, luetic, and Takayasu's aortitis

In years past, luetic (syphilitic) aortitis was a fairly common cause of thoracic aortic aneurysm, but since the introduction of penicillin it has become rare. Takayasu's disease is another form of aortitis which is seen, especially in women aged between 16 and 30 years. Arterial occlusions involve the proximal branches of the aortic arch, such as the brachiocephalic trunk, common carotid and subclavian arteries. In contrast to atherosclerosis, it is mostly young people that are affected. The disease is accompanied by signs of systemic illness and inflammation, such as a markedly elevated erythrocyte sedimentation rate. The disease has a tendency to progress. Treatment with anti-inflammatory agents including steroids is recommended, but their effectiveness has not been proven.

## 6.2  Aortic aneurysms

Aneurysmal enlargement of the aorta appears independently or in conjunction with other diseases. Aortic aneurysm is known to occur in Marfan's syndrome and with syphilis. More commonly, there is pressure-related enlargement due to hypertension, or there is atherosclerotic disease involving the collagenous and elastic tissue of the aortic wall. Modest aortic ectasia is frequent in the aged and, by itself, has no adverse significance. Aneurysms may also be found in the peripheral and coronary arteries. In these medium-sized vessels, progressive enlargement or perforation are not to be feared, but intra-arterial thrombi occasionally occur due to relative blood stasis. The aorta is at risk for perforation if the diameter of the aneurysm exceeds 6 cm. Surgical therapy is usually indicated at this stage, especially if progressive dilatation has been documented.

Another dangerous complication of aortic aneurysm is subintimal bleeding leading to intimal rupture (aortic dissection). The aortic wall layers are thus separated; the ensuing dissection may extend from the aortic valve to the bifurcation. If the intima is totally detached, a complete luminal occlusion may occur. In other cases, a second tear occurs, allowing intramural blood to re-enter distally.

Acute aortic dissection has to be differentiated from acute myocardial infarction. It is associated with equally severe chest pain. Absence of ECG changes and a lack of myocardial enzymes in the blood may hint at aortic dissection. With dissection near the cardiac valves the pain is predominantly precordial, but with dissection of the descending aorta the pain is located more in the back.

The diagnosis is made by echocardiography and x-ray. Contrast-enhanced computed tomography (CT) and transesophageal echocardiography are currently the most useful diagnostic techniques. The surgical outcome depends on the location of the rupture and the extent of the dissection. Occasionally, oversewing the proximal intimal tear is sufficient, while in other cases prosthetic aortic replacement is required (Figs. 71, 72).

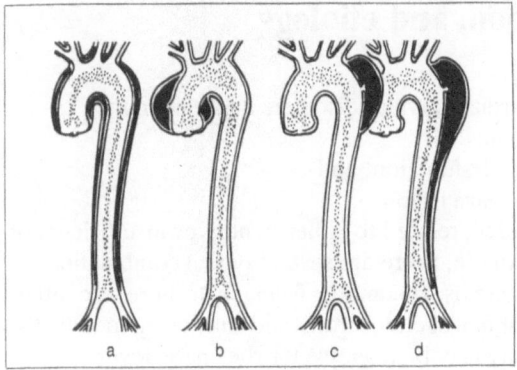

**Fig. 71.** Dissecting aneurysm **a** Type I, **b** Type II, **c** and **d** Type III after DeBakey [2].

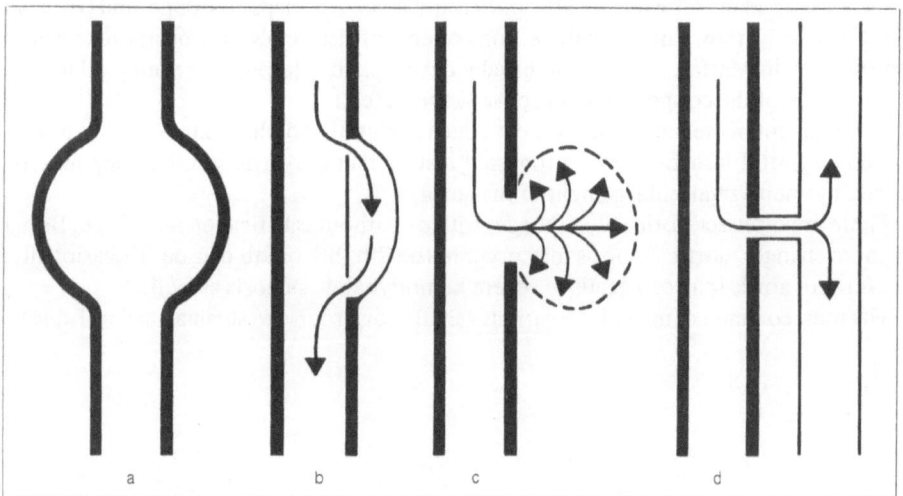

**Fig. 72. a** True aneurysm; **b** dissecting aneurysm with separation of wall layers. In this example distal reentry of blood into the vessel lumen can be seen; **c** "false" aneurysm. This is a pulsating hematoma without an intact vessel wall, which may occur, for example, after arterial puncture in the groin; **d** arteriovenous fistula, which may develop after trauma or vessel puncture.

# 7 Cardiac valvular disorders

## 7.1 Importance, classification, and etiology

The importance and classification of cardiac valvular disorders depends on the:
1) type and severity of the valve lesion;
2) degree of concomitant myocardial dysfunction, and
3) the underlying illness causing the valve lesion.

Eight valvular disorders may be considered, related to either stenosis or insufficiency of each of the four cardiac valves. Furthermore, there are several typical combinations.

A common cause of valvular disease is rheumatic fever, but there are other inflammatory causes, such as bacterial or fungal endocarditis and ankylosing spondylitis. In rheumatic valvular disease, the history may be negative for rheumatic fever.

Congenital valvular disorders are often the precursor of aortic valve stenosis (bicuspid aortic valve) and mitral valve insufficiency (mitral valve prolapse). Congenital tricuspid insufficiency is rare and usually a component of Ebstein's malformation. Aortic insufficiency in Marfan's syndrome usually develops in a juvenile or young adult as a consequence of the congenital connective tissue defect.

Enlargement of the valve annulus, e.g., due to dilatation of the ventricles, may lead to secondary mitral insufficiency or tricuspid insufficiency. Aortic insufficiency may be caused by aneurysmal enlargement of the aorta.

There are often sclerotic valve changes with or without calcification in old age. Based on these changes, aortic stenosis may occur in the 7th, 8th or 9th decade. Occasionally, this form of aortic sclerosis leads to severe hemodynamic stenosis as well.

The most common causes of the various valvular disorders are summarized in Table 9.

Table 9. Common valvular disorders and possible causes.

| | Rheumatic endocarditis | Bacterial endocarditis | Congenital | Malformation | Other causes |
|---|---|---|---|---|---|
| Mitral stenosis | + | | | | Atrial myxoma |
| Mitral insufficiency | + | + | + | Mitral valve prolapse | Papillary muscle dysfunction after myocardial infarction. Left ventricular dilatation |
| Aortic stenosis | + | | + | | Sclerotic or senile valvular stenosis |
| Aortic insufficiency | + | + | + | Marfan's syndrome | Ankylosing spondylitis, luetic aortic aneurysm |
| Pulmonary stenosis | | | + | | |
| Pulmonary insufficiency | | | | | Iatrogenic after commissurotomy |
| Tricuspid stenosis | + | | | | |
| Tricuspid insufficiency | | | + | Ebstein's syndrome | Endocarditis in drug addicts. Right ventricular dilatation |

# 7.2 Mitral stenosis

Worldwide, mitral stenosis is the most common valvular disorder. It occurs four times as often in women as in men. Rheumatic endocarditis is virtually always the cause of mitral stenosis. Some degree of mitral insufficiency is often an associated finding.

## 7.2.1 Etiology

Rheumatic endocarditis usually occurs between the ages of 5 and 15 years. It often causes mitral insufficiency which is hemodynamically not significant. Mitral stenosis will almost never be symptomatic in early childhood, but occurs much later after a latent period of 10–30 years. It appears that scarring and shrinking is responsible, but the diseased valve ring may also not grow appropriately for the increasing size of the heart. In the advanced stage the mitral valve will show grotesque changes with fibrous scars, calcification, growing together of commissures, fusion of chordae tendineae and papillary muscles. The valve leaflets may have shrunk back to a small collar. In deformations which are not so advanced, the valve tissue still exists and is flexible; stenosis in these cases is mostly caused by fused commissures.

## 7.2.2 Pathophysiology

The spectrum of hemodynamic effects seen with mitral stenosis is determined by the reduction in diastolic valvular opening. The normal mitral orifice is 4–6 cm$^2$, and is reduced to less than 1 cm$^2$ in severe mitral stenosis. Any disturbance of the diastolic blood inflow into the left ventricle increases the back pressure in the left atrium. The atrial myocardium becomes hypertrophied; the pressure eventually rises from the normal value of around 10 mm Hg to above 40 mm Hg. Initially, this pressure increase occurs only with exercise. Later on, left atrial and pulmonary hypertension develop at rest, with the result that the obstruction to blood flow eventually is of similar degree in the narrowed pulmonary bed as in the stenosed mitral valve. The right heart will suffer from the increased pressure load and will eventually decompensate. The left heart failure associated with mitral valve stenosis is not a function of myocardial failure, but is the consequence of reduced diastolic inflow into the left ventricle and a resulting high left atrial pressure. In contrast, the right heart failure which follows pulmonary hypertension is due to myocardial failure as a consequence of the increased pressure load.

## 7.2.3 Clinical manifestations and course

A prominent symptom is dyspnea, especially with exercise. Pulmonary congestion may be so severe that pulmonary edema occurs. Sputum may be tinged with blood, and when it is examined by microscopy, hemosiderin-laden macrophages ("heart-failure cells") are seen.

During examination of the patient a "mitral face", i.e., bluish-red cheeks may be noted; this is caused by dilatation of small blood vessels (telangiectasia). When mitral stenosis is severe there may be cyanosis of the lips due to increased peripheral oxygen extraction secondary to the low cardiac output.

During auscultation, depending on whether there is sinus rhythm or atrial fibrillation, four or five classical signs can be distinguished (Fig. 73):
1) Loud, first heart sound; this is associated with good left ventricular function.
2) Accentuated second heart sound over the pulmonary area (accentuated pulmonary component of the second heart sound). This is caused by pulmonary hypertension.
3) Mitral opening snap. This early diastolic extra sound is caused by impaired mitral valve excursion during its opening. Its occurrence depends on the mitral leaflets still being flexible; its origin can be compared to the "snap" which a sail produces when the wind catches it. The more severe the mitral stenosis, the higher the pressure is in the left atrium, and the earlier that the mitral valve opening snap occurs. The interval from the aortic component of the second heart sound to the opening snap varies from 0.04 to 0.12 s (measured by phonocardiography).
4) Diastolic murmur. The murmur is heard over the mitral region, sometimes more easily when the patient lies in the left lateral position. It may be augmented with physical exercise such as repeated sitting-up, or it may even only be heard then. Its loudness varies; in rare cases a diastolic thrill may be palpable. This low-frequency murmur is caused by turbulent diastolic inflow through the stenosed mitral valve.
5) Presystolic murmur. This murmur is caused by augmented blood inflow late in diastole, due to atrial contraction; it occurs only during sinus rhythm (see Fig. 73).

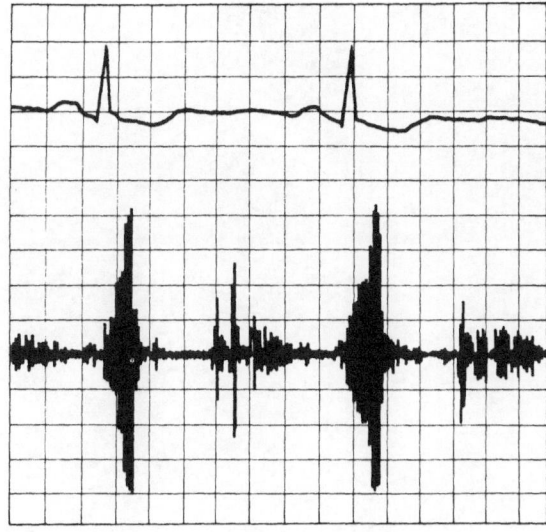

**Fig. 73.** Mitral stenosis: ECG (above) and phonocardiogram using filter frequencies similar to the human ear (below). During sinus rhythm a presystolic murmur, a loud, first heart sound, a mitral valve opening snap 0.06 s after the second heart sound, and a diastolic murmur are recorded on the phonocardiogram.

None of these signs is obligatory. Auscultatory findings may be absent even in severely diseased valves ("silent mitral stenosis").

The "mitral contour" on an x-ray of the heart may be recognized by a straightened left-heart silhouette, due to an enlargement of the pulmonary artery, left atrium, and left atrial appendage (Fig. 74). In the PA view, the enlarged left atrium is recognized by a double contour in the area of the right cardiac border and, also, by a filling in of the retrocardiac area on the lateral view. Often pulmonary venous congestion is found. The cardiac volume usually exceeds the upper normal values (in women 700, in men 800 ml/ 1.73 m$^2$).

During sinus rhythm a P-mitrale (P-wave with a double peak) is often recorded in Lead II, and an enlargement of the negative phase of the P-wave in V1 is seen on the ECG. Atrial extrasystoles and atrial fibrillation are also frequent.

The echocardiogram is very important for the noninvasive diagnosis of mitral stenosis. The motion of the anterior mitral valve leaflet can be observed very well in the echocardiogram, because it is clearly distinguished from the echo-poor, blood-filled left ventricle. This was the first cardiac structure to be reliably detected with echocardiography. One may estimate the impairment of mitral opening from the decrease of the velocity of diastolic valve leaflet motion. Reduction in total leaflet excursion also indicates an impairment of valve motion (Fig. 75). The thickness of the valve leaflets, the presence of calcification, and involvement of the chordae are also recognizable. Enlargement of the left atrium can be evaluated using the echocardiogram, as well as the size and contractility of the left ventricle. An atrial myxoma as cause of mitral obstruction is usually easily detected. Doppler gradient measurements and transesophageal imaging of the left atrium and mitral valve have refined the noninvasive assessment.

During intracardiac pressure recording, the diastolic pressure gradient between left atrium and left ventricle is the key to diagnosis (Figs. 74, 76, 77). The valve orifice area can be estimated from the magnitude of the pressure gradient and the cardiac output.

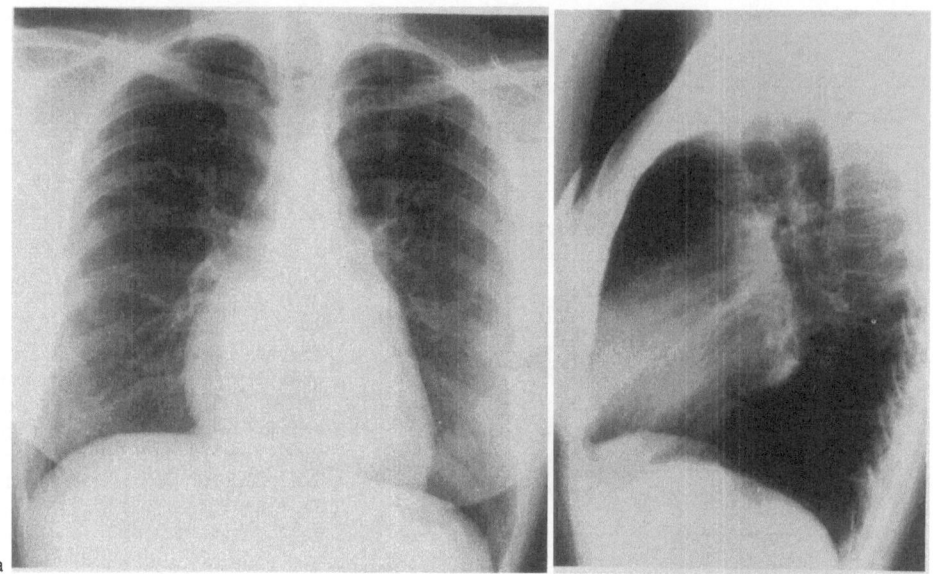

| | | | Pressure | | Mean pressure | | O$_2$ | |
|---|---|---|---|---|---|---|---|---|
| | | | mm Hg | norm. | p | norm. | Sat. % | norm. |
| SVC | superior v.c. | | | | | | | 70 |
| IVC | inferior v.c. | | | | | | | 75 |
| RA | right atrium | upper | | | | | | 70 |
| | | middle | 6 | | | 5 | | 72 |
| | | lower | | | | | | 75 |
| RV | right ventricle | IT | 54/8 | 25/5 | | | | 73 |
| | | OT | | | | | | 73 |
| PA | pulmonary artery | | 54/32 | 25/10 | 42 | 15 | 72 | 73 |
| PC | pulmonary capillary | | | | 30 | 10 | | |
| Ab | A. brachialis | | | 120/70 | | 90 | | 95 |
| Ao | aorta | | 80/56 | 120/70 | 64 | 90 | 95 | 95 |
| LV | left ventricle | | 80/8 | 120/10 | | | | 95 |
| LA | left atrium | | | | | 10 | | 95 |
| PV | pulmonary vein | | | | | 10 | | 95 |

Al. A. ♀ 25 y.

**Fig. 74. a** X-ray and **b** hemodynamics in severe mitral stenosis.

Since the advent of echocardiography, cardiac catheterization has become of less importance for evaluation of mitral stenosis and other valve disorders. It is now used mainly to exclude or recognize associated coronary artery disease in older patients. The existence of concomitant valvular insufficiency can also be easily assessed by angiography. Pulmonary hypertension is nearly always found. After removal of the stenosis even very elevated pulmonary arterial pressures, which may be higher than the systemic arterial pressure, will usually decrease; in rare cases however fixed pulmonary hypertension can remain after successful surgery.

102

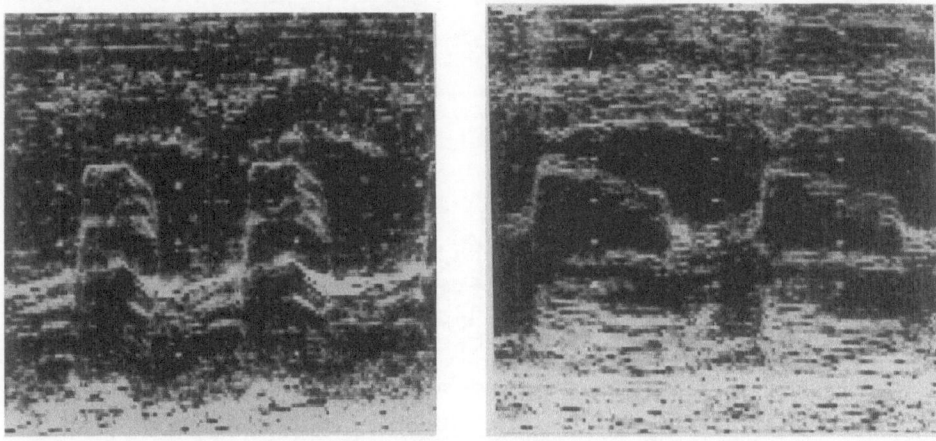

**Fig. 75.** M-mode echocardiogram in high-grade mitral stenosis before valvular dilatation with a balloon catheter (left). The stenosis was dilated significantly, yet not completely (right).

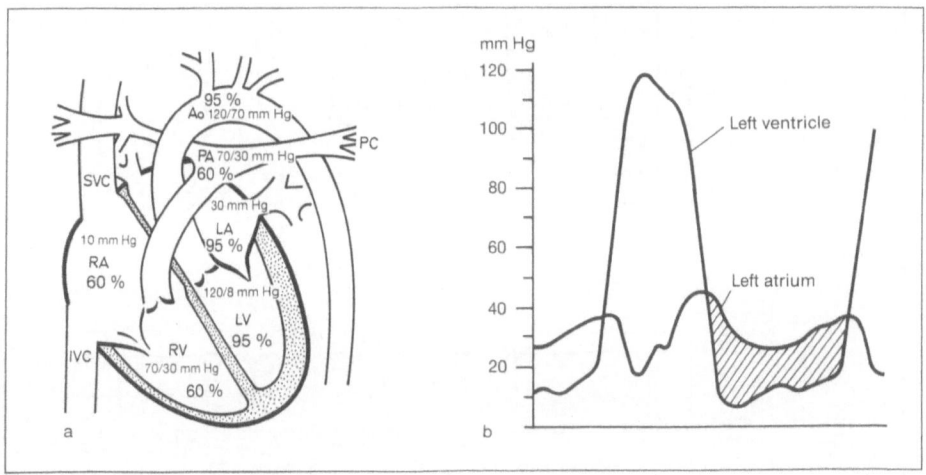

**Fig. 76. a** Cardiac parameters (pressure in mmHg and oxygen saturation in %), and **b** simultaneous recording of pressures from the left ventricle and left atrium in mitral stenosis. The shaded area corresponds to the diastolic pressure gradient associated with the stenosis.

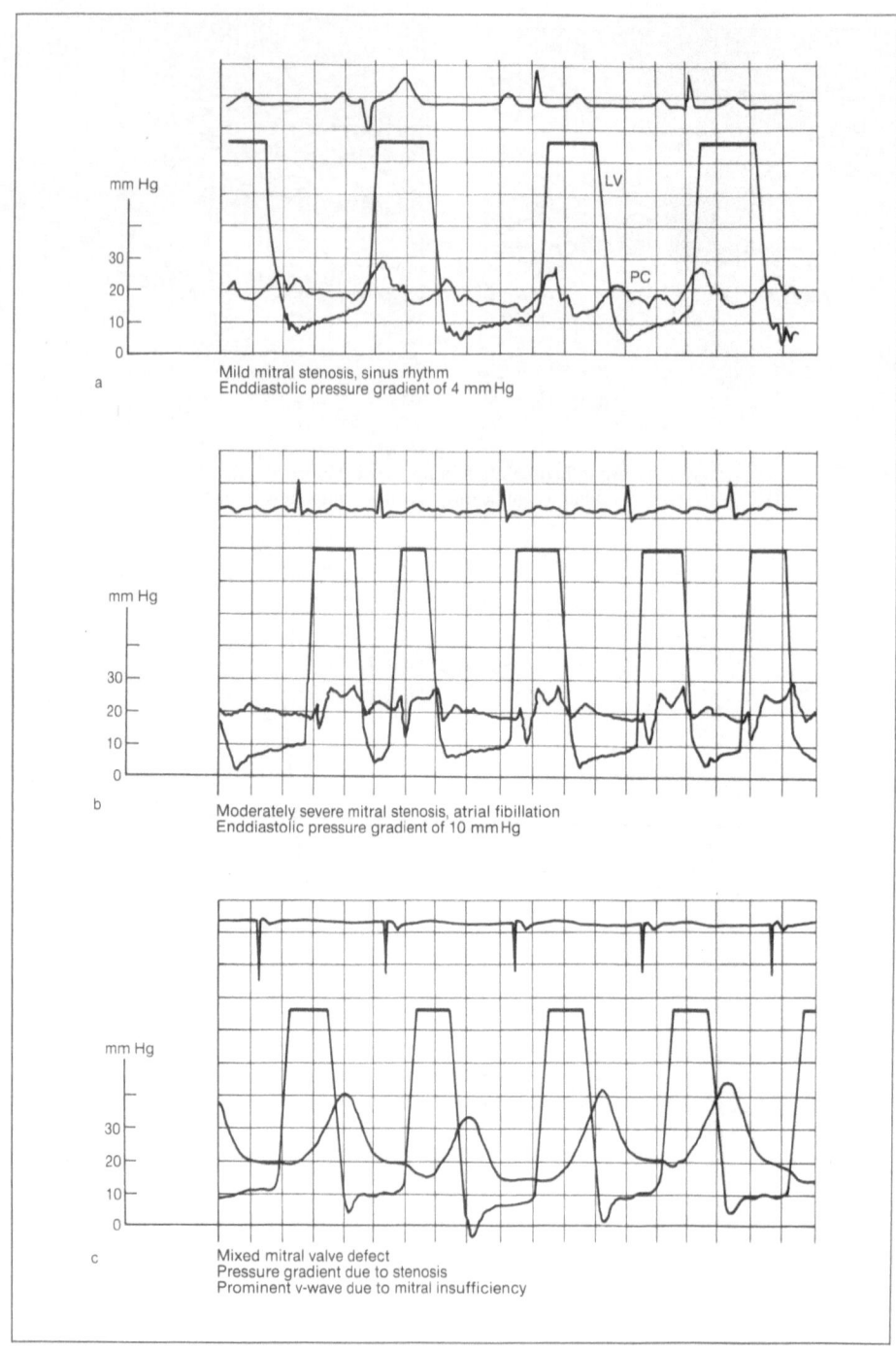

mm Hg

30
20
10
0

LV

PC

Mild mitral stenosis, sinus rhythm
Enddiastolic pressure gradient of 4 mm Hg

a

mm Hg

30
20
10
0

b

Moderately severe mitral stenosis, atrial fibillation
Enddiastolic pressure gradient of 10 mm Hg

mm Hg

30
20
10
0

c

Mixed mitral valve defect
Pressure gradient due to stenosis
Prominent v-wave due to mitral insufficiency

**Fig. 77.** Simultaneous pressure curves from the left ventricle (LV) and pulmonary capillaries (PC) in different mitral disorders.

## 7.2.4 Treatment

Mitral valve stenosis of minor degree may be relatively well tolerated for a long period, especially if the patient stays in sinus rhythm. Drug therapy includes digitalis and, if necessary, diuretics. Anticoagulants are indicated if there has been an episode of embolism, or if the patient develops atrial fibrillation. Surgical intervention is usually indicated in moderately severe or severe mitral stenosis. The indications for surgery also depend on whether a valve-conserving procedure is possible or whether valve replacement is necessary. This decision has to be made taking into account all available information. In some cases a final decision may be possible only during surgery. While balloon valve dilatation or reconstruction may be considered at a relatively early phase of the disease, valve replacement should only be performed when there are Class III (New York Heart Association Functional Classification) symptoms or significant pulmonary hypertension. In many cases, mitral valve dilatation may be performed without surgery using a balloon catheter; the evolution of this technique has been pioneered in Japan.

# 7.3 Mitral insufficiency

## 7.3.1 Etiology

Mitral stenosis or a combined mitral disorder are the usual late sequelae of rheumatic endocarditis. In some cases, however, isolated mitral insufficiency (incompetence) may be seen. As opposed to mitral stenosis, there is no increased frequency in women. Combined mitral valve disorders with a similar degree of severity of stenosis and insufficiency are rare; usually, either one or the other component is prominent. Mitral insufficiency may occur during bacterial endocarditis as a result of leaflet perforation or ruptured chordae tendineae. When it occurs, it is often a life-threatening complication. In papillary muscle dysfunction, valvular insufficiency is caused by ischemia or infarction of the papillary muscle, the anterolateral one with anterior myocardial infarction and the posterior papillary muscle with inferior infarction.

Mitral insufficiency in mitral valve prolapse is caused by myxomatous degeneration of the valve tissue, but it will only occur in a small percentage of patients with this relatively frequent syndrome. Usually, mitral valve prolapse does not produce any, or only hemodynamically insignificant, mitral insufficiency, but it may occur or become hemodynamically important during the course of the disease, especially with advancing age. Mitral valve prolapse is sometimes associated with an atrial septal defect. It is also often combined with atrial and ventricular arrhythmias even in the absence of any important mitral insufficiency.

Left ventricular dilatation often leads to mitral insufficiency due to dilatation of the valvular ring.

## 7.3.2 Clinical manifestations

The typical auscultatory finding in mitral valve insufficiency is a systolic murmur which radiates in the direction of the axilla. The murmur may be holosystolic, early or late systolic. A late systolic murmur and a systolic click are typical for valve insufficiency with mitral valve prolapse. A third heart sound due to increased early diastolic blood inflow into the left ventricle is frequent in severe mitral incompetence. It occurs 0.12–0.14 s after the second heart sound.

The x-ray reveals a general enlargement in cardiac size predominantly involving the left ventricle and the left atrium (Fig. 78). Left ventricular hypertrophy is typical on the ECG. Insufficiency, as opposed to valve stenosis, cannot be visualized directly by M-mode or 2D echocardiography. However, Doppler echocardiography does directly depict regurgitation of blood into the left atrium and may considerably facilitate noninvasive diagnosis.

Intracardiac pressure recordings often show an increase in left atrial systolic pressure due to regurgitation of the blood into the left atrium (see Fig. 77c; v-wave). Angiography with injection of contrast agent into the left ventricle is very useful. With severe mitral insufficiency, regurgitation often reaches back into the pulmonary veins. Visualization of the coronary arteries is especially important in older patients because mitral insufficiency may be caused by coronary occlusion with papillary muscle dysfunction and, despite severe valve insufficiency, the infarction may be so small that is is not detected on the ECG.

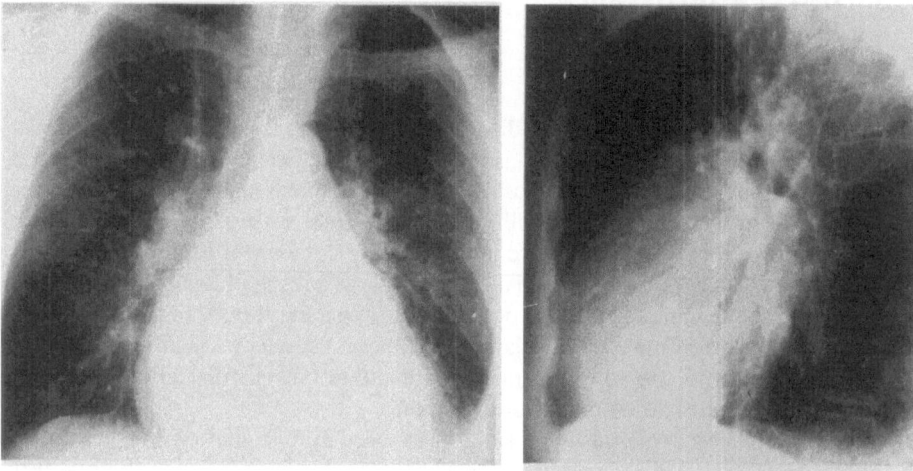

**Fig. 78.** X-ray of combined mitral valve disorder. Enlargement of the left atrium and left ventricle, signs of pulmonary venous congestion.

### 7.3.3 Clinical course, therapy

As in other cardiac disorders with predominant volume overloading, the course of mitral insufficiency may often be relatively stable for a long time. Sudden, unexpected decompensation is rare and, when it occurs, usually reflects valve or chordal rupture. Digitalis and diuretics are used for medical therapy. ACE inhibitors are also quite effective. Surgery is necessary if there is decompensation, documented deterioration, or increasing pulmonary hypertension. Usually, surgery involves valve replacement, but in some cases, surgical reconstruction of the mitral valve is possible. Concomitant or causative coronary artery disease may necessitate bypass grafting.

### 7.3.4 Anticoagulation in mitral valve disorders

Thrombosis prophylaxis is usually indicated in atrial fibrillation due to mitral stenosis or a combined valve disorder. The risk of thromboembolism is less in mitral insufficiency, as long as left ventricular function is not severely impaired. Anticoagulation is always necessary after valve replacement with a mechanical valve. This is not the case with bioprostheses if there is sinus rhythm and the left atrium is not greatly enlarged. Bioprostheses are not now implanted in juveniles, because of increased likelihood of valve degeneration in young age. They are, however, implanted in 20–40-year-old women who anticipate pregnancy, thus avoiding the fetal risk of oral anticoagulants. They are also used in patients for whom anticoagulants carry a significant risk of bleeding (the elderly or those with a history of bleeding disorder).

## 7.4 Aortic stenosis

### 7.4.1 Occurrence, etiology

Aortic stenosis is more frequent in men than in women. It is the most frequent valve disorder in men and is, in general, the second most frequent valve problem. It is caused by rheumatic endocarditis, or, equally frequently, by a dysplastic often bicuspid valve. In middle and old age, aortic stenosis may follow sclerosis due to an increase in fibrous tissue and calcification in the cusps and the valve ring. Congenital bicuspid valve is often associated with a particular type of coronary distribution, namely, a very dominant left coronary artery.

### 7.4.2 Clinical manifestations

Classical symptoms include exercise-induced dyspnea and angina pectoris. Exercise-induced dyspnea is caused by an increase of the diastolic pressure in the left ventricle and left atrium. Angina pectoris develops due to relative coronary insufficiency: the left ventricular hypertrophy necessitates an increase in coronary blood flow, but supply is impaired by a relatively low aortic pressure and simultaneous elevation of diastolic ventricular pressure and intramural pressure. Syncope associated with physical exercise may occur as a result of ischemia and, inadequate cardiac output. Prominent left ventricular hypertrophy is recorded on the ECG (Fig. 79). In some cases, however, the ECG may be normal despite severe aortic stenosis.

The carotid pulse tracing shows a slow upstroke with a pressure half-time (time from onset of upstroke to half peak pressure) of more than 0.05 s (Fig. 80). A cockscomb shape may be seen. Comparable to the ECG, normal findings may occasionally be recorded despite the presence of severe stenosis.

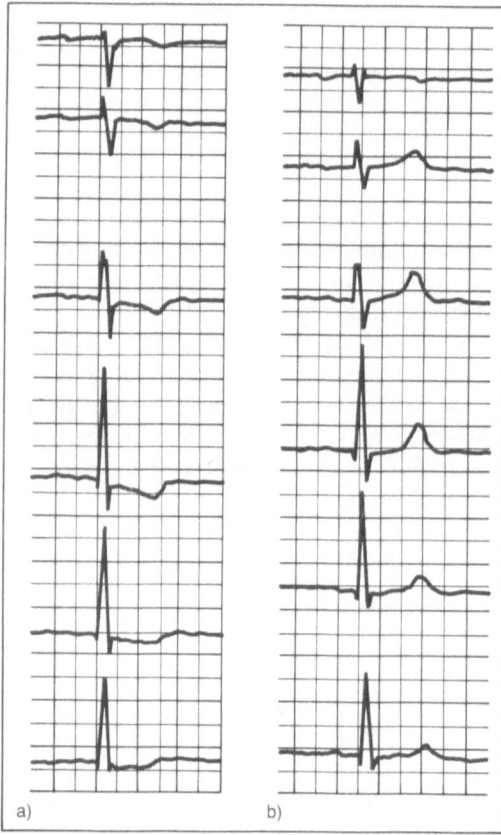

a)  b)

**Fig. 79.** ECG of a 72 year old physician with aortic valve disease. **a** Before surgery marked left ventricular hypertrophy. **b** After surgery with implantation of a bioprothesis, normalization of the ST-T-segment and reduction of the QRS-amplitude from 3.4 to 2.7 mV. Heart size and left ventricular volume decreased; heart volume determined from x-ray decreased from 1880 to 1240 ml.

With echocardiography, hypertrophy of the left ventricle and often a dilated left atrium can be documented. Thickening of the valve cusps and inadequate opening can be qualitatively assessed. Doppler echocardiography is of most help in estimating the severity. This method is also useful for recognizing or excluding concomitant aortic valve insufficiency, or mitral stenosis.

The x-ray reveals a heart which has a shoe-shape due to the enlargement of the left ventricle. If there is pressure loading alone, with concentric hypertrophy, cardiac enlargement cannot always be seen on the PA view. The cardiac volume is, however, usually already enlarged in this phase, because of some enlargement of the left atrium due to diastolic filling restriction.

Left heart catheterization provides key information for estimating the severity of aortic stenosis. The systolic pressure gradient between the left ventricle and the aorta is the most important parameter for the timing of surgery (see Fig. 80). When the gradient is above 50 mmHg, surgery is generally indicated in a patient with associated symptoms; above 100 mmHg it is indicated even when symptoms are absent. Similarly, surgery should be considered when the calculated valve area is less than 0.7 cm$^2$. Angina pectoris may be due to a high pressure gradient alone, or to concomitant coronary artery disease. The latter is common in the elderly and can only be recognized or excluded with coronary

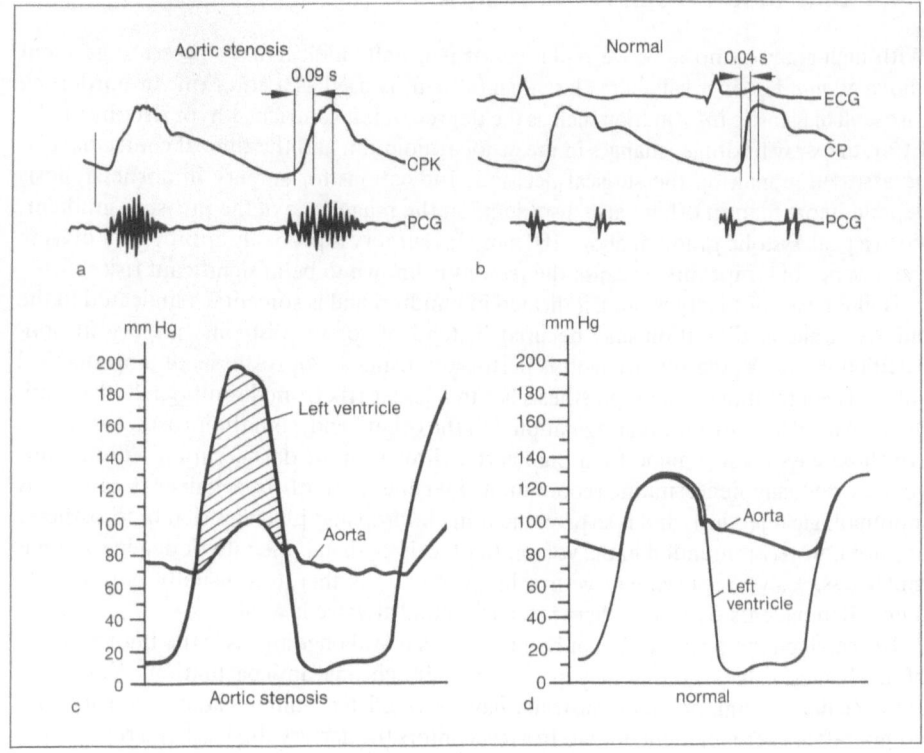

**Fig. 80. a** Pulse curve and phonocardiogram in aortic stenosis in comparison to the normal **b**. In aortic stenosis, the upstroke of the pulse curve is retarded, the pressure half-time is significantly prolonged at 0.09 s, and an acutely serrated cock's-comb shape can be seen. In the phonocardiogram a spindle-shaped murmur with peaking in late systole can be recorded. **c** A significant systolic pressure gradient between left ventricle and aorta of 100 mmHg is found on left-heart catheterization. **d** Comparison with a normal pressure curve.

arteriography. Aortography is used to assess the degree of aortic insufficiency; left ventriculography is done to evaluate concomitant mitral insufficiency. Left ventriculography also characterizes the contractile reserve of the left ventricle.

## 7.4.3 Clinical course, therapy

Mild aortic stenosis may be asymptomatic for years, but it may evolve quite rapidly into severe aortic stenosis. This holds true for congenital, post-endocarditic, and senile forms of aortic stenosis. Therefore, changes in symptoms have to be evaluated carefully, especially if there is exercise-induced dyspnea, angina or syncope. Cardiac arrhythmias may also be a sign of progression, but their occurrence is not as closely correlated with the hemodynamic course as is exercise-induced dyspnea and angina. Sudden cardiac death during the course of the disease is mostly due to ventricular fibrillation. It is more frequent in severe stenosis with a high pressure gradient.

### 7.4.4 Indication for surgery and surgical methods

With high-grade stenosis, valve replacement is usually indicated. A pressure gradient above 50 mm Hg or a valve area less than 0.7 cm$^2$ is used as a criterion. In borderline cases, all diagnostic information such as the degree of left ventricular hypertrophy on the ECG, the x-ray findings, changes in the echocardiogram, and the clinical course have to be assessed in making the surgical decision. Indications for surgery in aortic stenosis depend, more than in other valve disorders, on the magnitude of the pressure gradient. With a peak systolic gradient above 100 mm Hg, surgery is probably appropriate even in the absence of symptoms, because the patient is known to be at significant risk.

Balloon valvuloplasty is often indicated in children and is sometimes indicated in the elderly. Balloon dilatation may be used instead of, or to postpone surgery in non-calcified valves. Valve replacement is performed using a bioprosthesis or a mechanical valve. The advantage of a bioprosthesis lies in a lesser risk from thromboembolism and, thus, no need for chronic anticoagulation. On the other hand, some bioprostheses, which are these days mostly made from pig hearts, show signs of degeneration within a few years, eventually necessitating reoperation. Degeneration of these valves is caused by immunologic rejection, and is so prominent in children and juveniles that bioprostheses are not now recommended in the young. In elderly patients, the rate of degeneration is much less. Valve replacement with a bioprosthesis is therefore usually only recommended in patients over 60; otherwise, a mechanical valve is used.

Research on the preservation of bioprostheses is still ongoing, as is the improvement of mechanical valves, so that they may not require chronic anticoagulation. Workers in New Zealand, England, and Australia have refined the human cadaver aortic valve homograft as a replacement option. In a few centers the aortic valve has been replaced by the patient's own pulmonary valve while a homograft was put into pulmonary position. This procedure is too complicated for general application but has shown good long-term results. The ideal valve prosthesis is not yet available.

## 7.5 Aortic insufficiency

### 7.5.1 Etiology

Aortic insufficiency is usually caused by rheumatic or bacterial endocarditis. In rheumatic endocarditis, aortic stenosis may be the first to develop; later on, there is aortic insufficiency due to atrophy and loss of valve tissue. Bacterial aortic endocarditis usually occurs in a previously damaged valve with some degree of aortic stenosis leading to a combined valvular disorder due to valve tissue destruction or perforation.

The lack of aortic valve closure causes diastolic regurgitation of blood from the aorta into the left ventricle. The stroke volume is increased in compensation, which causes ventricular dilatation due to volume loading. If the degree of valve insufficiency does not increase, the disorder may remain well-compensated for a long time and physical exercise capacity may be normal. Therefore, this valve disorder is commonly found during a routine examination.

## 7.5.2 Clinical manifestations

In severe aortic incompetence a wide pulse pressure with elevated systolic and lowered diastolic pressure is characteristic. The degree of the valve insufficiency is correlated with the width of the pulse pressure. However, bradycardia may exaggerate the gradient, whereas tachycardia lessens it. Decreasing elasticity of central arteries with increasing age also leads to an increase in pulse pressure so that beyond the 50th year only the decrease in diastolic pressure is a reliable sign of severe aortic incompetence.

Patients often experience a pounding heart sensation. During examination, a bounding pulse is felt; it may also be seen in the carotids (Corrigan's sign). With severe valve incompetence, a pulse-synchronous nodding of the head may occur. Capillary pulsation can be recognized in the nail bed with slight pressure on the fingernail.

A diastolic murmur is auscultated over the aorta, left sternal edge, and down to the apex. With mild aortic insufficiency, the murmur is most prominent over the third left intercostal space near the sternum (Erb's point). The murmur is of high frequency and has a decrescendo character. With more severe aortic insufficiency a concomitant systolic murmur due to relative aortic stenosis is regularly heard (Fig. 81) even in patients without a systolic gradient.

Cardiac enlargement is seen at an early stage on the x-ray, especially involving the left ventricle (Fig. 82). The cardiac volume is also increased.

On echocardiography, the left ventricular cavity is enlarged due to the volume overload and a diastolic fluttering of the anterior mitral leaflet can be recorded. The

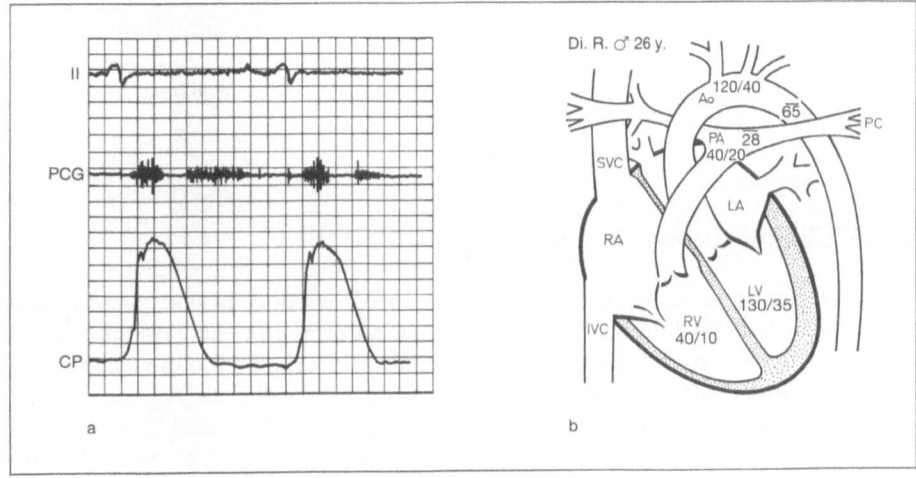

**Fig. 81. a** ECG, phonocardiogram, carotid pulse and **b** cardiac catheterization data in aortic insufficiency. Early systolic murmur due to relative aortic stenosis with augmented stroke volume and turbulence at the abnormal aortic valve and a diastolic decrescendo murmur on the phonocardiogram. There is a lack of dicrotic notch and rapid diastolic pressure drop in the carotid pulse. The heart catheterization shows a very low diastolic aortic pressure and an elevation in left-ventricular diastolic pressure with mild pulmonary hypertension. Angiocardiographically marked valve insufficiency was recorded, the left ventricle and the left atrium were both greatly enlarged. Surgical valve replacement was necessary in this 26-year-old symptomatic patient. A tilting-disc prosthesis was implanted.

111

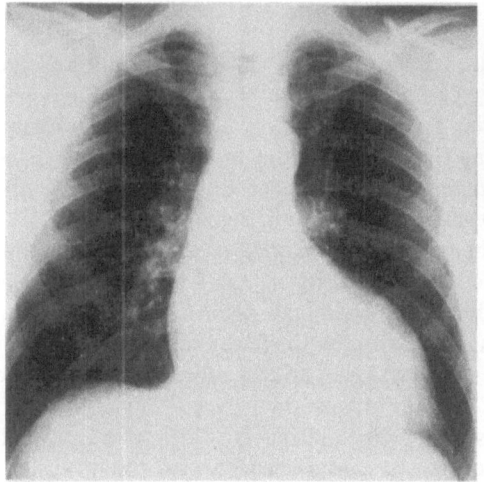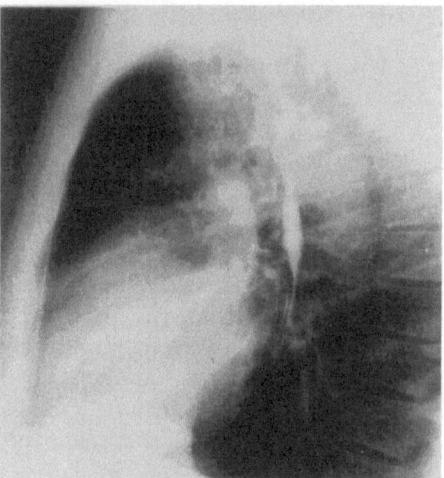

**Fig. 82.** Prominent heart silhouette with "boot-shape" of the cardiac contour, due to an enlarged left ventricle in aortic insufficiency.

regurgitant flow into the left ventricle can be visualized directly by Doppler echocardiography.

Heart catheterization is of additional importance for the qualitative and quantitative diagnosis. Aortography shows diastolic regurgitation of the contrast agent into the left ventricle. Sometimes anatomic abnormalities are seen only angiographically, such as aortic insufficiency due to dilatation of the valvular ring or due to perforation of a sinus of Valsalva aneurysm. Exact knowledge of the anatomic situation as well as of the coronary morphology may be of importance for surgery.

### 7.5.3 Clinical course, therapy

Whereas acute aortic insufficiency in bacterial endocarditis or dehiscence of an artificial valve usually leads to dramatic symptoms, chronic aortic insufficiency will often remain asymptomatic. The disorder may be detected only by chance on routine examination. Also, only clinical follow-up will provide hints on whether the disorder is progressive and necessitates surgery or whether it may be treated medically. Increasing left ventricular hypertrophy on the ECG, and in increase in cardiac size on the x-ray (cardiac volume) or an increase in left ventricular diameter on the echocardiogram may provide evidence for surgery. Approximation of the regurgitant fraction and the left ventricular ejection fraction using radionuclide ventriculography may be of further value in follow-up.

In chronic aortic insufficiency the physician and the patient have to face the problem that often only repeated and careful follow-up examinations provide the basis for a clear decision and, thus, for optimum timing regarding surgery. The aim is to perform surgery as late as possible, but as early as necessary to prevent irreversible ventricular damage.

# 7.6 Pulmonary valve disorders

## 7.6.1 Etiology

Severe pulmonary stenosis usually causes symptoms during infancy. It is therefore diagnosed early, and if possible, treated during that period. Less severe pulmonary stenosis is also often diagnosed during infancy, but may be recognized first in adults. Treatment is only necessary if the stenosis progresses or causes a gradient of more than 60 mmHg. Pulmonary valve insufficiency is infrequent and usually hemodynamically insignificant. It usually occurs only after surgical valvular dilatation.

## 7.6.2 Pathology, pathophysiology

Fusion of the pulmonary leaflets at the commissures occurs during middle or late gestation, while peripheral pulmonary artery stenosis may occur in late gestation due to rubella infection. An infundibular or muscular subvalvular stenosis may be associated with tetralogy of Fallot or with hypertrophic cardiomyopathy.

Pulmonary stenosis leads to pressure loading of the right ventricle which leads to concentric hypertrophy and, later, to ventricular dilatation and right-heart failure. Usually, pulmonary stenosis with a pressure gradient above 70 mm Hg leads to unfavorable hemodynamic consequences and the need for invasive therapy.

## 7.6.3 Clinical manifestations

A left parasternal precordial pulsation may be palpated due to enlargement of the right ventricle. On auscultation a spindle-shaped systolic murmur with maximum loudness above the left second intercostal space is prominent. Sometimes the murmur is so loud that it may be palpable as a buzzing sensation. As in aortic stenosis, the loudness of the murmur does not provide a reliable clue to the severity of the disorder. The timing of maximum loudness during systole is a better indicator. With mild pulmonary stenosis the murmur peaks early, while in severe pulmonary stenosis it peaks late.

The ECG is an important diagnostic method. Right-ventricular hypertrophy due to pressure loading leads to right-axis deviation and enlargement of the R-waves in $V_1$ and $V_2$, with reduction of S-waves in those same leads (Fig. 83). The findings of pressure loading differ from those of volume loading with widening of the QRS complex and incomplete right bundle branch block.

With echocardiography, right-ventricular hypertrophy and, eventually, right-ventricular dilatation can be visualized. Incomplete opening of the pulmonary valves can be visualized in some cases. the pressure gradient can be reliably assessed using continuous wave Doppler.

The x-ray often reveals poststenotic dilatation of the pulmonary artery, cardiac enlargement, and diminished peripheral pulmonary vessel markings (Fig. 84). With mild stenosis the x-ray may be normal.

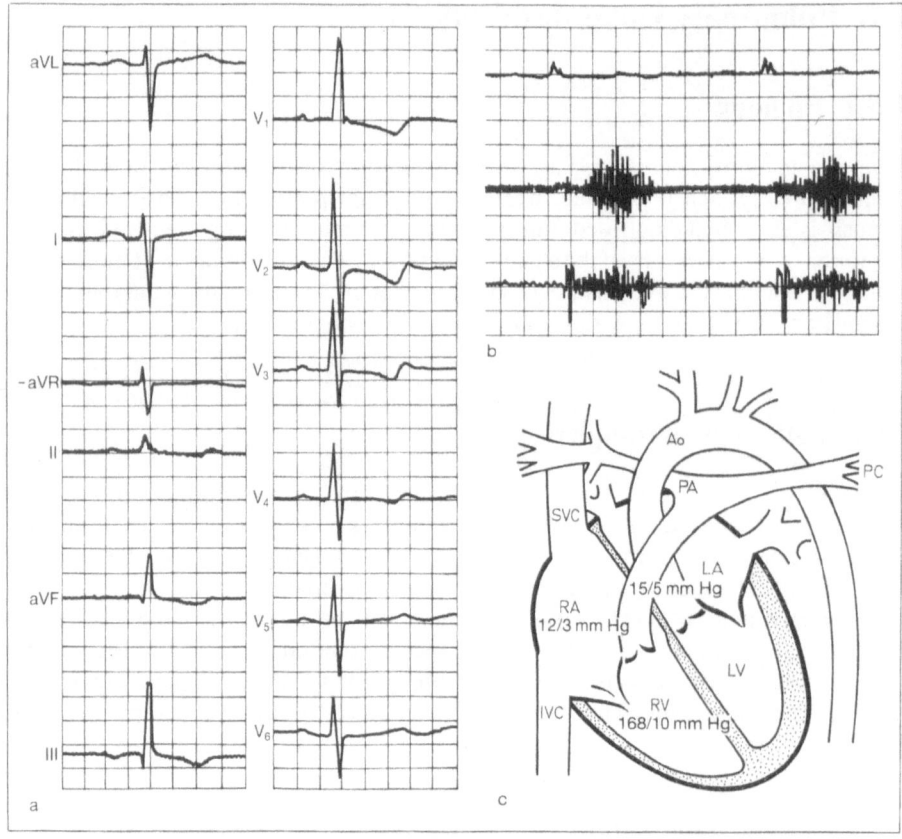

**Fig. 83.** Severe pulmonary stenosis with a peak systolic pressure gradient of 153 mmHg. **a** Right-ventricular hypertrophy on the ECG, **b** spindle-shaped ejection murmur on the phonocardiogram, **c** cardiac catheterization data. Valvular stenosis in this 36-year-old patient was dilated using a balloon catheter, which was introduced via the femoral vein. Three months after the procedure the systolic gradient was only 30 mmHg. For x-ray see Fig. 84.

The magnitude of the pressure gradient is measured at right-heart catheterization; with the help of a pressure recording during withdrawal of the catheter it can be seen whether it occurs at the level of the pulmonary valve, below (infundibular), or above (supravalvular). Comparable to aortic stenosis, the size of the pressure gradient is an important clue to the degree of severity and, therefore, to management.

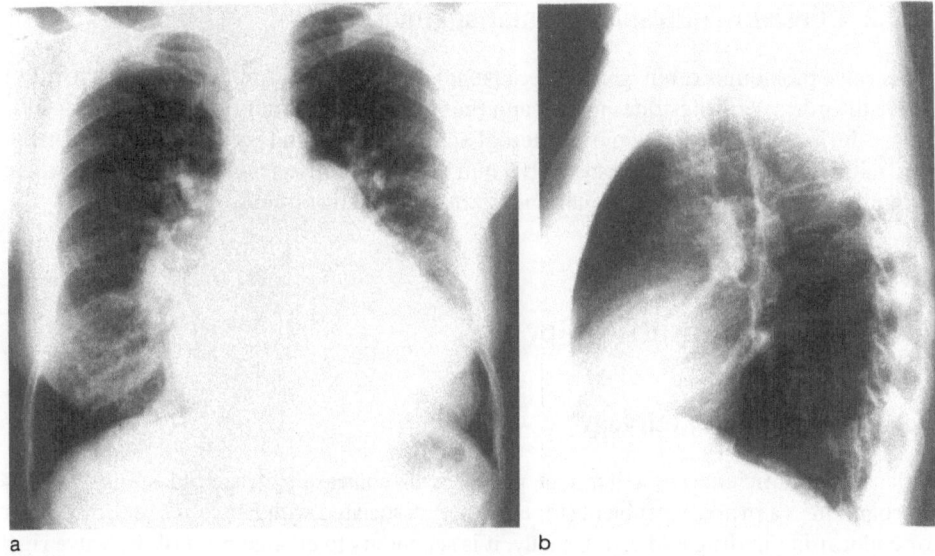

a           b

**Fig. 84.** Chest x-ray in severe pulmonary stenosis (same patient as in Fig. 83). The heart is enlarged, as is the pulmonary segment; the central pulmonary vessels are enlarged and the peripheral vessels reduced.

### 7.6.4 Therapy

No treatment is necessary with a pressure gradient of less than 60 mm Hg. Valvular dilatation is indicated with a higher gradient. Until 1985, this was possible only with surgery, but it has since been shown that dilatation with a balloon catheter will usually provide good results. Pulmonary valve insufficiency due to valve dilatation is only rarely seen using this method.

## 7.7 Tricuspid stenosis

### 7.7.1 Pathology, pathophysiology, occurrence

Tricuspid stenosis usually develops from rheumatic endocarditis. While involvement of the tricuspid valve by postrheumatic endocarditis is rare in western countries, for unknown reasons this valve disorder is more frequently found in Asia. It is usually associated with other disorders, such as mitral valve stenosis. When the tricuspid valve area is less than 1.5 cm$^2$ the impeded diastolic inflow into the right ventricle increases pressure in the right atrium, and thus causes liver congestion, peripheral edema, and, eventually, ascites.

### 7.7.2 Clinical manifestations, management

This valve problem is often ignored because it is disguised by symptoms related to other valve disorders. The diastolic murmur and the presystolic murmur of tricuspid stenosis is heard during sinus rhythm at the left sternal edge. The auscultatory areas of the tricuspid and mitral valve may overlap, especially when the right ventricle is enlarged. Either valve dilatation or prosthetic valve replacement are therapeutic options.

# 7.8 Tricuspid insufficiency

## 7.8.1 Occurrence, etiology

Tricuspid insufficiency is a frequent problem in contrast to tricuspid stenosis. It is uncommon as a primary problem (for example, associated with Ebstein's malformation or endocarditis in drug addicts). Usually, it is secondary to enlargement of the valve ring in a dilated right ventricle. This secondary type is most frequently caused by myocardial failure of the right ventricle as a result of mitral valve disease or other disorders causing right ventricular failure.

## 7.8.2 Clinical manifestations, management

The enlarged right ventricle may often be palpated over the precordium. A systolic venous pulsation and an enlarged pulsatile liver are characteristic findings. The systolic murmur may easily be mistaken for mitral insufficiency, but it may be differentiated from this disorder by absent radiation into the axilla, and the murmur being maximal at the left sternal border (Fig. 85). The murmur also often increases with each inspiration.

**Treatment**
Treatment depends on the underlying disorder. Frequently, all signs of tricuspid insufficiency vanish with medical correction of right-heart failure. With a severe irreversible lesion of the right ventricle (for example, secondary to end-stage mitral valve disease) surgical treatment of the tricuspid insufficiency may be necessary. Restoration of valve competence is attempted by surgical valvuloplasty involving a reduction in the size of the valve ring. Surgical implantation of a posthetic valve is applied to patients with severe valvular malformation or destruction.

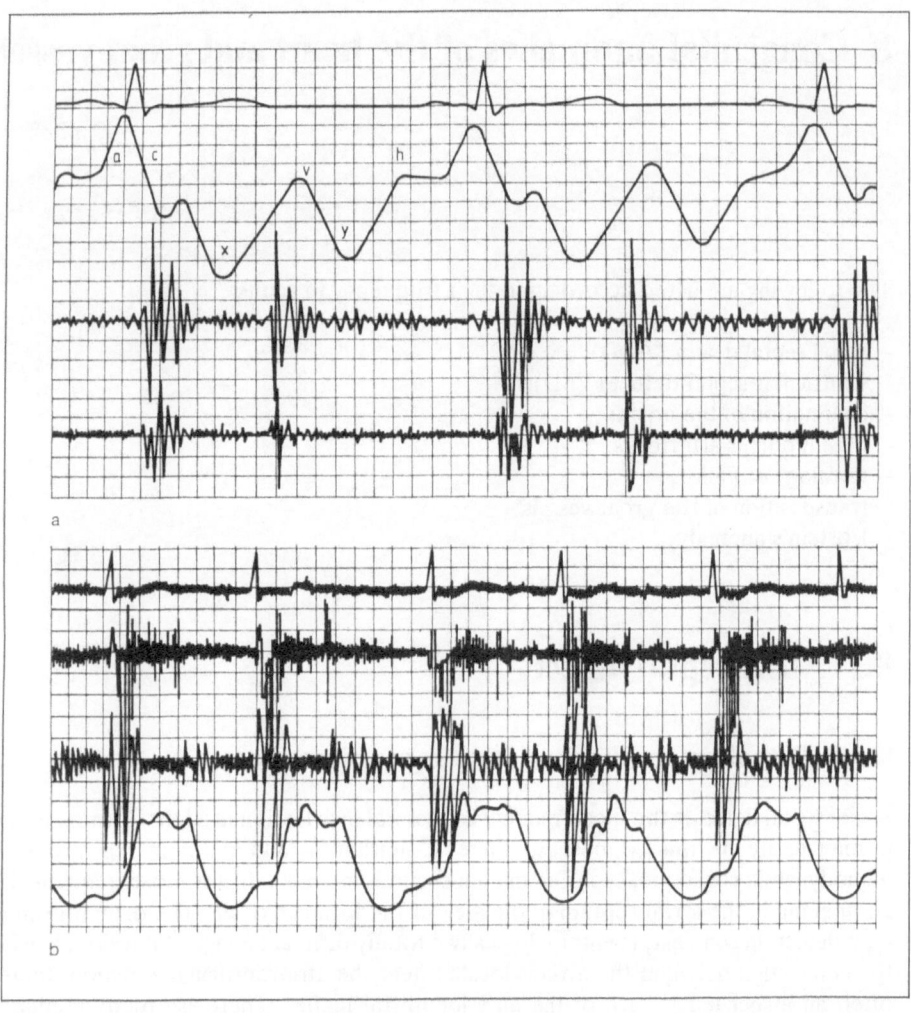

**Fig. 85. a** Normal venous pulse, **b** "ventricularized" venous pulse-wave form in tricuspid insufficiency.

# 8 Congenital anomalies of the heart and great vessels

The following are listed according to their frequency in adults:

– atrial septal defect (ASD);
– ventricular septal defect (VSD);
– coarctation of the aorta;
– patent ductus arteriosus;
– tetralogy of Fallot;
– transposition of the great vessels;
– Ebstein's anomaly.

## 8.1 Atrial septal defect

### 8.1.1 Pathology, pathophysiology, occurrence

Atrial septal defect is the most frequent congenital heart lesion in adults. During infancy it may easily be missed because there is neither a loud murmur nor prominent hemodynamic consequences. The ostium-secundum-type defect is most frequent, i.e., an opening in the atrial septum in the area of the foramen ovale. The ostium-primum-type defect, in contrast, is embryologically a totally different congenital lesion, in which the connection between the atria is located near the atrioventricular junction; there is often an associated fissure of the anterior mitral leaflet. There are many gradations between a minor valve fissure and a persistent wide atrioventricular canal.

An atrial septal defect higher in the septum and often incorporating the pulmonary veins is classified as a sinus venosus defect. Finally, and least common of all, a defect in the area of the coronary sinus may occur. In this case, both atria are connected due to an enlarged coronary sinus ostium which extends beyond the septum.

Isolated, anomalous, pulmonary venous connection into the right atrium leads to the same hemodynamic consequences as an atrial septal defect. Anomalous insertions of the upper and lower pulmonary veins usually drain into the superior vena cava, but may also drain into the inferior vena cava or portal vein. Finally, complete anomalous insertion of all pulmonary veins may occur. Anomalous pulmonary veins are often associated with a sinus venosus defect.

Atrial septal defect and/or anomalous pulmonary veins cause left-to-right shunting. The hemodynamic consequences depend on the size of the shunt. A shunt reversal or bidirectional shunting occurs only in large atrial septal defects and with marked increase in right atrial pressure.

118

With a left-to-right shunt, the pulmonary blood flow exceeds the systemic flow. A proportion of the pulmonary venous blood flows back into the pulmonary circulation after crossing the atrial septal defect (shunted blood). Pulmonary blood flow is, therefore, increased by a multiple of the systemic circulation. For example, the ratio of flow in the pulmonary circulation to the systemic circulation may be 3:1 (e.g. if the flow in the pulmonary circulation is 12 liters, and the systemic flow is 4 liters. The shunt flow in this example is 8 liters). Hemodynamic consequences of a shunt usually occur if the ratio of pulmonary to systemic flow is greater than 1.5:1 or, stated in another way, if more than 33% of the pulmonary blood flow is shunt blood. Smaller shunt volumes are usually without consequence. However, single estimates of the size of a shunt are open to question as there is some variability from day to day. Pulmonary hypertension is a rare complication of atrial septal defect; it is much more commonly a complication of large ventricular septal defects. Large atrial septal defects lead more to chronic right ventricular and right atrial volume overloading with right ventricular failure and atrial arrhythmias.

## 8.1.2 Clinical manifestations, course, management

Atrial septal defect is not uncommonly diagnosed in the adult, when its most prominent signs namely pulmonary plethora and cardiac enlargement are noted on routine x-ray.

A systolic murmur over the pulmonary artery due to turbulence produced by the high blood flow, is found on auscultation. Usually, there is fixed splitting of the second heart sound with no change in splitting correlated with breathing. Normally, the gap between aortic and pulmonary components of the second heart sound increases with inspiration and decreases with expiration. The fixed delayed splitting of the second heart sound in atrial septal defect is caused by late closure of the pulmonary valve due to a prolonged right ventricular ejection time. In a large shunt, i.e., where the ratio of pulmonary to systemic flow is greater than 3:1, a diastolic murmur may also be heard at the left sternal border, due to a relative tricuspid stenosis.

The ECG shows signs of volume loading of the right ventricle with an incomplete right bundle branch block pattern. In the ostium primum defect, the ECG characteristically shows extreme left-axis deviation.

The pulmonary artery segment is enlarged on the x-ray (Fig. 86), and arterial and venous vascular markings are augmented. During fluoroscopy a systolic "dancing" of the hilar vessels may be found. The cardiac volume is also increased.

The size of the shunt volume can be measured using indicator dye dilution curves (Fig. 87), but the shunt may also be visualized by echocardiography with injection of a contrast agent in the form of very fine echo-producing air bubbles. A secondary sign of the disorder is enlargement of the right ventricle. Left-to-right shunting can be seen with the help of color-flow Doppler studies. The actual septal defect is best visualized by transesophageal echocardiography.

Right-heart catheterization permits the noninvasive diagnosis to be verified. It also allows measurement of the shunt to be more accurately quantitated (Fig. 88) and for anomalous pulmonary venous connections, if present, to be seen with angiography.

If the shunt volume is large enough (pulmonary to systemic flow greater than 1.5:1) surgical therapy is indicated. A small atrial septal defect is closed by a suture; for larger

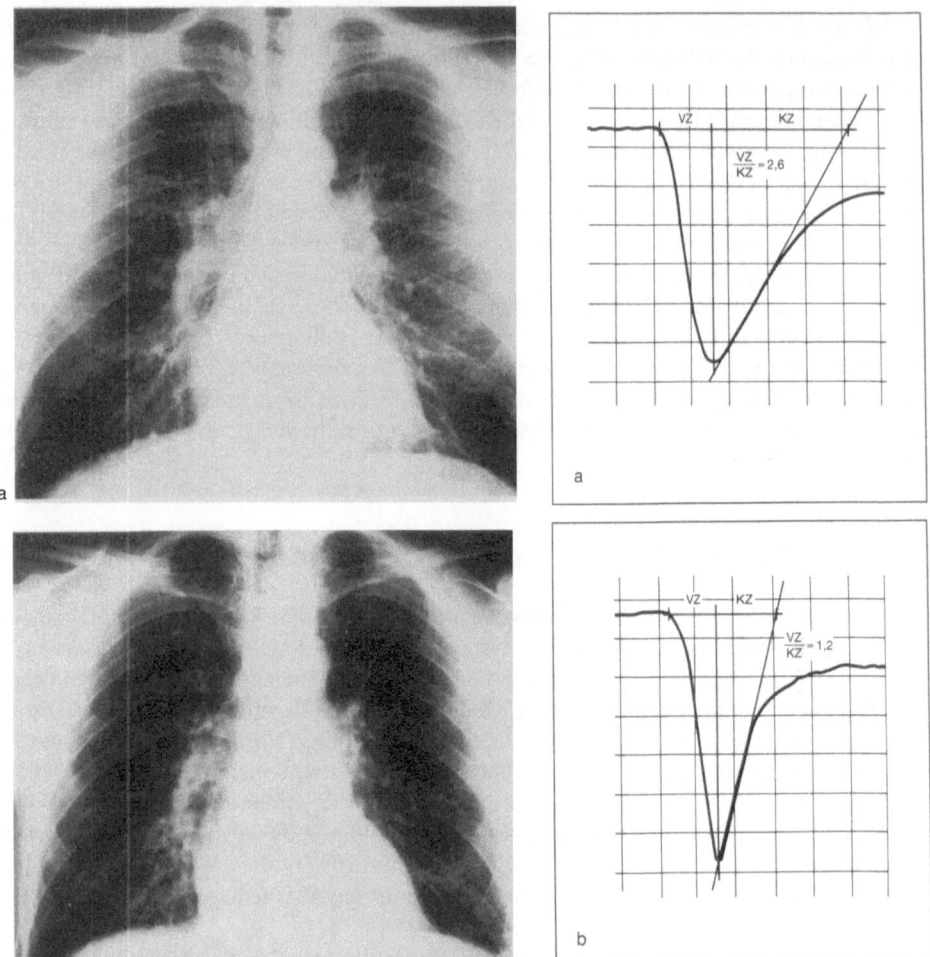

**Fig. 86. a** Atrial septal defect with cardiac enlargement. Enlargement of the pulmonary artery with augmented arterial and venous markings; **b** after surgical closure, decrease of cardiac size and vascular markings.

**Fig. 87. a** Indicator dye-dilution recorded from the ear after intravenous injection curve before and **b** after surgical closure of an atrial septal defect. Due to the left-to-right shunt, the preoperative dilution curve is prolonged and the ratio of dilution time (VZ) divided by concentration time (KZ) is increased.

defects, dacron or pericardial patches are used. A mitral valvuloplasty is frequently necessary in conjunction with an ostium primum repair. Anomalous veins may require reimplantation into the left atrium.

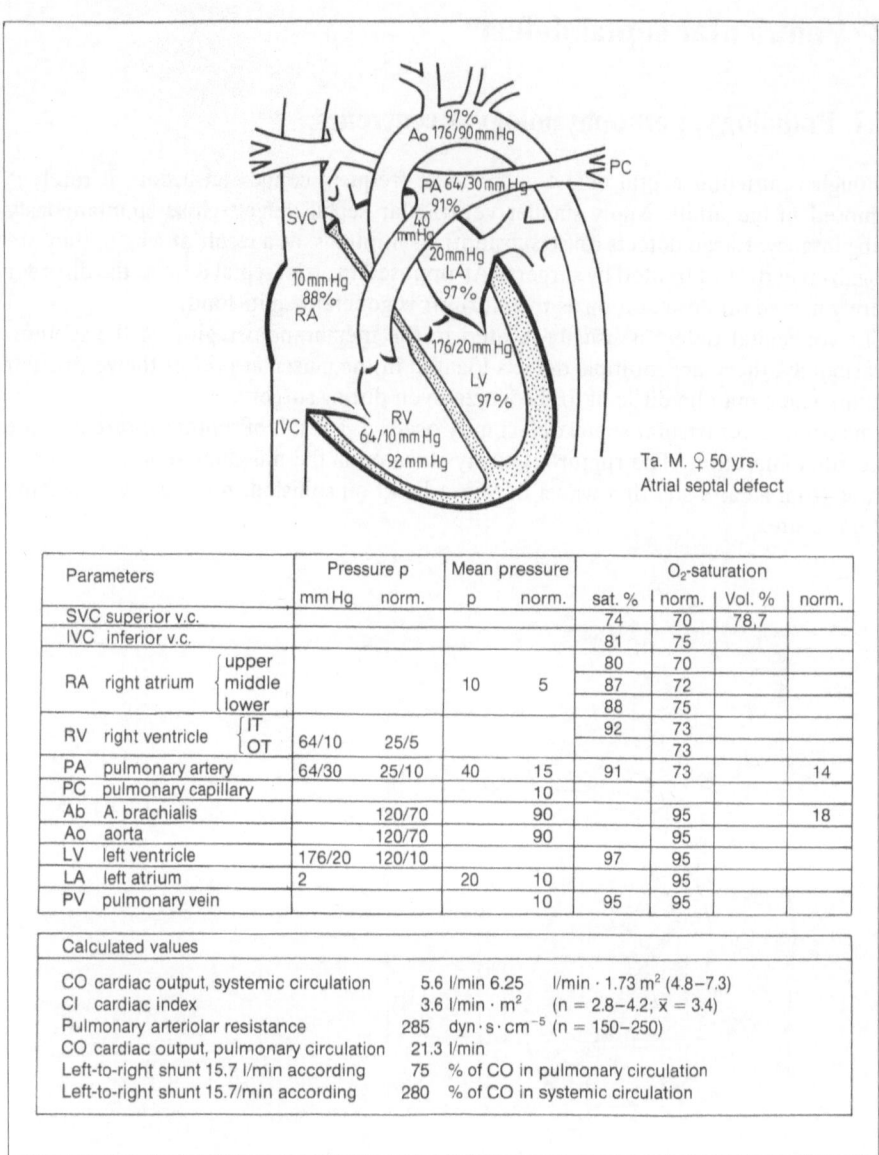

| Parameters | | Pressure p | | Mean pressure | | O₂-saturation | | | |
|---|---|---|---|---|---|---|---|---|---|
| | | mm Hg | norm. | p | norm. | sat. % | norm. | Vol. % | norm. |
| SVC  superior v.c. | | | | | | 74 | 70 | 78,7 | |
| IVC  inferior v.c. | | | | | | 81 | 75 | | |
| RA  right atrium | upper | | | 10 | 5 | 80 | 70 | | |
| | middle | | | | | 87 | 72 | | |
| | lower | | | | | 88 | 75 | | |
| RV  right ventricle | IT | 64/10 | 25/5 | | | 92 | 73 | | |
| | OT | | | | | | 73 | | |
| PA  pulmonary artery | | 64/30 | 25/10 | 40 | 15 | 91 | 73 | | 14 |
| PC  pulmonary capillary | | | | | 10 | | | | |
| Ab  A. brachialis | | | 120/70 | | 90 | | 95 | | 18 |
| Ao  aorta | | | 120/70 | | 90 | | 95 | | |
| LV  left ventricle | | 176/20 | 120/10 | | | 97 | 95 | | |
| LA  left atrium | | 2 | | 20 | 10 | | 95 | | |
| PV  pulmonary vein | | | | | 10 | 95 | 95 | | |

Calculated values

| | | |
|---|---|---|
| CO cardiac output, systemic circulation | 5.6 l/min 6.25 | l/min · 1.73 m² (4.8–7.3) |
| CI  cardiac index | 3.6 l/min · m² | (n = 2.8–4.2; x̄ = 3.4) |
| Pulmonary arteriolar resistance | 285 | dyn·s·cm⁻⁵ (n = 150–250) |
| CO cardiac output, pulmonary circulation | 21.3 l/min | |
| Left-to-right shunt 15.7 l/min according | 75 | % of CO in pulmonary circulation |
| Left-to-right shunt 15.7/min according | 280 | % of CO in systemic circulation |

**Fig. 88.** Large atrial septal defect with pulmonary hypertension. The pulmonary blood flow is four times the systemic flow. Secondary finding: systemic arterial hypertension.

121

# 8.2 Ventricular septal defect

## 8.2.1 Pathology, pathophysiology, occurrence

Although ventricular septal defect is the most frequent congenital lesion, it rarely is diagnosed in the adult. Many smaller ventricular septal defects close spontaneously during infancy. Large defects cause substantial symptoms, as a result of which, they are recognized early and treated by surgery. As opposed to atrial septal defect, the disorder is rarely missed on auscultation as the murmur is generally quite loud.

The congenital defect is usually located in the membranous region of the septum. Occasionally, there are multiple defects located in the muscular part of the ventricular septum. These may be difficult to recognize even during surgery.

An acquired ventricular septal defect may occur as a result of septal rupture in acute myocardial infarction. The rupture is always located in the muscular septum. Trauma, such as from a car's steering wheel during a head-on collision, may rarely also cause septal rupture.

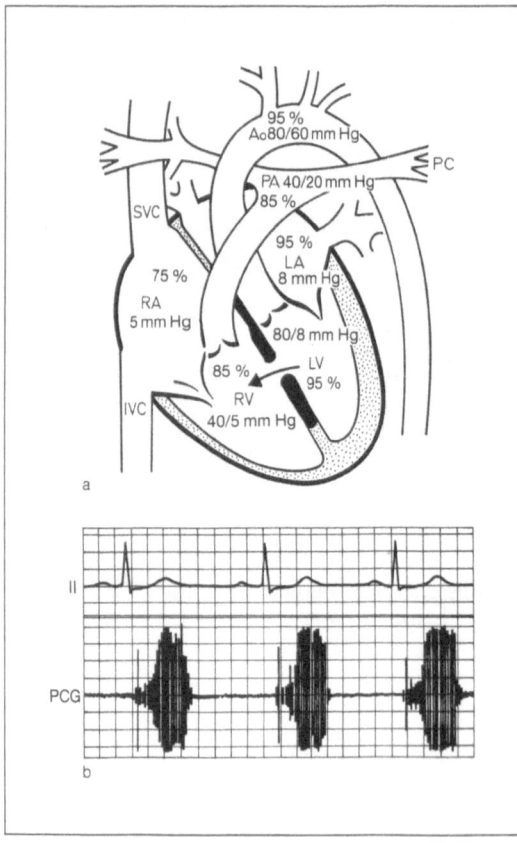

a

b

**Fig. 89. a** Findings from heart catheterization, **b** ECG and phonocardiogram in ventricular septal defect. The values for oxygen saturation are compatible with a pure left-to-right shunt. The pressure in the pulmonary circulation is mildly elevated. A loud systolic murmur is recorded on the phonocardiogram. Surgical closure of the defect was performed.

The consequences of a shunt at the atrial level are determined by volume overload, whereas in a shunt at the ventricular level it is also the pressure overload in the pulmonary circulation which determines the outcome. Hemodynamic consequences from a ventricular septal defect will usually occur if the ratio of pulmonary to systemic flow is greater than 1.5:1.

### 8.2.2 Clinical manifestations, course, management

A small ventricular septal defect without pressure loading of the right heart is well tolerated. There is increased susceptibility for endocarditis, but this is not enough to warrant surgery. Large septal defects may lead to severe fixed pulmonary hypertension in addition to volume overload of the left ventricle. Pressure in the pulmonary artery may exceed systemic pressure due to thickening and lumen obliteration of the small pulmonary resistance vessels. This may eventually lead to the Eisenmenger syndrome where there is right-to-left shunting at the ventricular level.

A loud holosystolic murmur maximal at the left parasternal third intercostal space (Erb's point) is heard (see Fig. 89). The size of the shunt may be estimated noninvasively using color-flow Doppler and/or micro-bubble contrast echocardiography. Echocardiography can also help evaluate further additional anomalies that may be present.

Depending on the size of the shunt and the hemodynamic consequences, signs of pulmonary hypertension, increased pulmonary flow, pulmonary artery ectasia, and enlargement of the right heart can be observed on the x-ray.

On the ECG there will be evidence of right-ventricular hypertrophy and left-ventricular volume overload.

The hemodynamic consequences are easily and accurately measured by heart catheterization (Fig. 89). The location of single or multiple defects is verified by left-heart catheterization with injection of contrast agent into the left ventricle and angiocardiography in the left anterior oblique view. In this projection, the ventricular septum is brought into line with the direction of radiation. The angle of projection is chosen with additional craniocaudal angulation so that the entire length of the septum can be visualized without any foreshortening.

The treatment of choice is surgical closure, unless the defect is hemodynamically insignificant or, at the other end of the scale, there is already severe fixed pulmonary hypertension. This latter problem is rare before the age of 2 years, thus making important to recognize a ventricular septal defect in infancy.

## 8.3 Coarctation of the aorta

### 8.3.1 Pathology

The disorder involves a collar-shaped stricture of the aorta near the orifice of the ductus arteriosus. A more proximal (pre-ductal) form can be distinguished from a more distal (post-ductal) one; in the former, the left subclavian artery has its origin distal to the stenosis, so that there is a difference in blood pressure between both arms, whereas in the latter the blood pressure is elevated in both arms. In both forms the blood pressure is decreased in the lower part of the body. To compensate for the stenosis, collateral blood vessels open up, especially the intercostal arteries, internal mammary arteries, and subscapular arteries.

### 8.3.2 Clinical course

In severe coarctation, complications such as heart failure and cerebral hemorrhage occur early in life. Without early surgery, more than half of these infants die within the first year. Later consequences of the congenital lesion are determined by the degree of arterial hypertension in the upper part of the body.

### 8.3.3 Clinical manifestations

Aortic coarctation is not common in adults, but it should always be considered in the evaluation of systemic arterial hypertension because of its therapeutic significance. It should be suspected if an elevated blood pressure is recognized, but the lower extremity pulses are not easily palpated. In such a case, blood-pressure measurements should be taken in both arms and legs. If only the usual arm cuffs are available then a systolic blood-pressure measurement in the legs may be estimated using the capillary pressure method (see blood pressure measurement). In order to obtain comparable values, blood-pressure measurements in the upper and lower limbs have to be performed during recumbency, with the arms and legs located at the same level with respect to the heart. Pressure measurements can best be obtained using the Doppler technique. Pre-ductal coarctation is rare in the adult and is associated with a blood-pressure difference between the arms.

A systolic murmur is heard in the area of the first and second intercostal space and, characteristically, can be found over the back, between the scapulae. There is often a concomitant bicuspid aortic valve which may produce signs of aortic stenosis.

Rib notching is often seen on the x-ray (Fig. 90). Under certain circumstances, the stenotic region may be visualized directly on a tomogram cut parallel to the aorta; it may also be seen on contrast-enhanced computed tomography (CT).

The pressure gradient across the stenosis is measured at heart catheterization (Fig. 91). It is the aim of aortography to document the degree and length of the stenosis. A concomitant congenital lesion of the aortic valve should also be ruled out. If a lesion of the aortic valve and additional vessel anomalies can be ruled out reliably, imaging of coarctation by intravenous subtraction angiography may be sufficient.

### 8.3.4 Therapy

Usually, a coarctation is repaired by surgery. Surgery should preferably be performed between the 7th and 14th years of life, that is at a sufficiently young age to avoid

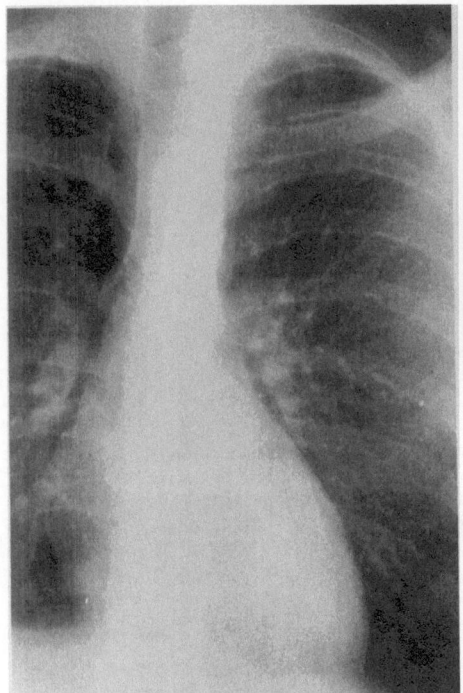

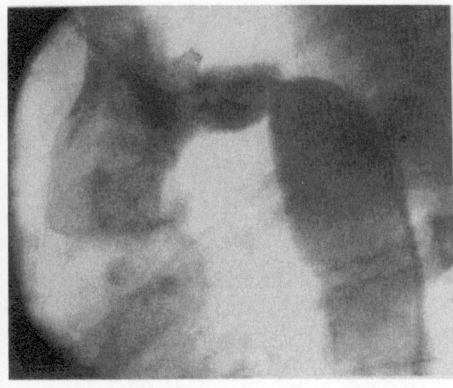

a

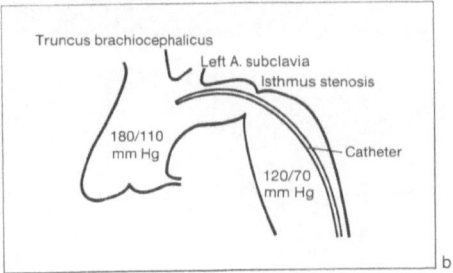

b

**Fig. 90.** Coarctation of the aorta in a 29-year-old man with prominent rib notching of the left dorsal ribs.

**Fig. 91. a** Angiocardiogram, and **b** corresponding anatomic illustration of an aortic coarctation with a systolic pressure gradient of 60 mmHg. The stenosis was dilated with a balloon catheter and the gradient reduced to 10 mmHg.

irreversible or fixed hypertension. In some cases dilatation is possible using a balloon catheter (Fig. 92).

# 8.4 Patent ductus arteriosus

## 8.4.1 Occurrence, pathology

Patent ductus arteriosus is a not uncommon defect and is the consequence of persistent opening of a fetal vessel communication between the aorta and the pulmonary artery. Physiologically, closure of the ductus occurs within the first week after birth. A persistent ductus arteriosus is especially frequent in premature babies.

While a large patent ductus leads to early symptoms such as heart failure, a small ductus is without consequences. In the adult, it is usually a small- or medium-sized ductus that is found, but occasionally, a larger ductus with a luminal diameter of more than

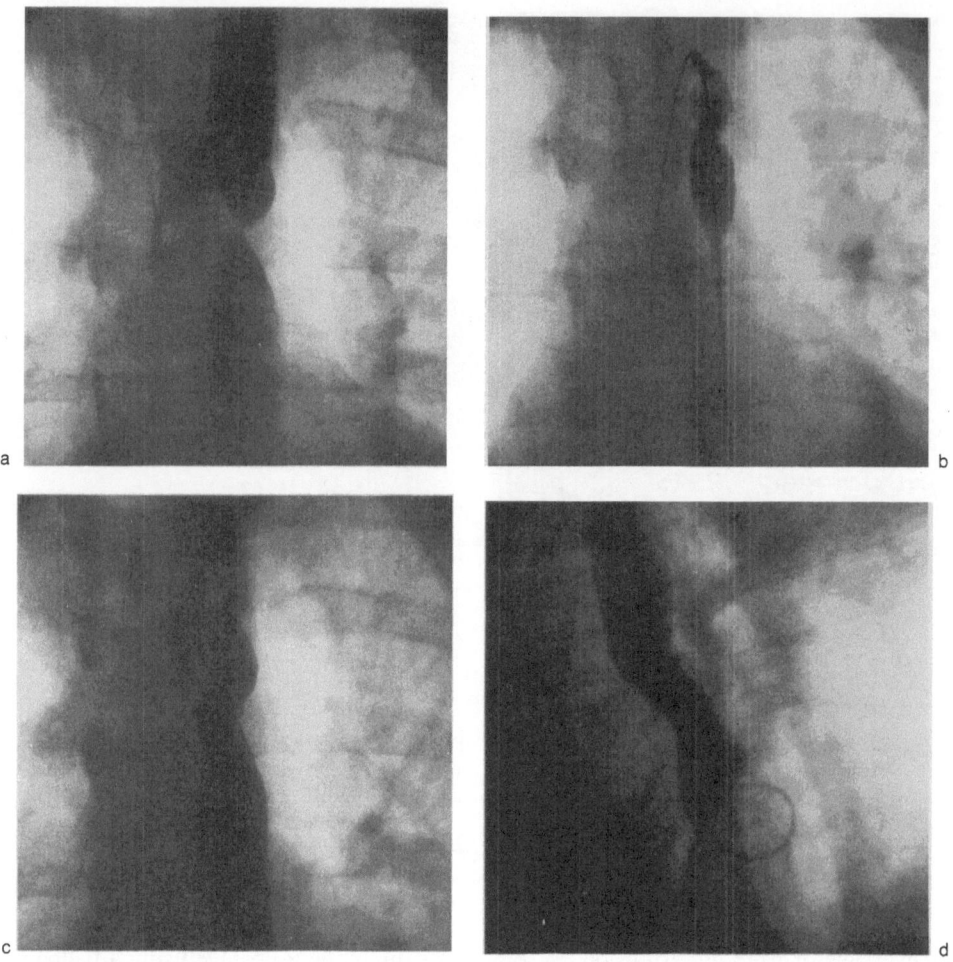

**Fig. 92.** Stenosis of the aortic isthmus in a 27-year-old woman. The gradient was 75 mmHg (**a**). A ballon catheter was introduced and the stenosis dilated (**b**). After the procedure the gradient was reduced to 20 mmHg, the stenosis is now widely open in PA view (**c**) and oblique view (**d**). The irregular contour within the stenosis is probably due to an intimal dissection which had already occured before dilation in this patient. It has been seen in other patients occuring during the procedure – usually without clinical consequences.

10 mm is discovered. A patent ductus leads to a left-to-right shunt, producing increased pulmonary flow and pulmonary hypertension. There is a risk of endocarditis in the area of the ductus, but its occurrence is so rare that, by itself, this is not a sufficient indication for surgery.

## 8.4.2 Clinical manifestations

Characteristically, there is a systolic-diastolic (continuous) murmur in the second left intercostal space; it is sometimes compared to the sound of a machine or a train (Fig. 92 A). It is caused by blood flowing into the pulmonary artery under high pressure from the aorta; because of the constant pressure difference between these two arteries the

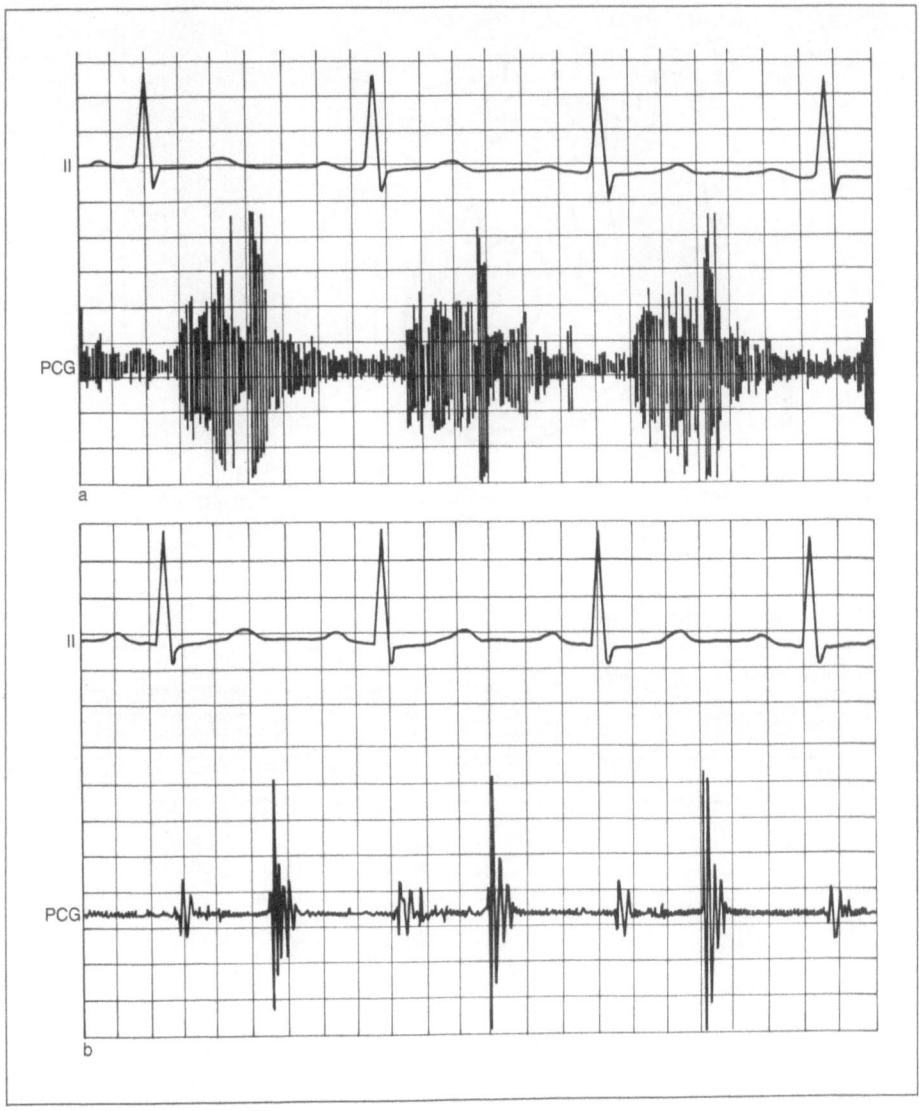

**Fig. 92 A. a** Systolic-diastolic "machinery murmur" in an 11-year-old girl with a patent ductus, **b** after noninvasive closure with an ivalon plug, placed into the ductus using a catheter technique the murmur has disappeared.

shunt occurs, not only in systole, but also during diastole. In some patients, especially those with a small ductus, one may hear only a systolic murmur. The symptoms and signs are determined by the width of the ductus (which ranges from 2–12 mm) and the resulting degree of left-to-right shunt. A large ductus may eventually lead to fixed pulmonary hypertension and right-to-left shunting.

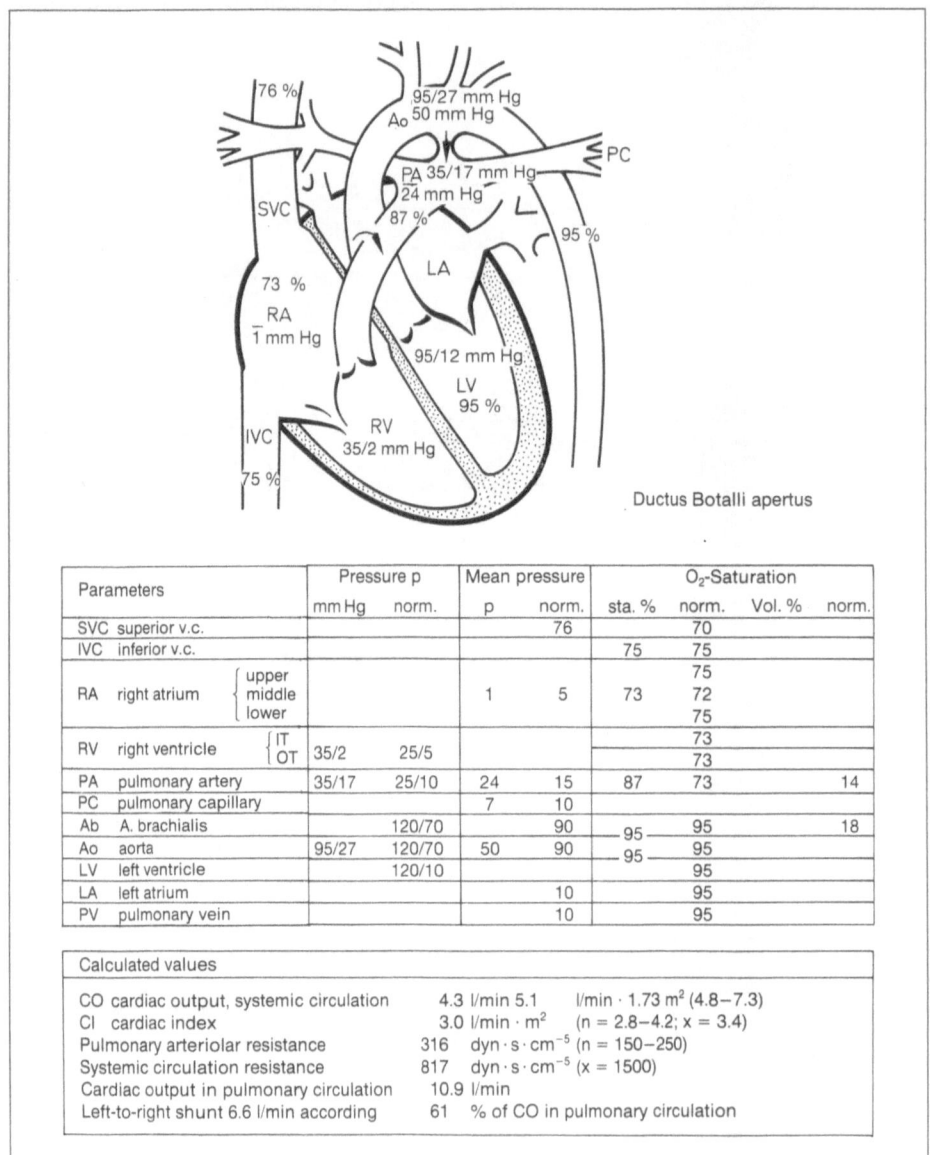

| Parameters | | | Pressure p | | Mean pressure | | O₂-Saturation | | | |
|---|---|---|---|---|---|---|---|---|---|---|
| | | | mm Hg | norm. | p | norm. | sta. % | norm. | Vol. % | norm. |
| SVC superior v.c. | | | | | | 76 | | 70 | | |
| IVC inferior v.c. | | | | | | | 75 | 75 | | |
| RA right atrium | upper | | | | | | | 75 | | |
| | middle | | | | 1 | 5 | 73 | 72 | | |
| | lower | | | | | | | 75 | | |
| RV right ventricle | IT | | | | | | | 73 | | |
| | OT | 35/2 | 25/5 | | | | | 73 | | |
| PA pulmonary artery | | 35/17 | 25/10 | 24 | 15 | 87 | 73 | | | 14 |
| PC pulmonary capillary | | | | 7 | 10 | | | | | |
| Ab A. brachialis | | | 120/70 | | 90 | 95 | 95 | | 18 | |
| Ao aorta | | 95/27 | 120/70 | 50 | 90 | 95 | 95 | | | |
| LV left ventricle | | | 120/10 | | | | 95 | | | |
| LA left atrium | | | | | 10 | | 95 | | | |
| PV pulmonary vein | | | | | 10 | | 95 | | | |

Calculated values

| | | |
|---|---|---|
| CO cardiac output, systemic circulation | 4.3 l/min 5.1 | l/min · 1.73 m² (4.8–7.3) |
| CI cardiac index | 3.0 l/min · m² | (n = 2.8–4.2; x = 3.4) |
| Pulmonary arteriolar resistance | 316 | dyn · s · cm⁻⁵ (n = 150–250) |
| Systemic circulation resistance | 817 | dyn · s · cm⁻⁵ (x = 1500) |
| Cardiac output in pulmonary circulation | 10.9 l/min | |
| Left-to-right shunt 6.6 l/min according | 61 | % of CO in pulmonary circulation |

**Fig. 93.** Findings at heart catheterization with a patent ductus arteriosus and a large left-to-right shunt. Mild pulmonary hypertension and a decreased diastolic aortic pressure are hemodynamic consequences of the disorder. Closure of the ductus was performed without surgery using a catheter-introduced plug.

The ECG and x-ray may be normal with a small ductus. In a large ductus signs of right-heart strain develop on the ECG and right-heart enlargement and increased pulmonary vessel markings are found on the x-ray.

The size of the shunt can be estimated using indicator dye-dilution curves. Verification of the diagnosis can be obtained with the help of right- and left-heart catheterization (Fig. 93). The degree of pulmonary hypertension and the degree of left-to-right shunting are of importance. Direct angiographic visualization of the ductus by injecting contrast agent into the aorta or directly into the ductus is important in planning non-surgical closure. Since high flow vessels are often difficult to outline exactly with contrast injections they can be visualized more accurately by a very compliant dye-filled balloon brought into the ductus.

### 8.4.3 Therapy

Closure of a patent ductus arteriosus may be done using surgical ligature and division of the ductus. Surgery is usually not difficult, but there is some danger of bleeding in the adult due to degenerative changes in the wall of the ductus.

Closure may also be performed non-surgically with the help of a catheter using a method developed by Porstmann. The ductus is approached from the aorta and a guide wire is advanced through the ductus into the pulmonary artery. With the help of a right-heart catheter this guide-wire in the pulmonary artery is grasped with a loop and withdrawn to the femoral vein. A connection is thereby established between the femoral artery via aorta and ductus into the pulmonary artery, then back into the right ventricle, right atrium, and inferior vena cava to the femoral vein. An ivalon plug is advanced along this guide wire from the femoral artery into the ductus and tightly fixed there. The ivalon plug selected has to be matched in size, shape, and width against the size of the actual ductus. Experience with this procedure, over many years, has shown that reliable closure is possible without surgery (Fig. 94). Recently umbrella-like devices are also being used.

## 8.5 Fallot's tetralogy

This congenital disorder usually leads to prominent symptoms, such that it is diagnosed and treated in early infancy. The therapy of choice is surgical correction. In infancy and when the pulmonary arteries are very small, a palliative connection between the systemic and pulmonary circulations can be created by surgically connecting a subclavian artery with a pulmonary artery. Tetralogy of Fallot is seen in adults when surgical correction was rejected or was not possible in infancy.

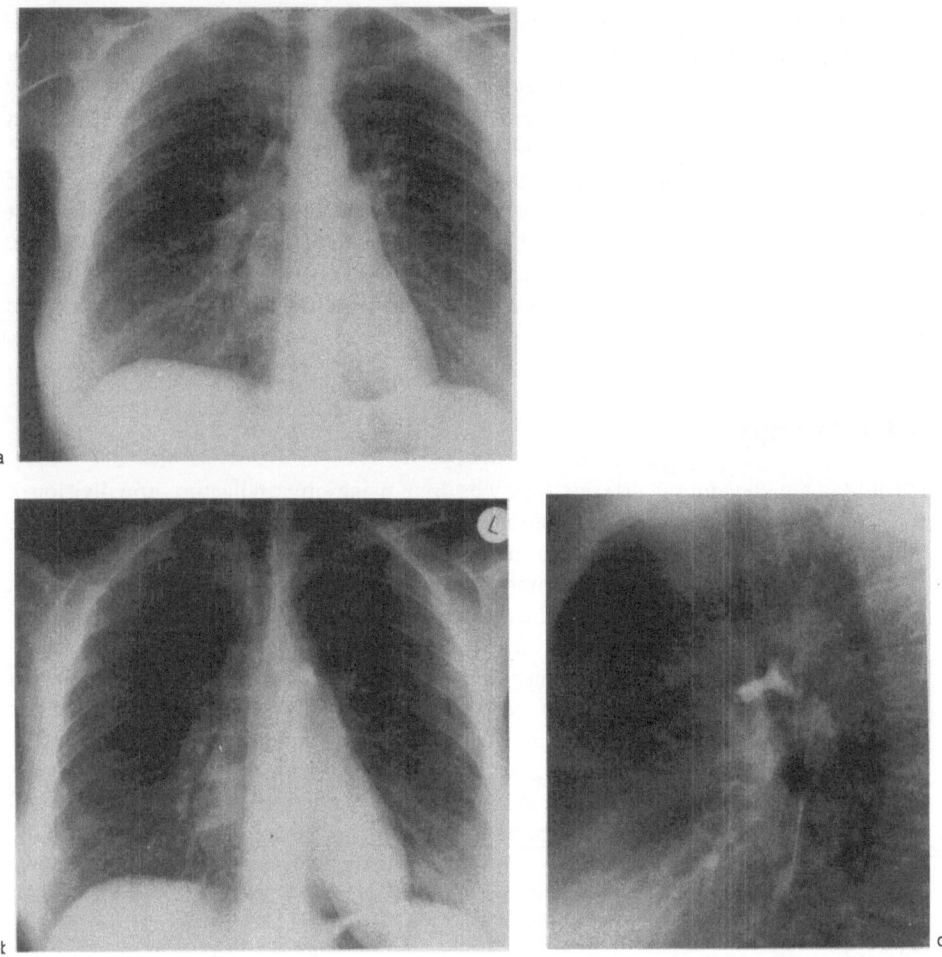

a

b

c

**Fig. 94.** 26-year-old woman with ductus arteriosus. Marked left-to-right shunt: Flow in pulmonary circulation 8 l/min; in systemic circulation 4 l/min. The chest x-ray (**a**) shows increased pulmonary vessel markings. The ductus was occluded by the catheter technique. After occlusion (**b**) pulmonary vessels appear normal. The ductus was occluded with an ivalon plug, introduced over an arterial catheter after introduction of a wire through the ductus. This wire formed a track from the femoral artery through the ductus to the femoral vein. In the lateral view (**c**) the plug can be seen in position.

## 8.5.1 Pathology

The disorder consists of a ventricular septal defect, infundibular and sometimes also valvular pulmonary stenosis and an overriding of the aorta over the ventricular septum. Hypertrophy of the right ventricle is the fourth component of the tetralogy and develops due to equalization of the right and left ventricular pressures.

The degree of hypoplasia of the pulmonary arteries is of importance for satisfactory surgical correction.

## 8.5.2 Clinical manifestations

There is prominent right-to-left shunt-induced cyanosis. Children may relieve symptoms by squatting. Digital clubbing is often found.

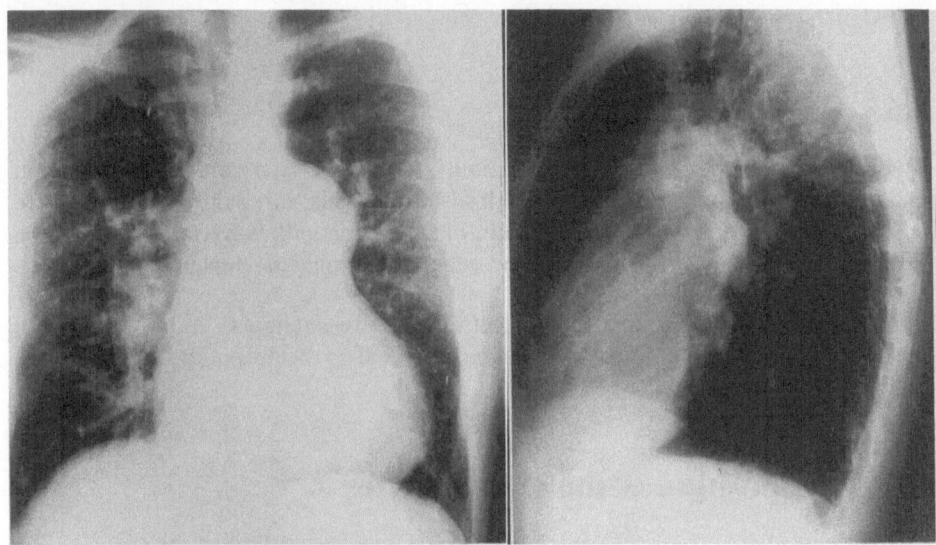

**Fig. 95.** X-ray of an adult with tetralogy of Fallot.

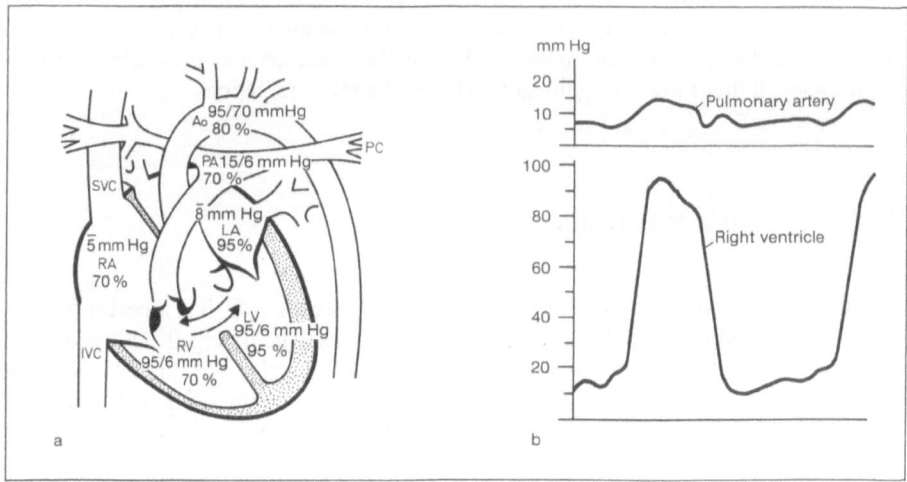

**Fig. 96.** Findings at heart catheterization in Fallot's tetralogy. **a** Pressure equalization in both ventricles, bidirectional shunting at the ventricular level, subpulmonic stenosis. **b** Pressure curves from the pulmonary artery and the left ventricle shows a gradient of 80 mmHg.

Auscultation reveals evidence of pulmonary stenosis and ventricular septal defect. There are signs of severe right-heart hypertrophy on the ECG.

On x-ray cardiac enlargement, especially of the right heart and a paucity of peripheral pulmonary vessel markings is seen. The aortic arch is frequently located on the right side (Fig. 95).

A complete diagnosis is possible by echocardiography, but verification by heart catheterization is usually performed (Fig. 96).

### 8.5.3 Therapy

If possible, a "complete" surgical correction is attempted by closure of the VSD and resection of the infundibular stenosis. If this is not possible, for example, due to severe hypoplasia of the pulmonary vessels, right-heart failure and polycythemia have to be treated symptomatically. For the latter, venesection may be indicated (e.g., if the hemoglobin level exceeds 18 g/dl).

In contrast to isolated ventricular septal defect, Eisenmenger's syndrome does not develop, because the pulmonary vessels are protected by the pulmonary stenosis.

## 8.6 Transposition of the great arteries

Transposition of the great arteries usually occurs in the adult in the "corrected" form. In this form, the aorta originates from the anatomic right ventricle and the pulmonary artery from the anatomic left ventricle. However, systemic venous blood drains from the right atrium into the anatomic left ventricle and thus out the pulmonary artery (hence the term "corrected"). Both ventricles are quite capable of sustaining their reversed ("inverted") roles. Accordingly, corrected transposition of the great arteries may not shorten life expectancy, if there are no significant additional congenital lesions.

## 8.7 Ebstein's anomaly

While tricuspid atresia occurs only in infancy, Ebstein's anomaly has a better prognosis and is seen occasionally in the adult. In Ebstein's disease, the tricuspid valve is displaced from the atrioventricular ring into the right ventricle. An "atrialized" part of the ventricle is thus developed. An intracardiac ECG may be helpful for diagnosis, but today echocardiography is usually diagnostic. Surgical repair of the abnormal valve is often possible.

# 9 Myocardial disease (except myocarditis, see 5.2)

## 9.1 Terminology, etiology, classification

These are diseases of cardiac muscle, the causes of which are largely unknown. In only a few patients can the myocardial lesion be traced back to a known underlying disease. Variations in nomenclature reflect the rapid increase of knowledge in this disease category. For the hypertrophic form of myocardial disease alone there are literally dozens of different terms that have been used.

Instead of cardiomyopathy, the term myocardiopathy might be more appropriate for referring to a degenerative disease of the myocardium, just as to myocarditis as used for inflammatory myocardial disease (not "cardiomyositis").

Classification based on the gross ventricular morphology has been widely accepted. It distinguishes a dilated form from a hypertrophic one (Fig. 97). Dilated cardiomyopathy is associated with ventricular enlargement, whereas hypertrophic cardiomyopathy has myocardial wall thickening especially in the septal area and an increase of cardiac muscle mass with cavity encroachment. Restrictive forms of myocardial disorder are diagnosed when impaired diastolic distensibility is the most prominent feature.

### 9.1.1 Pathology, pathogenesis, pathophysiology

Both the dilated and hypertrophic forms are disorders with an increase in muscle mass. In dilated cardiomyopathy, myocardial hypertrophy is associated with contractile impairment and dilatation, and the ventricular cavity is enlarged, whereas in hypertrophic cardiomyopathy, the contractility is normal or increased and thus, the cavity-encroaching myocardial hypertrophy is associated with a normal or small ventricle. The decrease in cardiac output in this latter disorder is mainly caused by a decrease of inflow into the left ventricle, due to reduced ventricular compliance whereas in the dilated form a decrease in systolic function is responsible. Pathophysiologically dilated cardiomyopathy is associated with a decrease in myocardial contractility, while hypertrophic cardiomyopathy has normal or increased contractility. In the dilated form the dysfunction is mostly systolic, while in the hypertrophic form it is diastolic, except when there is a large intraventricular or outflow gradient.

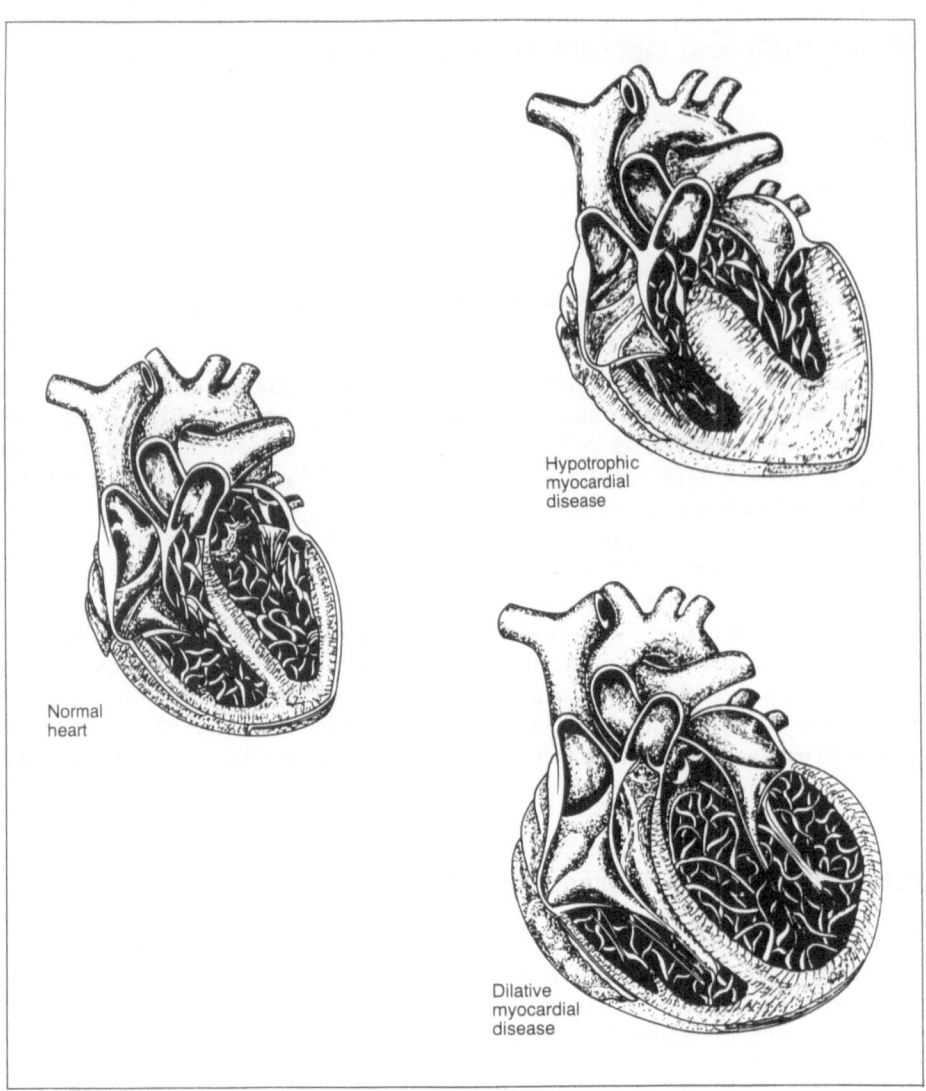

Normal
heart

Hypotrophic
myocardial
disease

Dilative
myocardial
disease

**Fig. 97.** Different forms of cardiomyopathy.

## 9.2 Dilated cardiomyopathy

### 9.2.1 Definition, occurrence

The disorder is characterized by decreased contractility of the myocardial fibers. There is ventricular dilatation and often, an increase in end-diastolic pressure. The ejection fraction is decreased, and the end-systolic volume increased.

The disorder has been more frequently recognized during the last two decades, but it is doubtful whether this represents a true increase in disease incidence. Better diagnosis is probably responsible for the increased frequency, especially because the distinction from coronary artery disease has been improved by coronary arteriography and, with echocardiography, the disease is often diagnosed in an early stage.

## 9.2.2 Pathology, pathogenesis, pathophysiology

The cardiac chambers are dilated and there is a large increase in myocardial mass, documented by an increase in heart weight. The average cardiac fiber diameter increases as a histologic sign of hypertrophy, as does the nuclear volume. There is a loss of myofibrils and electron microscopic studies show degenerative changes in individual cell organelles, especially the mitochondria. Significant fibrosis occurs in approximately one-third of all patients (Fig. 98).

The cause of the disorder is usually unknown. A viral myocarditis etiology has repeatedly been claimed.

In some cases a familial clustering can be documented. If two siblings are affected, the characteristics of the disorder are usually quite similar and they differ only in the severity or the time-course of evolution.

A possible triggering of the disease by alcohol, especially heavy consumption of beer is generally accepted. Some patients show a regression of the disorder and of the cardiac enlargement after abstinence. A causal connection with cardiotoxic substances such as adriamycin has also been recognized.

## 9.2.3 Clinical manifestations

Loss of energy, dyspnea, and edema of the lower limbs are frequent symptoms. The disorder may be first detected on echo or found by chance due to enlargement of the cardiac silhouette on the x-ray. The first symptoms may occur during or after an infection or fever. A causal connection with viral myocarditis is often suspected, but uncommonly proven. Usually it is found, after a careful history, that the symptoms are not new, and that cardiac enlargement existed prior to the infection.

Cardiac arrhythmias occur frequently, predominantly ventricular or supraventricular extrasystoles. Atrial fibrillation is also frequent. All forms of atrioventricular and intraventricular conduction disturbance may occur, as may sustained or nonsustained ventricular tachycardia.

When the disease is advanced, physical examination shows signs of right- or left-heart failure. On auscultation a third heart sound or a murmur of mitral insufficiency is found.

In addition to arrhythmia, the ECG shows different forms of conduction disturbances, sometimes even suggesting myocardial infarction. Left bundle branch block is the most typical abnormality. Signs of left ventricular hypertrophy are frequent.

A characteristic enlargement of the cardiac chambers is found on the echocardiogram, where the left ventricle is the chamber most enlarged and it has markedly impaired contraction.

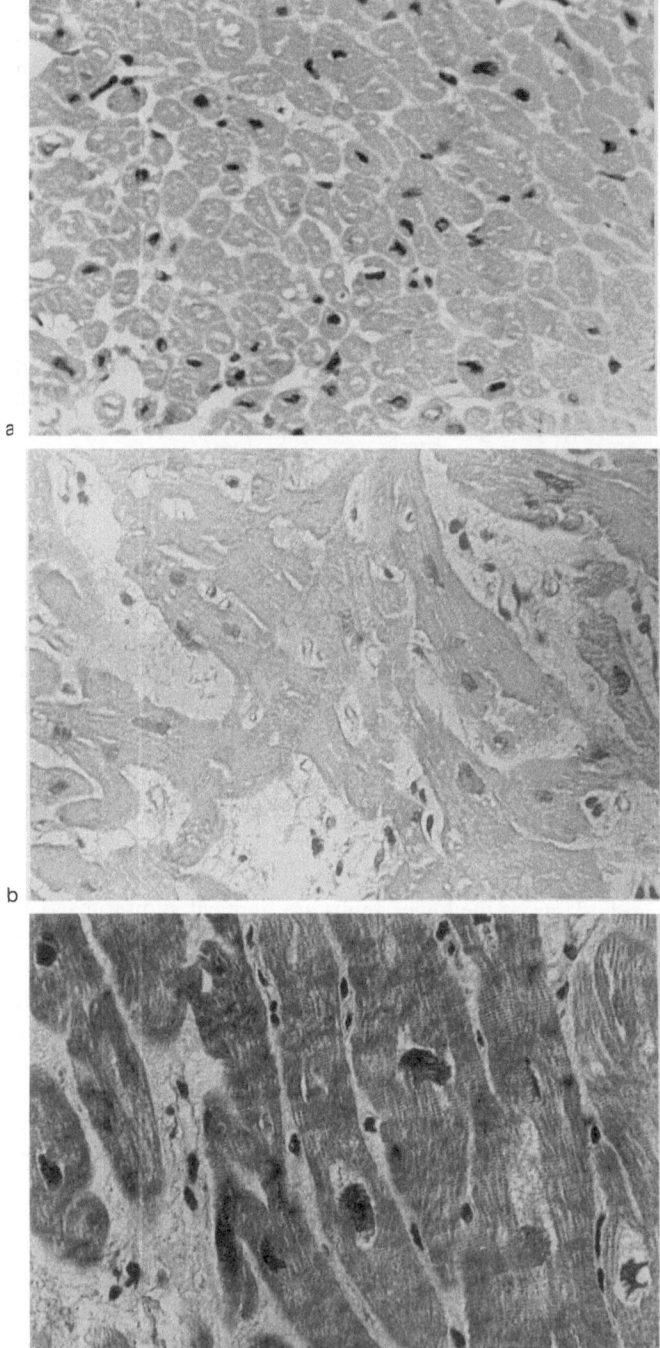

a

b

c

**Fig. 98.** Myocardial biopsies from the left ventricle. **a** normal myocardium; **b** fiber disarray in hypertrophic cardiomyopathy; **c** cellular hypertrophy and interstitial fibrosis in dilated myocardiopathy (histologic preparation by the Senckenbergisches Pathologisches Institut der Universität Frankfurt).

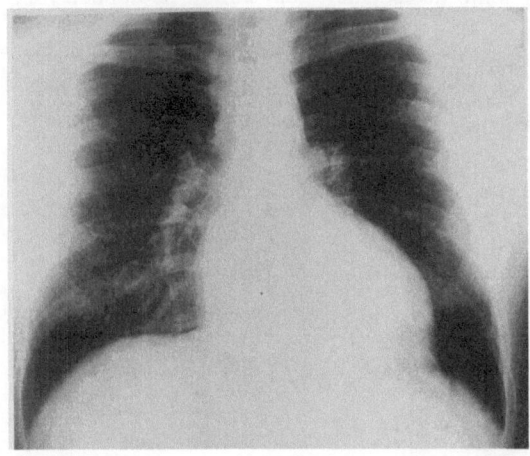

**Fig. 99.** Moderate cardiac enlargement in dilated cardiomyopathy.

Cardiac enlargement occurs early on the x-ray. The cardiac silhouette differs from the normal and approaches a ball shape (Fig. 99). The cardiac volume is greatly increased. In early cases, determination of the cardiac volume commonly allows distinction from other disorders.

With radionuclide imaging methods, a reduced ejection fraction and an enlarged ventricular volume are seen.

Coronary artery disease has to be ruled out, as this may also lead to global and regional contractile disturbances.

The degree of elevation in filling pressure is determined by right- and left-heart catheterization, but even in advanced phases of the disorder there may be only slight or no elevation in filling pressure. The ruling out of coronary artery disease is important. Even after careful noninvasive diagnostic evaluation, one may be surprised to find coronary artery disease as the culprit. But the reverse also occurs where depressed ST-segments during exercise or Q-waves were thought to be caused by coronary artery disease, but catheterization reveals dilated cardiomyopathy.

At the time of heart catheterization biopsies of the left or right ventricle may be obtained. They will provide further clues to the degree of destruction of contractile myocardial tissue, the degree of cellular hypertrophy, of subcellular degeneration and the occurrence of fibrosis (see Fig. 98). Rarely, a florid myocarditis can be documented. Endocardial fibrosis, amyloidosis, hemochromatosis, sarcoidosis, and other disorders can also be ruled out or recognized.

### 9.2.4 Therapy

Therapy for idiopathic dilated cardiomyopathy is palliative; usually, digitalis is indicated. Impulse formation or conduction disturbances occasionally necessitate the implantation of a pacemaker. With gross ventricular dilatation and reduced ejection fraction, thrombosis prophylaxis with oral anticoagulants is appropriate. Therapy with vaso-dilators, especially ACE inhibitors, has been found beneficial. Calcium antagonists may possibly help. β-blockers are used by some investigators, but should be applied very cautiously, if at all.

There are marked differences in clinical progression. Usually there is slow progression, or a standstill, but, occasionally, improvement may occur. Early phases are more likely to be stationary. In patients with severe heart failure, heart transplantation may be indicated (Fig. 100).

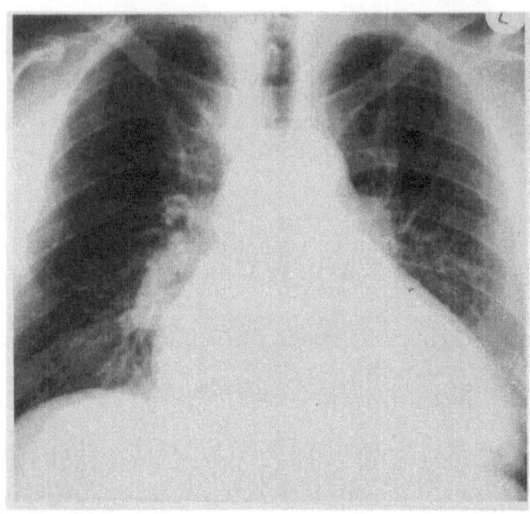

a

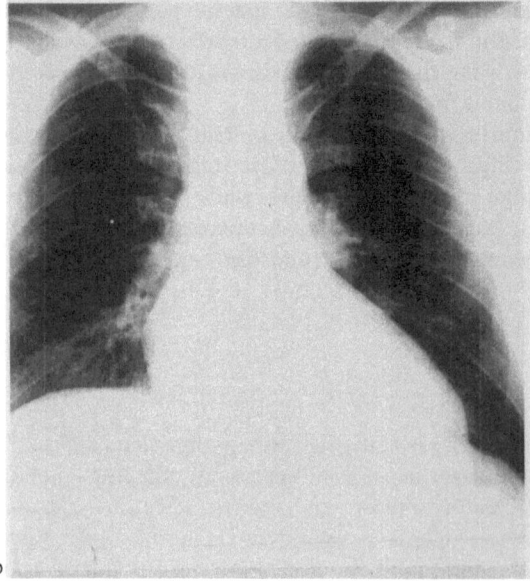

b

**Fig. 100. a** Severe cardiac enlargement with dilated cardiomyopathy in a 44-year-old male with New York Heart Association Class-IV failure; **b** normal heart silhouette after cardiac transplantation.

## 9.3 Hypertrophic form of myocardial disease – Hypertrophic cardiomyopathy

### 9.3.1 Definition

The disorder is characterized by normal or increased contractility of the myocardial fibers and concentric hypertrophy with reduction of the left ventricular cavity. The increase in myocardial mass in the septal area and outflow tract, and the hypercontractility as well, may lead to intraventricular obstruction (obstructive form). The non-obstructive form is of equal clinical importance as the obstructive one.

### 9.3.2 Occurrence, pathology, pathogenesis

The disease was first described at the beginning of this century, but has only been diagnosed clinically since the 1950s. Since the introduction of echocardiography the frequency of the diagnosis has increased rapidly, although there has probably been no real increase in frequency. The disorder occurs sporadically, but there clearly is, in some cases, a familial clustering. Some families seem to suffer from a specially severe form. Examination of relatives may also reveal asymptomatic forms and minor manifestations of the disease.

An increase in thickness of the ventricular septum is prominent. The remainder (free wall) of the left ventricle is usually also hypertrophied, but to a lesser degree. In a small number of patients the right ventricle is affected as well.

Often the cardiac valves themselves are not affected, but the mitral leaflets may be thickened and complete closure of the mitral valve is often limited by a thickening of the myocardium in the septal area, resulting in mitral insufficiency.

There are muscular regions, especially in the septum, where the direction of the fibers is irregular and overlapping. Similar changes have also been seen in left ventricular hypertrophy due to other diseases such as hypertension or aortic stenosis; the degree of myocardial fiber disarray is however especially severe in hypertrophic cardiomyopathy. The median diameter of myocardial fibers is increased in some patients; in others it is normal. In some cases the increase in cardiac muscle mass is due to an increased number of fibers (hyperplasia) while in others thickening of the fibers (hypertrophy) alone may account for the increased mass.

Myocardial fibrosis may be marked, especially in advanced cases, but it may also not be present.

The pathogenesis of this disorder is unknown, but it is probably genetically determined. There are various hypotheses. A disorder of the sympathetic nervous system was once suspected and a hormonal factor (nerve growth factor) was implicated. Such an explanation might also explain why the disease is sometimes associated with neurofibromatosis (von Recklinghausen's disease). A conduction disturbance of the ventricle was once proposed with initial excitation at the base instead of at the cardiac apex and consequent treatment with pacemaker electrodes located at the ventricular apex. Newer findings focus on increased calcium activity of the myocardial cell, possibly due to an increase in calcium channels.

There has been no convincing evidence for any of these theories. According to current knowledge, all we can say is that there is a genetic predisposition, whereby the manifestations may occur during infancy or in early adult life.

### 9.3.3 Pathophysiology

The increased contractility of the myocardial fibers leads to a rapid increase of ventricular pressure and an increase in velocity of blood ejection from the left ventricle. The first phase of ventricular emptying is not disturbed in the obstructive form of the disease, but later during ventricular systole, an increasing stenosis of the outflow tract develops, such that the later phases of ventricular emptying are impeded. Intraventricular pressure gradients over 100 mmHg may develop. Despite normal or hypernormal contractility of the ventricular muscle, the stroke volume and cardiac output may be reduced. Whereas formerly the disturbance of ejection was considered the primary and sufficient cause of the functional disturbance, it is today recognized that there is also disturbed diastolic filling of the left ventricle. The ability of the ventricular muscles to stretch and relax is impaired leading to a marked rise in left ventricular filling pressure with secondary hypertrophy and dilatation of the left atrium.

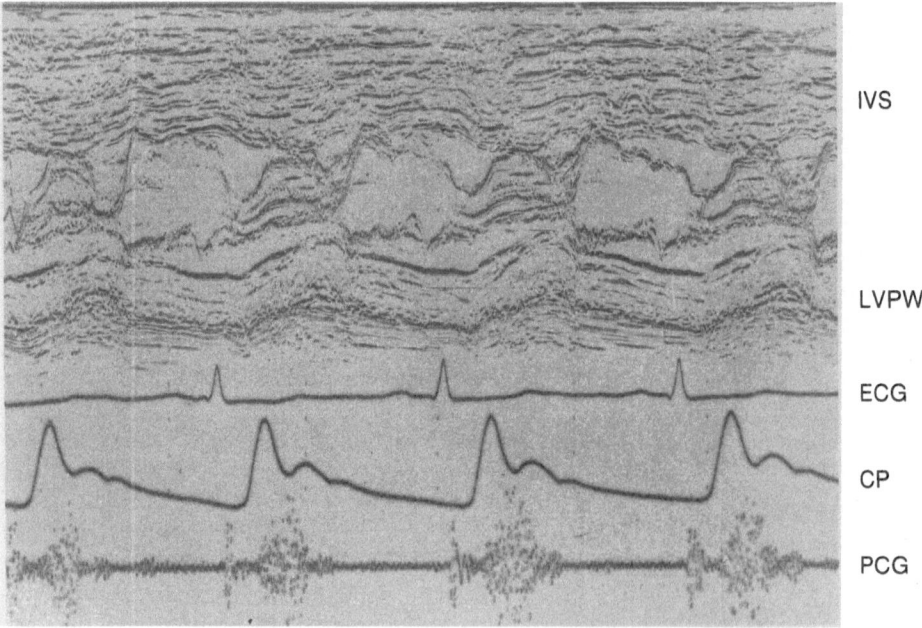

**Fig. 101.** Hypertrophic obstructive cardiomyopathy. Echocardiographic thickening of the septum and a decreased ventricular cavity size. Systolic anterior motion of the anterior mitral leaflet at the time of the second peak in the carotid pulse curve and the systolic murmur (modified after [3]). (*IVS* septum; *LVPW* posterior wall of the left ventricle; *CP* carotid pulse; *PCG* phonocardiogram)

The role of the intraventricular systolic pressure gradient has been debated in the 1980s. Is the gradient the cause or a consequence of the disorder? Doppler echocardiographic findings indicate that the increased contractility leads to an increased outflow blood flow velocity and consequent suction of the anterior mitral leaflet onto the septum. This systolic anterior movement of the mitral leaflet towards the septum leads to impeded outflow in the second half of systole. Septal hypertrophy further narrows the left ventricular outflow tract exacerbating the high outflow blood velocity induced during contraction.

### 9.3.4 Clinical course

This serious disorder has a mortality of 3–5% per year. It is usually diagnosed during infancy and early adulthood. Unexpected sudden death of apparently healthy people is often caused by this disease. Sudden cardiac death in athletes is also not infrequently caused by undiagnosed hypertrophic cardiomyopathy. Ventricular fibrillation is the usual mechanism, but deaths may also be due to profound hypotension due to poor left-ventricular filling and left-ventricular outflow obstruction. Hypotension might be precipitated by peripheral vascular dysregulation. On the other hand, there are also less severe forms which remain asymptomatic for many years. A correlation between the size and presence of the pressure gradient and mortality is not clear for this disease, in contrast to valvular aortic stenosis. Atrial fibrillation can lead to acute failure due to reduced ventricular filling when atrial contraction is lost.

### 9.3.5 Clinical manifestations

The most common complaints are dyspnea, arrhythmias, angina pectoris, dizziness and/or syncope.

Auscultation reveals a systolic murmur over the second intercostal space. It is maximal in late systole in the obstructive form. The murmur may also be heard over the aorta and may radiate into the carotids. Concomitant mitral insufficiency is likely when a systolic murmur over the apex radiates into the axilla.

A double peak of the arterial pulse wave (bisferiens pulse) is often found in the obstructive form. In the carotid pulse curve, this is seen as a second peak before the dicrotic notch.

An increase in ventricular free wall thickness and of the septum is characteristically found on the echocardiogram (Fig. 101). The ratio of septal thickness to the thickness of the free wall is above normal and > 1.3:1.

In patients with the obstructive form, abnormal forward movement of the anterior mitral leaflet is seen during systole, leading to constriction of the outflow tract. In the right ventricle an increase in thickness of the free wall can sometimes be seen.

The diagnosis is usually established noninvasively and verified invasively (Fig. 102). Concomitant coronary artery disease may be excluded or verified by coronary angiography in patients with symptoms of angina pectoris.

A disturbance in muscle structure is recognized by myocardial biopsy, but the findings are nonspecific. Hypertrophy with increase of the mean myocardial cell diameter is

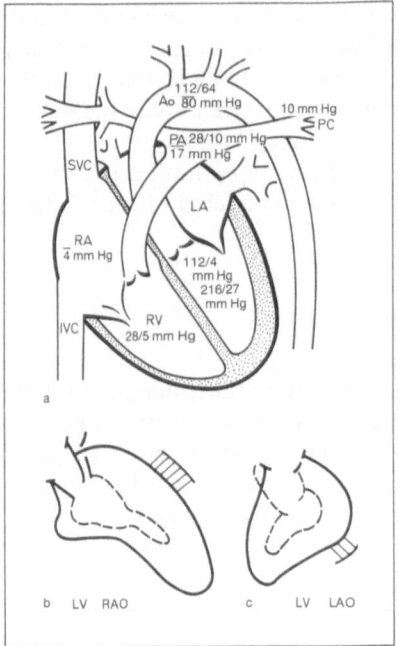

**Fig. 102.** Findings at heart catheterization in hypertrophic cardiomyopathy. During Valsalva maneuver a systolic pressure gradient of 104 mmHg (216 minus 112) is recorded across the left ventricular outflow tract. **a** Decreased systolic volume on the ventriculogram; **b** a "banana-shaped" bend in the left ventricular cavity shape (**c**).

found in a number of patients, while in others, fibrosis may be a striking feature. The nonobstructive form may be mimicked by Fabry's disease, a genetic disorder of lipid-storage which causes myocardial abnormalities readily recognized by biopsy.

### 9.3.6 Therapy

Positive inotropic agents such as catecholamines and digitalis are contraindicated and may lead to acute deterioration. Vasodilators, especially nitroglycerin, may aggravate the symptoms and signs, because venous dilatation leads to reduced ventricular filling and exacerbation of the outflow obstruction (Fig. 103). Treatment with β-receptor blockers was based upon the concept of an adrenergic-mediated hypercontractility, but the long-term results of this therapy on mortality are disappointing.

In comparison, the effects of high-dose calcium antagonist therapy with verapamil may be more favorable. The agent reduces outflow obstruction and increases diastolic ventricular filling. The patient's complaints diminish and physical exercise capacity increases. The mortality in a 10-year study at Frankfurt University Hospital was only 1.5% in contrast to 3–5% with long-term follow-up of other types of therapies (Fig. 104).

Disopyramide has been suggested as another alternative. It decreases the gradient, however, at least partially, by increasing peripheral resistance. Surgical correction with septal myectomy may be performed in resistant patients suffering from the obstructive form. This usually leads to substantial clinical improvement.

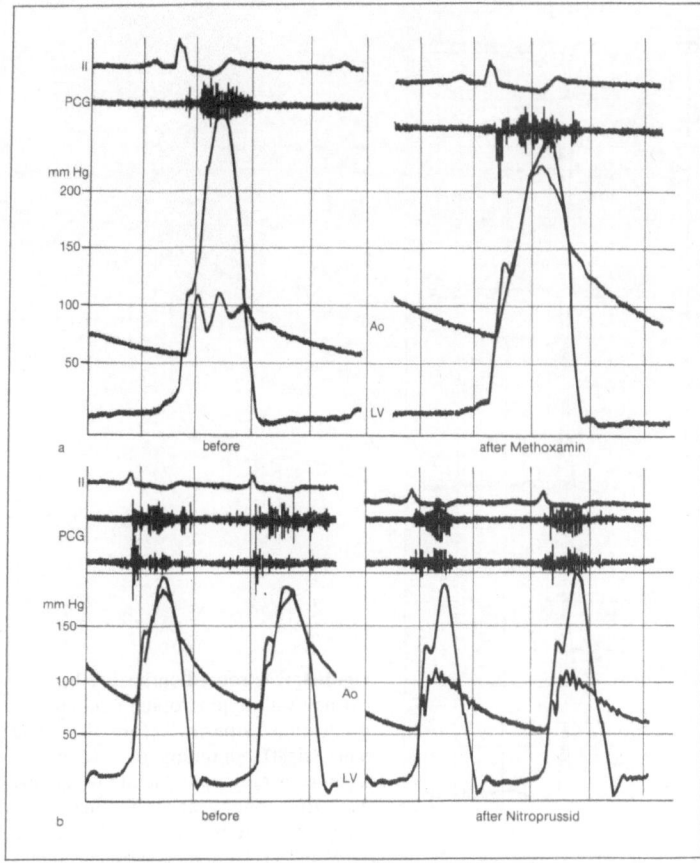

**Fig. 103. a)** Decrease in pressure gradient with the vasoconstrictor methoxamine, and **b)** reappearance with the vasodilator nitroprusside (after [3]).

## 9.4 Restrictive cardiomyopathies

Impaired diastolic ventricular filling is prominent, but in contrast to the hypertrophic form, this is not caused by myocardial hypertrophy and is also not associated with hypercontractility. The ventricular chambers are reduced, normal or enlarged, and the systolic function is normal at least during the early phase. A storage disease may be the underlying cause, namely, amyloidosis or hemochromatosis. Similar abnormalities can be found in Fabry's disease and in hypertrophic nonobstructive cardiomyopathy. Endocardial fibrosis or eosinophilic myocarditis may also cause a restrictive pattern, as can sarcoidosis or lymphogranulomatosis.

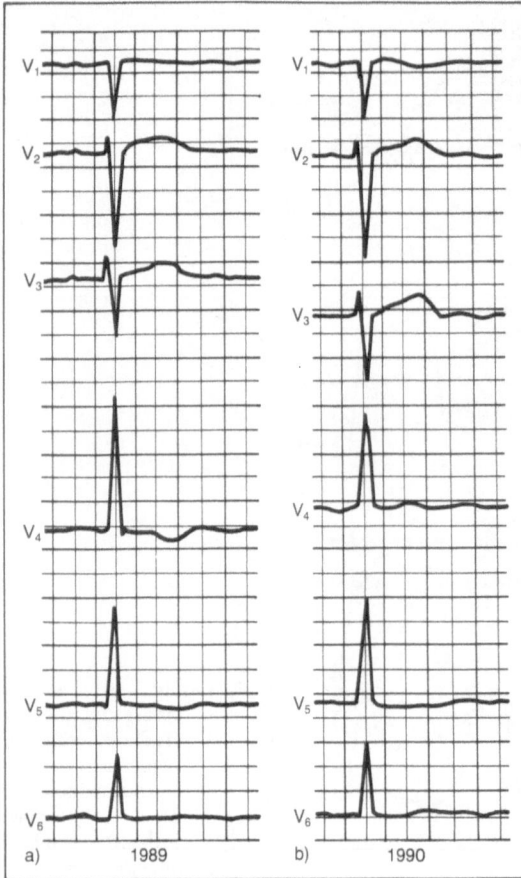

a) 1989    b) 1990

**Fig. 104.** Electrocardiogram of a 14-year-old boy with hypertrophic non-obstructive cardiomyopathy before (left) and after (right) beginning of calcium antagonist therapy with 280 mg verapamil/day. After one year of treatment the QRS-amplitude has decreased from 5 to 4 mV and ST-T-changes show a tendency toward normalization.

# 10 Systemic and pulmonary hypertension

## 10.1 Systemic hypertension

### 10.1.1 Definition of high blood pressure

A value of 140/85 mmHg is accepted as the upper limit of a normal blood pressure. Systolic or diastolic values just above this are borderline; values from 150/90 onward are definitely elevated. Only repeated measurements may help in deciding whether there is sustained hypertension or whether there is intermittent ("labile") hypertensive episodes, or stress-related hypertension ("white-coat hypertension"). With physical exercise and mental stress, there may be substantial pressure increases up to systolic values of 300 mmHg. Just as with a measurement at rest, a single measurement of blood pressure on exertion is not enough. Reliable diagnostic information is however provided by 24 hours ambulatory monitoring. Chronic observations have shown that patients with borderline hypertension and elevated arterial pressure with exercise often develop persistent hypertension. However, also complete normalization over time is not uncommon.

It is important to know that patients with borderline hypertension or labile hypertension are also at an increased risk of developing coronary artery disease. Curiously, the risk is not apparently caused directly by high blood pressure and is independent of its degree of elevation. Recent studies suggest that another associated abnormality in hypertensives, namely hyperinsulinemia and insulin-resistance, may be another genetically determined marker for coronary artery disease. Chronic elevation of blood pressure leads to cardiac hypertrophy and damage to other organs; these changes do show a positive correlation with the degree of hypertension. Besides the heart, the kidneys, the brain, and the retina are affected.

### 10.1.2 Pathogenesis

A familial predisposition exists for essential hypertension. Several pathogenetic mechanisms have been suggested such as increased sensitivity to salt in the diet, altered hormonal release, and abnormal baroreceptor control of resistance vessels, but no satisfactory mechanism has yet been defined. There is little doubt about the unfavorable and additive effect of obesity, alcohol intake, psychosomatic factors, and increased salt (sodium chloride) intake.

### 10.1.3 Manifestations of blood pressure elevation

Predominant systolic blood pressure elevation can be distinguished from that with both elevated systolic and diastolic values or simply high diastolic readings.

Renal hypertension due to parenchymatous renal disease is usually associated with diastolic blood pressure elevation. The same holds true for renovascular hypertension. Both forms are caused by an increased renin effect.

Blood-pressure elevation associated with hyperthyroidism and fever is characterized by a large pulse pressure and tachycardia with isolated systolic hypertension. Similarly, stroke volume hypertension also causes systolic pressure elevation; it can be regarded as a physiological adaptation to bradycardia (e.g., in complete heart block). The elevation of the blood pressure seen with aortic insufficiency usually has elevated systolic, but substantially decreased diastolic, values.

There is a loss of elasticity of the aorta and the large arteries with increasing age. This lack of vessel compliance leads to elevation of the systolic pressure with usually little change in diastolic pressure.

### 10.1.4 Clinical manifestations

Symptoms such as headache and tiredness may occur, but they are not very characteristic. A pale hypertensive patient, characteristic of high systemic resistance hypertension (e.g., associated with renal disease) can be distinguished from the "red" hypertensive patient, as seen with increased blood volume, plethora, and obesity. However, such clear distinctions are unusual.

Blood-pressure measurement has to be performed carefully, using the guidelines listed in section 2.2.3. When elevated values are found in one arm, measurements should be taken in the other arm. If the leg pulses are diminished, the measurements should also be performed in the lower limbs. The aortic component of the second heart sound (aortic valve closure sound) is often increased. An accentuated second heart sound with auscultation above the second right intercostal space compared to the left side may suggest that the ascending aorta is also enlarged. 24-h recordings can be very helpful in the diagnostic and therapeutic evaluations of patients with hypertension. The ECG and echo demonstrate the degree of left ventricular hypertrophy. Evaluation of the ocular fundi is part of the investigation.

### 10.1.5 Therapeutic principles, general measures

In secondary hypertension, one should try to treat the cause. This is possible, for example, in aortic coarctation or renovascular hypertension; dilatation of stenosed renal arteries can often be achieved with a balloon catheter. Adrenalin producing tumors may be removed, hyperthyreoidism treated.

After a diagnostic evaluation the need for chronic therapy has to be discussed with the patient. The patient is usually instructed in the technique of performing blood-pressure measurements. A double stethoscope with two pairs of ear pieces is suitable for instruction. Patients should keep a record of their blood pressure and also of their body weight. Their general lifestyle should include ample sleep and regular exercise. A reduction in sodium chloride intake is generally recommended, but a very strict low salt diet only makes sense for some patients.

### 10.1.5.1 Drug therapy

There are many classes of drugs that can be used today. If possible, the most effective agent with the least side-effects is chosen. The coexistence of other problems such as coronary artery disease, pulmonary and renal disease has to be taken into account.

#### 10.1.5.1.1 Calcium antagonists (Fig. 105)

Dihydropyridines (nifedipine-like) have their primary effect on the smooth muscle of peripheral arteries. Others (verapamil, diltiazem) have both cardiac and peripheral effects. Nifedipine is preferable in patients with bradycardia, while verapamil would be better in those with tachycardia. Adverse effects include edema formation (nifedipine and verapamil), flushing (nifedipine), and constipation (verapamil). Patients with rhythm disturbances of supraventricular origin and anginal complaints usually benefit from verapamil. Verapamil should be applied in doses of 240–480 mg daily. For gallopamil (not available in the USA), which has more or less the same effect as verapamil, a dose of 100–200 mg is equivalent; constipation is a less frequent side-effect. Nifedipine is usually given in a dose of 30 mg daily.

#### 10.1.5.1.2 β-receptor blocking agents

The antihypertensive effect is usually seen only after 1 or 2 weeks of treatment. However, patients with β-adrenergic stimulation respond more rapidly. Agents with partial agonist effect (e.g., pindolol) will induce less bradycardia than those with a pure β-blocking effect (e.g., propranolol).

Adverse effects include lethargy, depression, nightmares, muscular fatigue, and impotence. AV-conduction disturbances may be aggravated or induced; severe brady-cardia, AV-block, and sinus arrest may occur. Bronchial obstruction may worsen in patients with preexisting airway disease. Usually, angina pectoris is reduced, but there are patients with an angiospastic component, who react to β-blockade with an increase in angina pectoris.

#### 10.1.5.1.3 α-blocking agents, peripheral vasodilators

α-blocking agents such as prazosin, and vasodilators such as hydralazine are effective in that they decrease peripheral resistance. Agents of the labetolol type have both α- and β-blocking activities.

#### 10.1.5.1.4 Clonidine and methyldopa

These agents act centrally via α-2-receptor stimulation, to reduce sympathetic nerve traffic. The lessened catecholamine release induces a decrease in blood pressure and bradycardia.

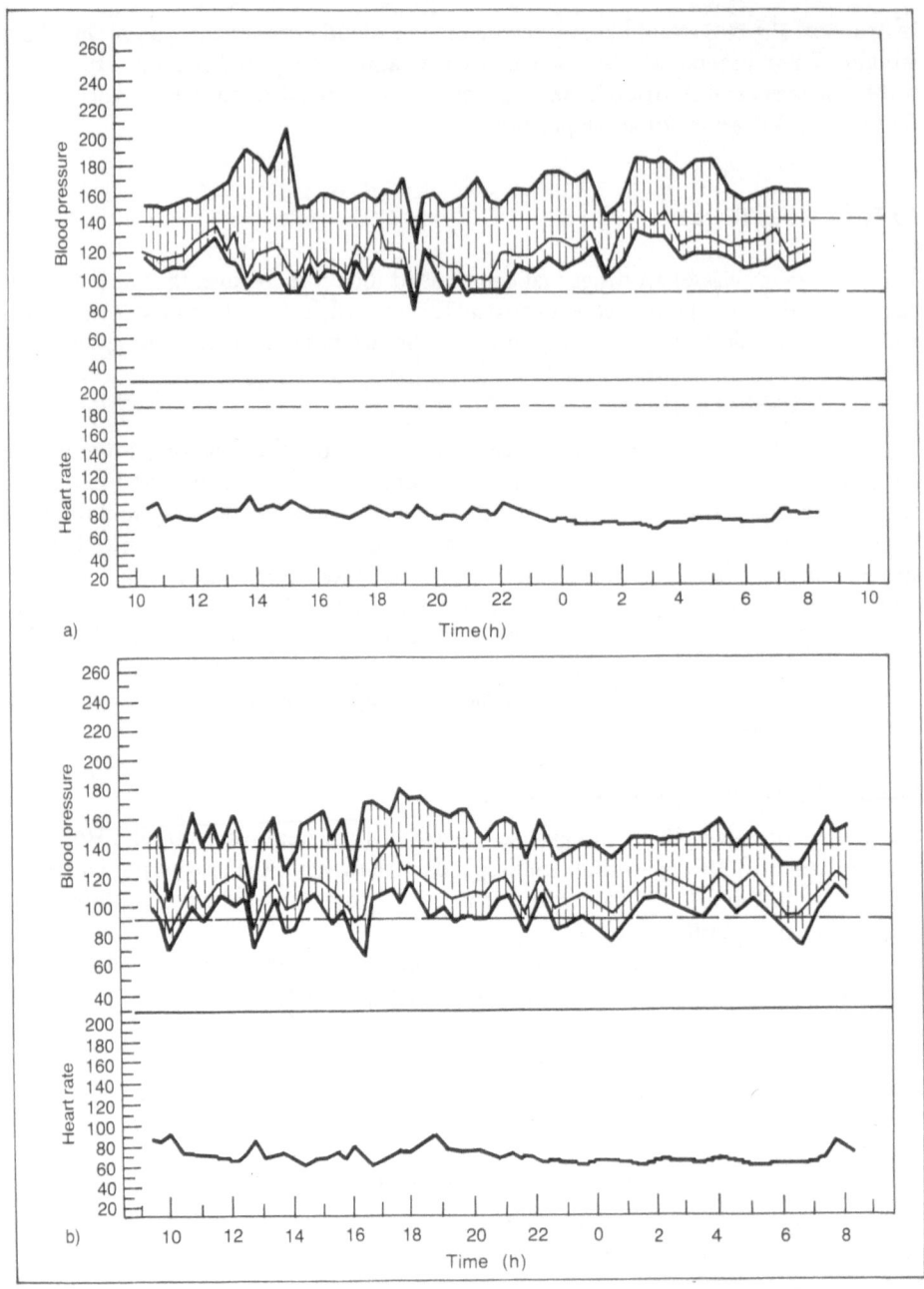

**Fig. 105.** Ambulatory 24-h blood pressure recordings (Spacelabs) of a 52-year-old man with essential hypertension. **a** Before therapy marked elevation of systolic and diastolic pressure, particularly during sleeping hours. **b** After initiation of therapy with calcium blockers there is marked improvement.

#### 10.1.5.1.5 Angiotensin converting-enzyme (ACE) inhibitors

Their effect is most prominent if an overactive renin-angiotensin mechanism is responsible for the hypertension. Inhibition of this mechanism is only rarely risky, but may cause problems if critical renal artery stenosis already exists and renal hypoperfusion results from the marked reduction in blood pressure.

#### 10.1.5.1.6 Diuretics

The use of diuretics as first-line agents does not seem warranted today, because of adverse effects such as aggravation of or, diabetogenic effect, and an adverse effect on lipid metabolism. But diuretics may have to be used if there is fluid retention, or if blood-pressure reduction has not been sufficient with other medications. A major advantage of these agents is their low cost.

### 10.1.5.2 Management of hypertensive crisis

Marked blood-pressure elevation often occurs in connection with emotional and other stress, e.g., high salt intake or antihypertensive drug withdrawal. A rapid, but not abrupt blood-pressure decrease may be achieved using nitroglycerin. The blood pressure can be reduced without the risk of collapse if one starts with a small sublingual dose. Repeat sublingual application at 10-min intervals, later, 20–30-min intervals, leads to good regulation. In difficult situations, the titration may be performed by intravenous infusion. Nifedipine or nitroprusside may be used in a similar manner.

# 10.2 Pulmonary hypertension

## 10.2.1 Etiology, clinical course

Primary pulmonary hypertension may manifest itself during infancy or youth, but in most cases becomes apparent in early adulthood. In Europe an epidemic of acquired forms occurred after use of amphetamine appetite suppressants. Symptomatic pulmonary hypertension often occurs secondary to ventricular septal defect. Diseases of the left heart such as mitral or aortic valve disease may also lead to pulmonary hypertension by way of pulmonary venous hypertension. A frequent cause in the adult is pulmonary embolism, often due to multiple small emboli which have not been noticed by the patient.

In some patients pulmonary hypertension proceeds from a phase of labile, reversible hypertension to a phase with fixed irreversible hypertension. Pulmonary arteriolar resistance vessels of the lung show a gradual increase in wall thickness due to the hypertensive effect, and later show irreversible proliferative changes (plexiform lesions) which obliterate the vessel lumen.

## 10.2.2 Clinical manifestations

A prominent second heart sound is characteristic during auscultation over the pulmonary valve. There is wide, fixed splitting of the second heart sound, as can also be found with other causes of right heart strain. Advanced pulmonary hypertension leads to cyanosis, frequently accompanied by polycythemia. Drumstick ("clubbed") fingers and "watch-glass" nails may appear. Right-heart failure may develop in the severe forms.

The ECG shows right-ventricular hypertrophy, and the echocardiogram shows hypertrophy and dilatation of the right ventricle. Continuous-wave Doppler measurements confirm the pulmonary hypertension.

The central pulmonary vessels are enlarged on the x-ray, but the peripheral pulmonary vessels are of normal width or narrow. A prominent drop in luminal size can be seen ("amputation of the hilar vessels").

## 10.2.3 Treatment

Symptomatic pulmonary hypertension is best treated by therapy of the causative disease. Even when pulmonary systolic pressures exceed 100 mmHg they will usually return normal after surgical correction of aortic or mitral valve disease.

Drug therapy is used for primary pulmonary hypertension, if the causal factor is untreatable, and advanced secondary pulmonary hypertension (Eisenmenger's syndrome). Unfortunately, drugs are rarely of much help. It is recommended that any drugs employed be initiated during right-heart catheterization to determine if there is a pulmonary pressure decrease and whether the drug has detrimental hemodynamic effects on the systemic circulation. Vasodilators such as nitroglycerin, calcium antagonists, and α-blockers may be tried. In patients with secondary polycythemia, phlebotomy may lead to symptomatic improvement. Anticoagulation, and occasionally embolectomy surgery is indicated when recurrent pulmonary embolism is the cause of pulmonary hypertension. At an advanced stage, chronic oxygen therapy may be symptomatically helpful. Heart-lung transplantation is increasingly being applied when all else fails.

# 11  Disorders of circulatory regulation

## 11.1  Hyperkinetic and hypertensive regulatory disorders

### 11.1.1  Definition

The hyperkinetic heart syndrome is characterized by tachycardia and by an increased cardiac output with a decreased arteriovenous oxygen difference. It is often associated with a tendency for an elevated blood pressure. It is characterized by an excess increase in exercise heart rate for the corresponding workload (Fig. 106).

### 11.1.2  Occurrence

The hyperkinetic heart syndrome is not uncommon. It occurs more often in females, and it is often associated with symptoms of anxiety, neurasthenia, or other psychological symptoms.

### 11.1.3  Pathogenesis

The symptoms reflect increase β-adrenergic activity. A decrease in vagal activity may also play a role. Most authors focus on an increased responsiveness of the cardiac β-1-adrenergic receptors. However, as research has found no evidence for cardiac hyper-responsiveness, nor a decreased vagal activity a central nervous system dysfunction has to be considered.

### 11.1.4  Clinical manifestations

Lack of energy and exercise-induced tachycardia are characteristic symptoms. There may be frequent palpitations. Sudden attacks of anxiety, restlessness, and cardiac arrhythmias are common. The symptoms are similar to those which appear with infusion of β-adrenergic agents.

Tachycardia may be present at rest, but usually the heart rate is only increased during and after exercise. The blood pressure is often mildly increased; with auscultation, a systolic murmur at the cardiac base may be heard.

Exercise testing provides diagnostic information. One finds an overshoot in heart rate, which is easily recognized if one compares the heart rate with normal values for a corresponding age, sex, workload, and body surface area (see Fig. 106).

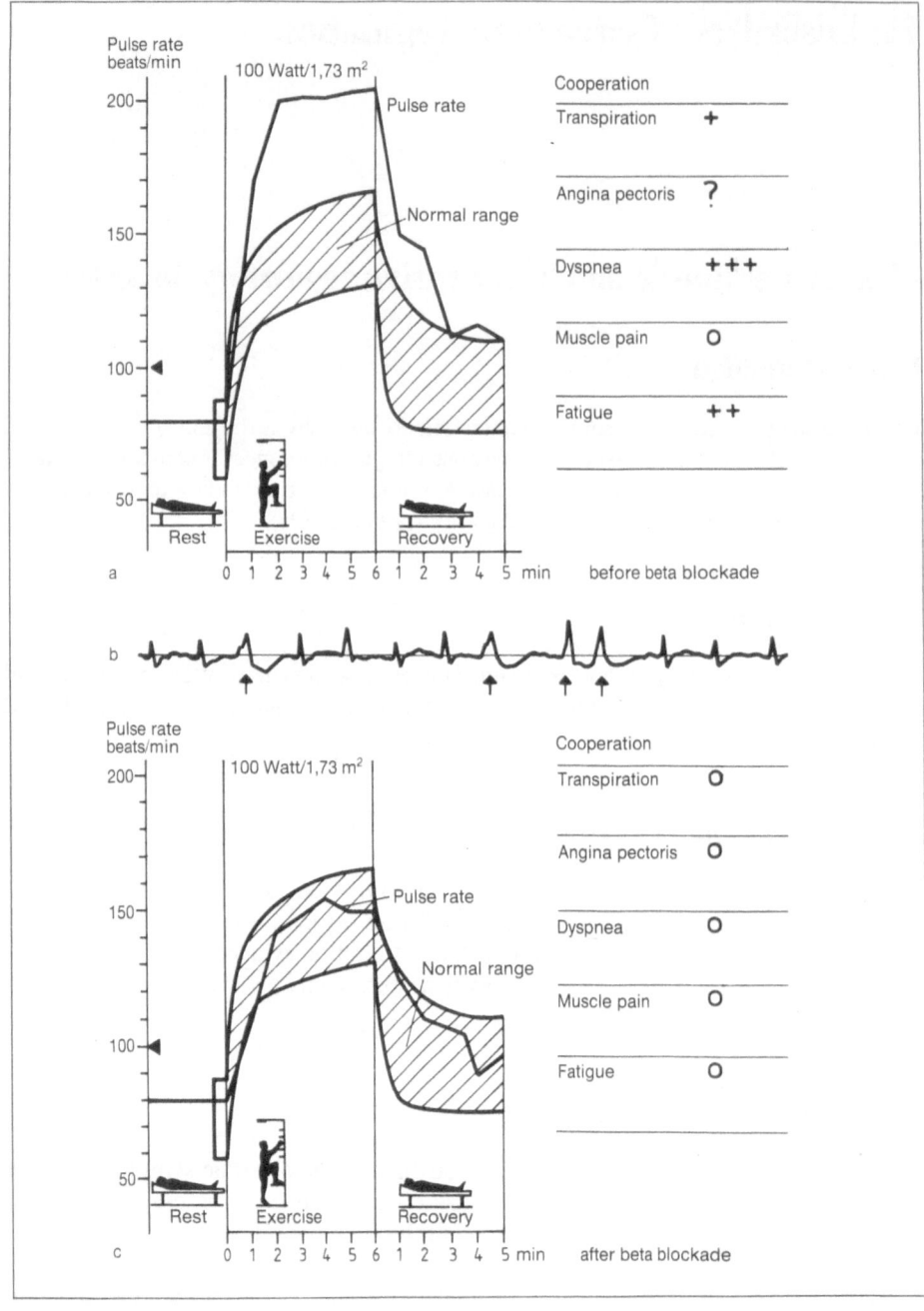

**Fig. 106. a** Exaggerated increase in heart rate during exercise and slow return to normal after exercise in a 28-year-old female with hyperkinetic heart syndrome. **b** Multiple ventricular extrasystoles recorded on the ECG during exercise. **c** Normalization of heart rate response after administration of a β-blocker (40 mg propranolol orally). With β-blockade extrasystoles disappeared, fatigue and dyspnea were considerably less (see right side of protocol; see also next figure).

When other possibilities such as hyperthyroidism, inflammatory disorder and systemic disease have been ruled out, the diagnosis may be verified by right-heart catheterization. However, this is rarely justified. There will be normal to upper-normal pressures in the pulmonary artery. The mixed venous oxygen saturation in the pulmonary artery is elevated, and the arteriovenous oxygen difference decreased. The cardiac output is elevated at rest and on exertion (Fig. 107).

The increased muscle blood flow with decreased oxygen extraction can be verified by venous occlusion plethysmography which enables quantitative measurement of the blood flow in the extremities (Fig. 108).

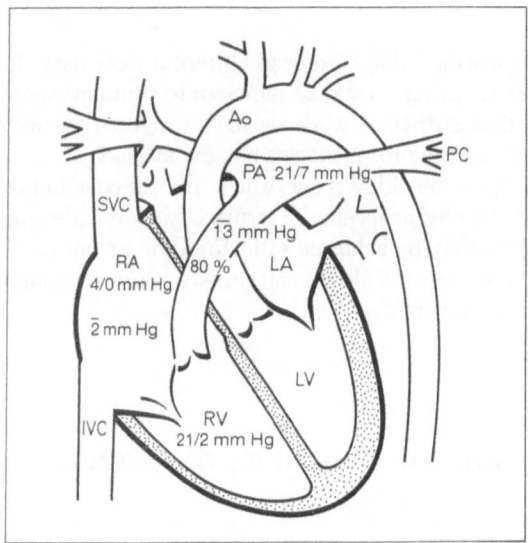

**Fig. 107.** Findings at right-heart catheterization in a 28-year-old woman with hyperkinetic heart syndrome. The oxygen saturation in the pulmonary artery (PA) is elevated to 80% due to an increased cardiac output; pressure measurements are normal. After administration of the β-receptor blocker pindolol the PA saturation and cardiac output returned to normal.

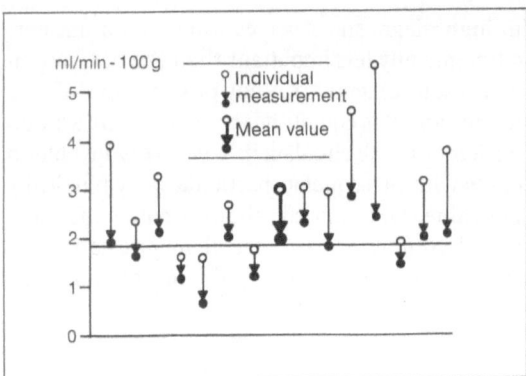

**Fig. 108.** Muscle blood flow in the leg in 14 patients with hyperkinetic heart syndrome. Most values are clearly above normal. After β-blockade by propranolol there is a tendency for normalization of individual measurements and the mean value. The horizontal line represents the mean normal value of 1.85 ml/min × 100 g muscle.

### 11.1.5 Differential diagnosis, prognosis

Distinguishing this disorder from physical deconditioning can be difficult, especially if the syndrome occurs for the first time after a period of bedrest. Usually, careful history-taking will reveal long-standing symptoms in the hyperkinetic heart syndrome. Where symptoms are due to a lack of exercise, it will show that physical exercise capacity was normal before the onset of symptoms. The hyperkinetic heart syndrome will remain for years, often for life, while a deconditioning-effect will completely resolve within a few weeks. The prognosis is good even if the disorder persists over many years.

### 11.1.6 Therapy

Prior to therapy the patient has to be informed that chronic treatment is necessary. In mild cases, an individually adapted exercise program may be sufficient to stimulate vagal activity and to curb tachycardia, so that sufficient work capacity can be regained. Psychotherapy may also be helpful, for example for managing anxiety attacks.

Drug therapy is primarily with β-receptor blocking agents which are effective in low doses. Normalization of exercise-induced tachycardia may be verified by exercise testing (Fig. 106). Comparably beneficial effects may be achieved with clonidine or one of its derivatives (amilidin – not available in the USA). Calcium antagonists of the verapamil type may also reduce exercise-induced tachycardia.

## 11.2 Hypodynamic and hypotonic circulatory disorders, hypotension

### 11.2.1 Definition

These are quite frequent problems, although diagnostic classification is often unclear. The decrease in blood pressure is hemodynamically less important than the decrease in cardiac output in relation to physiological requirements. It is not possible to define a precise lower limit of normal blood pressure, and it is equally not possible to fix a blood pressure value below which there is insufficient tissue circulation. Even very low blood pressures may be tolerated by some patients without sequelae, particularly by physically fit athletes, whereas others with the same values will complain about dizziness, fatigue, lack of initiative and energy. Orthostatic hypotension is a special manifestation accompanied by dizziness and a tendency to collapse when assuming the upright position.

### 11.2.2 Clinical manifestations

The affected patients complain about fatigue, lack of energy, and a tendency for dizziness and collapse. It is found more often in females and underweight persons.

In contrast to the hyperkinetic syndrome, there is great variation over time in the complaints. They may rapidly regress or progress, for example, under the influence of hormones, emotional and nutritional factors.

An asthenic body habitus is often seen. Commonly there is skin pallor and a tendency for hypovolemia. Blood pressure may be very low during recumbency, or it may only decrease in the upright position. The most prominent changes are found with tilt-table examination and a passive change to the upright position. Heart sounds are soft and murmurs are not usually heard.

The x-ray may reveal a surprisingly small cardiac silhouette in the upright position and a right cardiac border often located within the vertebral shadow, both due to orthostatic disturbances. The heart volume, however, is normal in recumbency. A comparison between the heart volumes in recumbency and in the upright position shows large volume differences of 30–50% (see also 3.5).

### 11.2.3 Therapy

The prognosis is good and the treatment is largely symptomatic. Spontaneous improvement can be seen during growth. Mild fluid retention due to increased sodium chloride intake may bring a marked relief, especially if hypovolemic-orthostatic disturbances are most prominent. Improvement is often experienced when the patient gains weight.

If there are emotional factors, they should be adequately treated. Exercise therapy requires individual prescription with a preference for short-term rather than endurance training. Drug therapy is not likely to work and is not necessary. Patients often seek drug therapy, however, although it has no real effect. Drugs even may be harmful, especially if adrenergic agents, ergot alkaloids, and amphetamines are prescribed.

# 11.3 Hyperventilation, pseudo dyspnea

Beside the typical hyperventilation syndrome which can lead to tetany, there is a form of nervous dyspnea characterized by a feeling of "not being able to take a full breath". The patients feel upset although there is no sign of real dyspnea. Apparent "gasping for breath" is often already clear when the patient presents. Dyspnea occurs during quiet sitting and vanishes with physical exercise. Therapy is usually not difficult, as the patient is usually reassured when informed about the harmless nature of the disorder.

# 12 Cardiac arrhythmias

## 12.1 Classification

The manifestations of cardiac arrhythmias may be remarkably varied. On the one hand, they may be an expression of physiologic function, and therefore may be documented in healthy subjects. On the other hand, they may be a manifestation of severe cardiac disease and, finally, they are the most frequent cause of sudden cardiac death. It is possible to classify them according to where they originate and also within the following four categories.

### 12.1.1 Classification by underlying disease

a) Cardiac arrhythmias may be the consequence of heart diseases where a positive correlation exists between the severity of the underlying disease and cardiac arrhythmia. It has been proven for coronary artery disease that the degree of left ventricular dysfunction, not the degree of ischemia, is correlated with the severity of cardiac arrhythmias. There are comparable findings in dilated cardiomyopathy. Abnormalities of other organs may trigger cardiac arrhythmia, for example, endocrine disturbances such as hyperthyroidism, renal disorders with electrolyte changes, and central nervous system problems such as subarachnoid hemorrhage.

b) In other cases cardiac arrhythmias occur, but there is no correlation in severity between the heart disease and the arrhythmia. Mild myocardial disease may thus be associated with severe life-threatening arrhythmias. In hypertrophic cardiomyopathy the hemodynamic consequences may be minor, but tachyarrhythmias life-threatening. In coronary artery disease, there are some patients who suffer from life-threatening arrhythmias, despite only a small hemodynamically-insignificant myocardial infarct. Similar findings are seen in mitral valve stenosis, where sometimes severe mitral valve stenosis may be associated with sinus rhythm, while hemodynamically unimportant stenosis may be associated with chronic atrial fibrillation.

c) Finally, there are arrhythmias which occur without any underlying cardiac disease. Even complex-looking arrhythmias are usually harmless in the healthy and do not require drug therapy.

### 12.1.2 Classification by heart rate

a) Tachycardias such as paroxysmal supraventricular tachycardia, atrial fibrillation, ventricular tachycardia, and ventricular fibrillation;

b) Bradycardias such as sinus bradycardia, sinus arrest, and atrioventricular (AV) block;
c) Combinations of bradycardia and tachycardia in the same patient often classified as the bradycardia-tachycardia ("brady-tachy") syndrome or sick sinus node syndrome.

### 12.1.3 Classification by occurrence

a) Arrhythmias which occur with sudden onset such as paroxysmal supraventricular tachycardia and paroxysmal atrial flutter or fibrillation.
b) Chronic arrhythmias such as chronic complete AV block or chronic atrial fibrillation, supraventricular and ventricular premature beats.

### 12.1.4 Classification by need for therapy

a) Most arrhythmias do not need any therapy; antiarrhythmics may even be harmful.
b) Life-threatening arrhythmias with or without known heart disease usually have to be treated. A clear need for therapy is seen, for example, in total AV block with Stokes-Adams attacks (due to periods of ventricular asystole).
c) If the arrhythmias are not life-threatening, the potential benefits of drugs have to be weighed against their possible harm. Most antiarrhythmics may aggravate arrhythmias ("pro-arrhythmic" effect). This risk/benefit relationship also has to be considered with every pacemaker implantation. Implantation of a pacemaker requires a thoughtful consideration of these issues because the patient has to cope, not only with the implant procedure, but the long-term follow-up, need for replacement or revision, and a long-term sense of "dependency".

## 12.2 Diagnostic procedures

### 12.2.1 Electrocardiography

The recognition and analysis of arrhythmias belongs to the domain of electrocardiography. In some cases, an ECG with extremity leads may suffice, but atrial waves are sometimes better seen in the chest leads, especially $V_1$ and $V_2$. Esophageal leads augment the atrial potentials and may therefore be tried in selected cases. Supraventricular tachycardias are occasionally diagnosed only with such a lead.

Potentials may be amplified by averaging many single ECG signals which are not normally recognized ("signal-averaged ECG"). With such an ECG, late potentials of ventricular excitation are recordable; this may be of diagnostic importance for the evaluation of ventricular arrhythmias.

## 12.2.2 Holter monitoring

With tape-recording devices, ECGs may be recorded for long time periods. Holter ECGs are mostly used for periods of 12 to 24 h. The evaluation of these recordings is assisted by computers. Many brief unsuspected or previously undocumented arrhythmias may be documented by this method. It has been shown by this procedure that virtually any type of arrhythmia can occur in the clinically healthy subject.

## 12.2.3 Ergometry, exercise electrocardiography

ECG recording during exercise reveals whether or not the heart rate response is physiologic. An exaggerated heart rate increase is often found in patients with hyperthyroidism, atrial fibrillation, and the hyperkinetic heart syndrome. An inadequate heart rate response is seen in sick sinus syndrome and in high-grade AV block. First degree AV block may often resolve during exercise. Exercise testing may be used to evoke suspected serious arrhythmias, e.g., ventricular tachycardia. It may also be used in evaluating the effectiveness of medications.

## 12.2.4 His bundle electrocardiography

With the help of a catheter positioned across the tricuspid valve, an ECG recording is obtained which shows the timing of conduction through the His bundle. It helps in deciding whether an AV-conduction disturbance is caused by conduction block above, below, or within the His bundle. It has been shown that AV block of the Mobitz I (Wenckebach) type is usually caused by conduction block in the AV node, while AV block of the Mobitz II type is located in, or below, the His bundle.

## 12.2.5 Sinus node recovery time

By stimulation of the right atrium at increasing rates, it can be determined at what rate physiologic AV block develops ("Wenckebach point"). One may further test how long it takes for the sinus node to resume its activity after a period of stimulation at high rate (sinus node recovery time). Prolongation of this recovery time is characteristic for the sick sinus syndrome.

## 12.2.6 Programmed stimulation

Ventricular tachycardias may be provoked by single or multiple premature beats induced artificially through ventricular electrodes. The method can also be used to find out whether the inducibility of ventricular tachycardias is reduced by drug therapy or by surgical procedures.

### 12.2.7 Intracardiac mapping

Arrhythmogenic areas in the ventricular myocardium can be located with the help of electrode catheters. The method is of special importance in coronary heart disease and is used pre- or intraoperatively to determine which parts of the ventricular myocardium are responsible for triggering life-threatening ventricular tachycardias. Surgical excision or ablation of these areas can cure severe tachyarrhythmias.

## 12.3 Ventricular extrasystoles, ventricular tachycardia, ventricular fibrillation

### 12.3.1 Clinical manifestations

Ventricular premature beats (extrasystoles) are the most frequent manifestations of arrhythmia (Fig. 109). If Holter monitoring is done over 24 h, some ventricular extrasystoles are almost always seen, even in healthy persons. The more frequently that these premature beats occur and the greater number of different morphologies (indicating multiple origins), the more seriously they are considered. If premature beats occur early in diastole (e.g., on the T-wave), they may be harbingers of ventricular tachycardia. After a ventricular premature beat there is usually a post-extrasystolic pause; only rarely are extrasystoles truly "interpolated" between consecutive normal QRS complexes.

Many consecutive ventricular extrasystoles are classified as "runs"; one speaks of couplets or triplets, sustained or nonsustained ventricular tachycardia, if there are more beats (Fig. 110). Ventricular tachycardia may end spontaneously or persist. There is sometimes a grey zone between ventricular tachycardia and ventricular flutter. In ventricular flutter, the pulse rate is above 200 beats/min, the ventricular complexes are continuous, without interruption and the cardiac output is consequently markedly reduced. In ventricular fibrillation, the ECG shows an erratic wave form changing in amplitude and frequency. Complete circulatory arrest occurs (Fig. 111).

### 12.3.2 Therapy

Premature ventricular beats occurring occasionally do not require any therapy. Frequent extrasystoles can cause unpleasant sensations. If they occur so early that the additional contraction of the heart does not contribute much to cardiac output and they are very frequent, then the effective heart rate may be substantially reduced. Extrasystoles in salvos may progress to ventricular tachycardia. Underlying disease has to be treated accordingly. Before institution of drug therapy, one should search for possible causes. Digitalis glycosides and intracellular loss of potassium are frequent causes of ventricular arrhythmia. Diuretics and laxatives may be the cause of potassium loss.

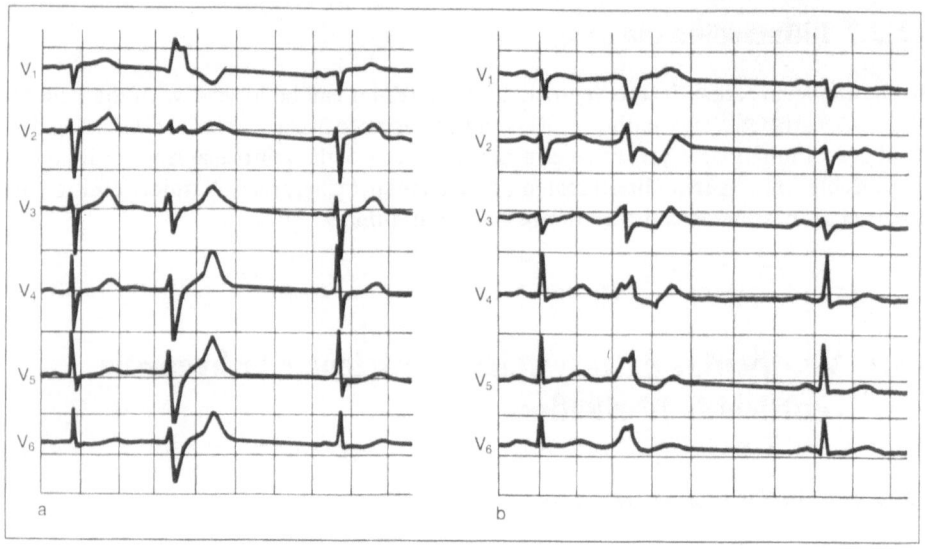

**Fig. 109.** Ventricular premature beat in the chest leads **a)** with complete right bundle branch block morphology indicating left-ventricular origin, and **b)** with complete left bundle branch block morphology indicating right-ventricular origin.

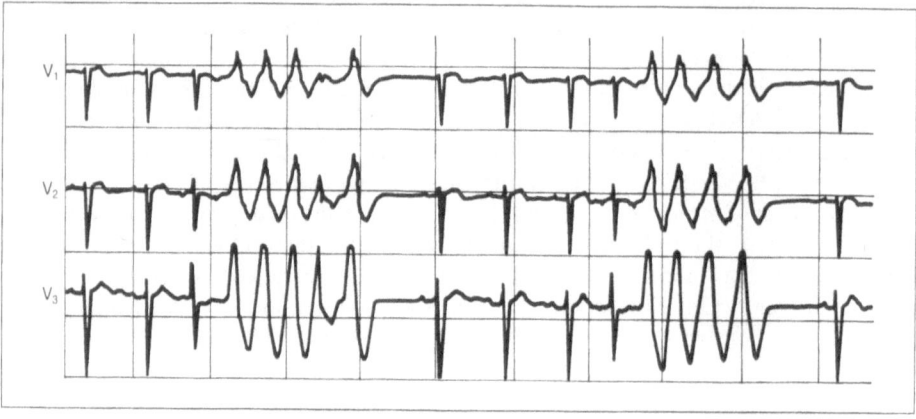

**Fig. 110.** Two short episodes of ventricular tachycardia.

Medical therapy with a sedative alone is occasionally very effective. Ajmaline bitartrate (not available in the USA), quinidine, procainamide, mexiletine, and amiodarone are among the antiarrhythmic agents sometimes used. With antiarrhythmic therapy, the indications and potential risks have to be thought through very carefully.

Ventricular flutter is treated with defibrillation, where usually a relatively low-energy shock (50 joules) is sufficient. High energy (200–400 joules) is used for defibrillation in ventricular defibrillation. Analgesia is, of course, not necessary because the patient loses consciousness within a few seconds of the onset of fibrillation.

160

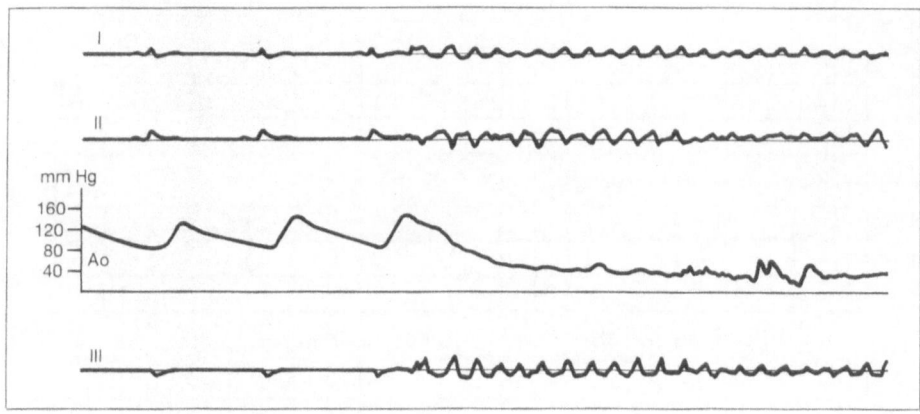

**Fig. 111.** ECG and aortic pressure curve during onset of ventricular fibrillation. An immediate drop of pressure is seen with the onset of tachyarrhythmia. Ventricular fibrillation occurred in this patient during heart catheterization and could be managed immediately by defibrillation.

Because ventricular arrhythmias may also be promoted by a prolonged QT time, it is helpful to determine the rate-corrected QT duration on the ECG (see chapt. 12.7).

For patients with severe ventricular arrhythmias such as those surviving cardiopulmonary resuscitation due to ventricular tachyarrhythmias, the implantation of an automatic defibrillator may be considered.

## 12.4 Supraventricular extrasystoles, atrial fibrillation and flutter, paroxysmal supraventricular tachycardia

Supraventricular premature beats are also frequent. Atrial extrasystoles can usually be recognized by the occurrence of a P-wave of different morphology (Fig. 112). Occasionally, the QRS complexes will also have a different morphology due to changes in conduction. If a extrasystole originates from the AV node area, the P-wave may be negative and may either follow the QRS complex or be hidden in it.

Atrial premature beats commonly precede the onset of atrial fibrillation or flutter. In atrial fibrillation, there is usually an erratic ventricular rate due to changing AV conduction. In atrial flutter, a saw-toothed shaped atrial activity at about 300/min is recorded on the ECG. Erratic ventricular rhythm may occur, but more usually there is regular conduction in a ratio of 3:1 or 4:1. If the ratio is 2:1 or 1:1 the ventricular rate may become very high.

In atrial ectopic tachycardia, the atrial rate is slower than in atrial flutter. One may recognize single atrial complexes, separated from each other, with rates between 150 and 250/min. In AV nodal reentrant tachycardia, the atrial potentials may be hidden in the QRS complex or may follow the QRS complex with retrograde atrial activation.

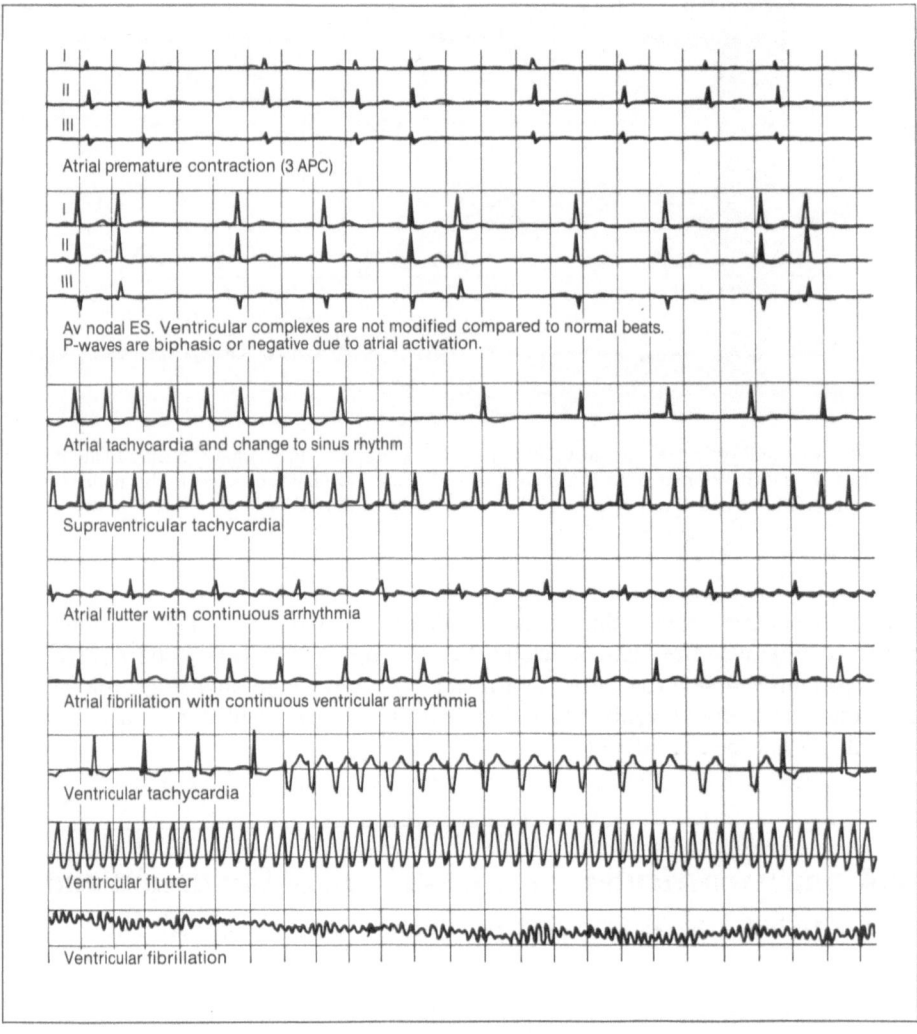

**Fig. 112.** Frequent manifestations of tachyarrhythmias (after [8]).

## 12.4.1 Therapy

In the case of underlying cardiac disease, atrial premature beats and paroxysmal atrial fibrillation or flutter are treated preferably with quinidine and verapamil. Quinidine induces conversion to sinus rhythm, while verapamil slows AV conduction. Digitalis glycosides have the same AV node effect, but they only uncommonly induce conversion to sinus rhythm. Paroxysmal atrial fibrillation also occurs in the healthy. It is not uncommonly triggered by excessive alcohol intake.

Thrombosis prophylaxis with anticoagulants is necessary in chronic or recurring atrial fibrillation, if the left atrium and/or ventricle is enlarged.

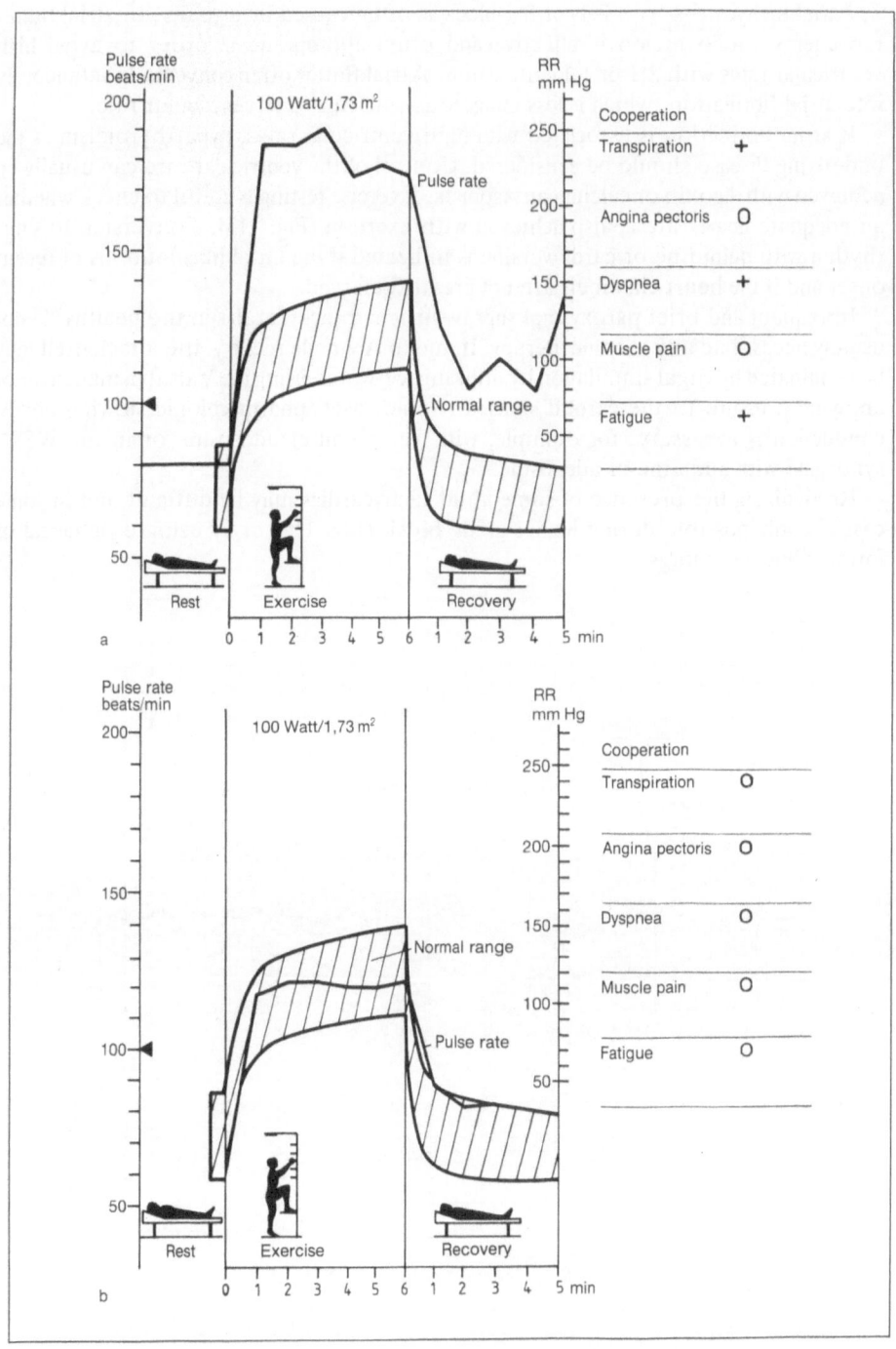

**Fig. 113. a** Large overshoot in heart rate increase and dyspnea during physical exercise in chronic atrial fibrillation. **b** Normalization after cardioversion with restoration of sinus rhythm.

163

Atrial tachycardia with 2:1- or 3:1-block is often caused by digitalis. In atrial flutter low-energy cardioversion is effective and often appropriate in order to avoid high ventricular rates with 2:1 or 1:1 conduction. Atrial flutter often converts spontaneously into atrial fibrillation, which is less dangerous with regard to ventricular rate.

If atrial fibrillation is associated with high ventricular rates, hyperthyroidism as the underlying disease should be considered. Control of the ventricular rate can usually be achieved with digoxin or calcium antagonists. Exercise testing is useful to check whether an adequate heart rate is also achieved with exertion (Fig. 113). Conversion to sinus rhythm with quinidine or cardioversion is indicated if the atrial fibrillation is of recent onset and if the heart chambers are not greatly enlarged.

Infrequent and brief paroxysmal supraventricular tachycardias in the healthy do not usually necessitate any chronic therapy. If due to AV node reentry, the attack itself may be terminated by vagal stimulation by drinking ice-water, using the Valsalva maneuver or applying pressure to the carotid sinus. In some cases, pharmacologic slowing of AV conduction is necessary, for example, with verapamil or adenosine or in the WPW-syndrome with ajmaline or adenosine.

Recognizing the presence of some atrial tachycardias may be difficult and in some cases is only possible during higher-grade block (Fig. 114) or by using esophageal or intracardiac recordings.

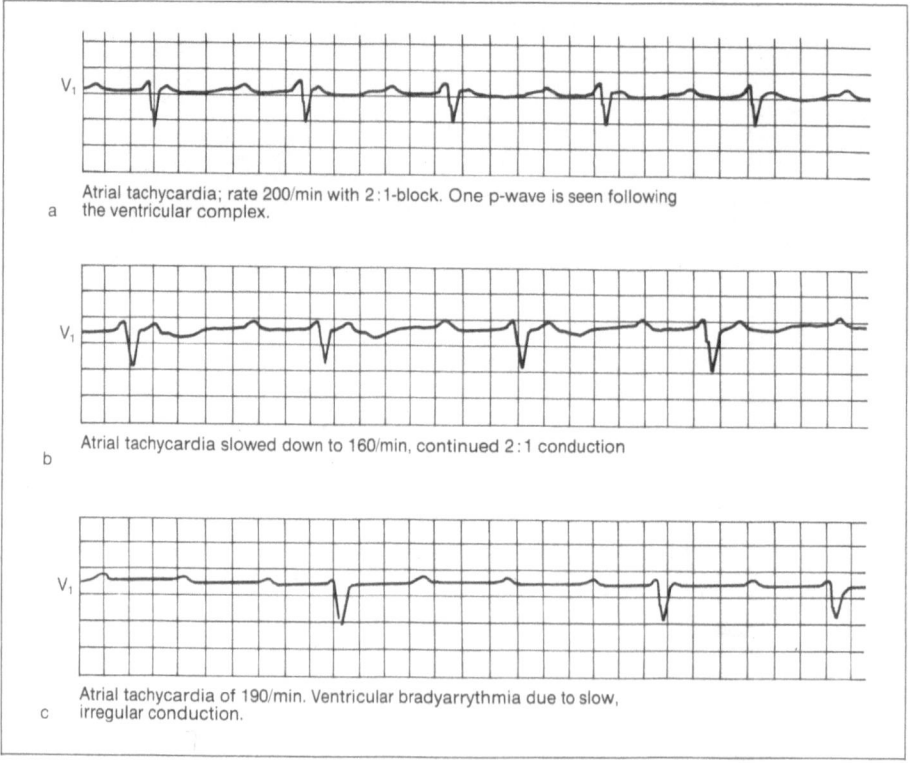

a    Atrial tachycardia; rate 200/min with 2:1-block. One p-wave is seen following the ventricular complex.

b    Atrial tachycardia slowed down to 160/min, continued 2:1 conduction

c    Atrial tachycardia of 190/min. Ventricular bradyarrythmia due to slow, irregular conduction.

**Fig. 114.** Atrial tachycardia with different rates and degrees of AV conduction. All three ECGs were recorded within a few days in the same patient. The underlying disease was mitral stenosis.

## 12.5 Bradyarrhythmias

### 12.5.1 Definition, occurrence, manifestations

Sinus bradycardia and a change from sinus rhythm to AV nodal or "junctional" rhythm are common findings, especially in trained athletes, and do not of themselves require any treatment (Fig. 115).

First-degree AV block is defined as a PR interval prolonged to more than 0.22 s (Fig. 116). A slight PR prolongation is often associated with increased vagal tone; this usually vanishes when the ECG is repeated with the subject in the upright position.

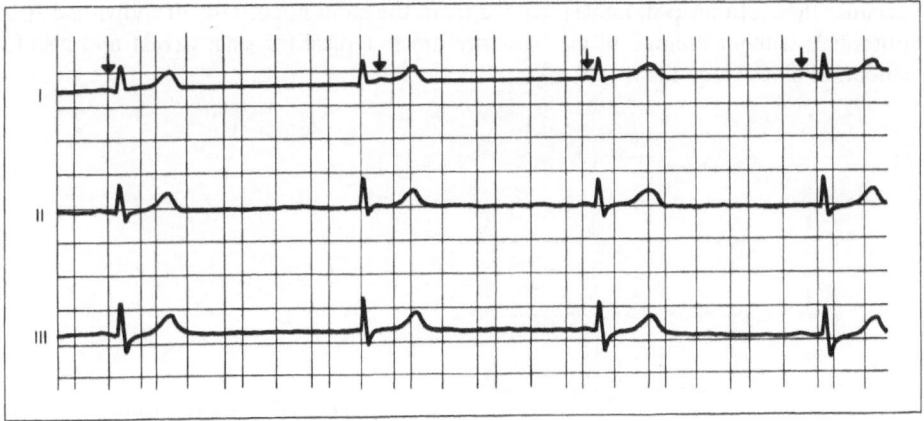

**Fig. 115.** Nodal ("junctional") rhythm in a healthy athlete. Because the sinus rate is slower than the AV nodal rate, the AV node takes over. The P-wave "walk through" the QRS complex.

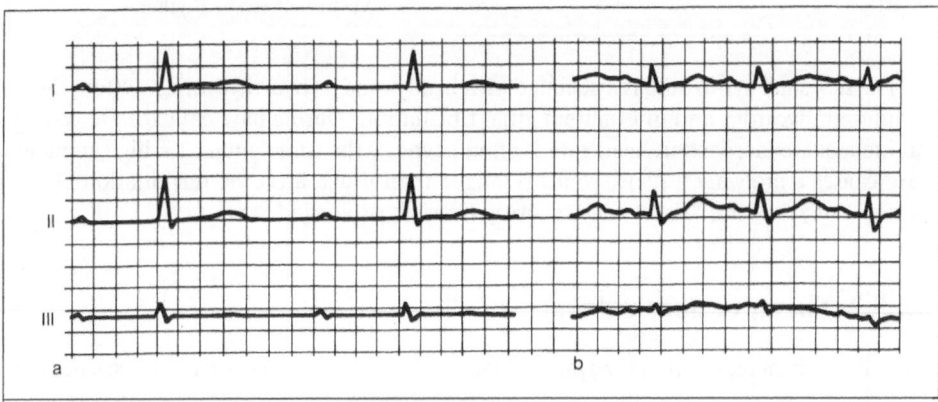

**Fig. 116.** First-degree AV block in an athlete with endurance training (**a**), which disappears in the upright position (**b**).

165

Second-degree AV block leads to intermittent loss of AV conduction. In Wenckebach periodicity (Mobitz I) there is a gradual prolongation of the PR interval from beat to beat, until a beat is not conducted ("dropped beat"). In second-degree AV block of the Mobitz-II type, there is a sudden loss of conduction, without prior prolongation of the PR interval. In Wenckebach morphology the conduction block occurs in the AV node and has a better prognosis than that of Mobitz-II block, where the block occurs below the AV node.

Third-degree AV block is characterized by a complete loss of conduction of atrial activity to the ventricles. Atrial potentials and ventricular potentials are independent of each other on the ECG. Ventricular activation results from an escape rhythm which, when of junctional origin, shows a QRS complex of normal morphology; when of ventricular origin, a wide QRS complex is seen.

Disorders of sinoatrial conduction can only be read indirectly from the surface ECG, because there are no potentials recorded from the sinus node. Loss of individual atrial potentials without change in the basis rhythm is typical for sinus arrest and also for sinoatrial block (Fig. 117).

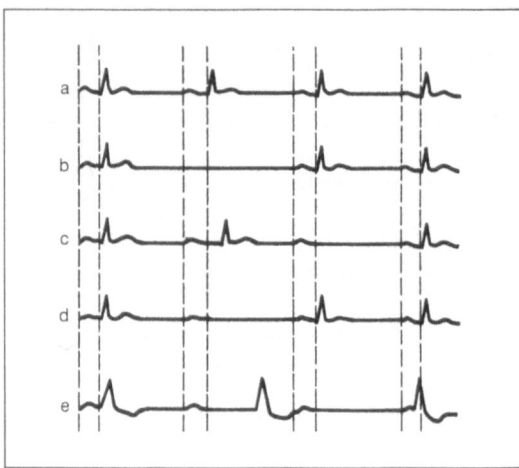

**Fig. 117.** Bradyarrhythmias: **a** sinus rhythm, **b** loss of atrial action due to SA block, **c** second-degree AV block (Wenckebach type) with preceding AV prolongation, **d** second-degree AV block Mobitz II type without preceding AV prolongation, **e** complete AV block with ventricular escape rhythm.

The sick sinus syndrome is associated with brady- and tachyarrhythmias. Often, there is sinus bradycardia and intermittent atrial fibrillation. During physical exercise testing an inadequate increase in heart rate is often seen. Atrial stimulation at a high stimulus rate causes a prolonged pause which is longer than usual, after the termination of the stimulation; i.e., the "sinus node recovery time" is prolonged.

## 12.5.2 Therapy, pacemakers

The clinical management of bradyarrhythmias has become much more effective since the introduction of pacemaker therapy. Pacemaker therapy is usually indicated in complete AV block, especially if it is associated with Stokes-Adams attacks. The same can be said for second-degree AV block of the Mobitz-II type. Pacemaker therapy is indicated for

166

sick sinus syndrome if during bradyarrhythmias (< 40 beats/min) there are symptoms of syncope or near-fainting. Occasionally, pacemaker therapy is necessary in order to be able to administer drugs for tachycardia.

Drug therapy of bradycardias is indicated when the problem is likely to be temporary, for example, when heart block accompanies an acute inferior myocardial infarction. Vagolytic agents, such as atropine, are first-line interventions. A temporary transvenous pacemaker may also be used.

The type of pacemaker chosen should be correlated with the patient's needs. When there is AV block but adequate atrial activity, implantation of a pacemaker that is triggered by atrial impulses may be considered. Alternatively, in the case of normal AV-conduction, pacemakers with exclusive atrial stimulation can be considered (AAI pacemakers). But for most purposes, the pacemaker systems that are used lead to activation in the apex of the right ventricle (VVI pacemakers). Units which provide sequential activation of the atrium and ventricle (DDD) are increasingly being used (Table 10).

**Table 10.** Code for implantable pacemakers

| *AAI:* | Atrium sensed<br>Atrium paced<br>Inhibition on sensing | *DDD:* | Atrium or ventricle sensed<br>Atrium or ventricle paced<br>Inhibited or triggered |
|---|---|---|---|
| *VVI:* | Ventricle sensed<br>Ventricle paced<br>Inhibition on sensing | *R:* | Rate adaptive |

The ability of the heart rate to increase with stress is useful for patients who are physically active. One may check the patient's heart-rate response to exercise by ergometry prior to implantation. In cases of severely impaired rate adaptation (see also Fig. 40, p. 51) the pacemaker systems implanted should allow the pacing rate to increase in proportion to physical activity (VVIR, DDDR). Today, this type of control is achieved via exercise-induced elevation of the blood temperature, shortening of the QT interval, increase in rate with respiration or body movement. Each of these methods of rate control has advantages and disadvantages (Fig. 118).

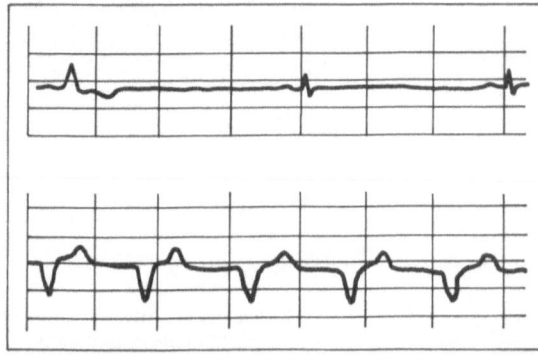

Fig. 118. Sick sinus syndrome in a 60-year-old woman. The patient complained about dizziness and dyspnea during effort. There were no signs of underlying heart disease, left ventricular function was normal. **a** The ECG shows sinus bradycardia at a rate of 30/min and an extrasystole. **b** After pacemaker implantation regular rhythm. A DDDR pacemaker was implanted. One can see the atrial and ventricular stimulation impulses.

Implantation of antitachycardia pacemaker systems is indicated in several types of cardiac arrhythmia. These pacemakers are programmed such that, in the case of tachycardia, a burst, scanning or premature stimulation is produced to terminate the arrhythmia. Implantable cardioverter-defibrillators are now used in patients to interrupt life-threatening ventricular arrhythmias which are not otherwise manageable.

## 12.6 Intraventricular conduction disorders

Bundle branch block morphology on the ECG is often an indication of an intraventricular conduction disturbance. A bundle branch block morphology of the QRS complex is also a typical finding for ventricular extrasystoles, although there is no actual bundle branch block in that case. For example, with a right ventricular premature beat, the right ventricle will be activated first and the left ventricle later, consequently giving rise to the morphology of complete left bundle branch block. In the case of left-ventricular premature beats, the QRS morphology is that of complete right bundle branch block (see Fig. 109, p. 160).

The QRS complex is prolonged to > 0.10 s in a bundle branch block. With "incomplete" right bundle branch block the QRS width is between 0.10–0.12 s, and right precordial lead rSr complexes are seen. Usually, (in the "physiologic" form) the second R-wave of the rSr complex is smaller than the first, but when there is associated volume

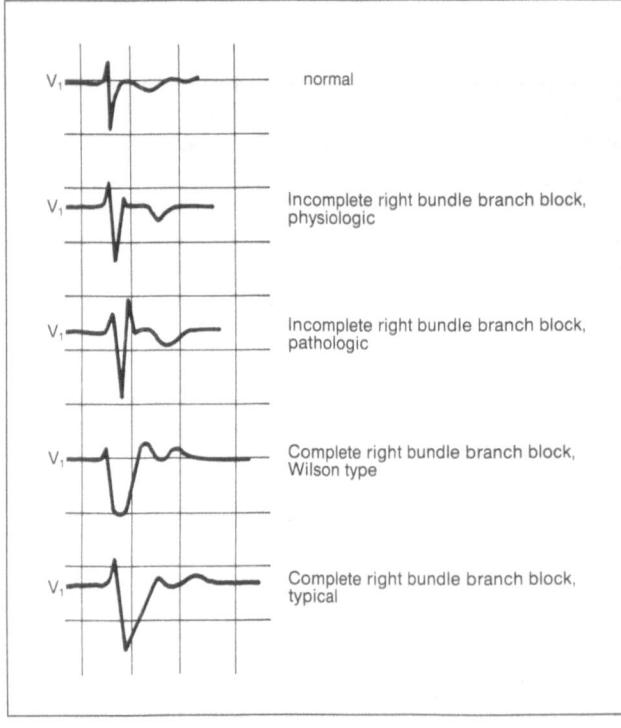

Fig. 119. Different forms of right bundle branch block.

168

overloading of the right heart, the second R-wave is higher. "Physiological" incomplete right bundle branch block is frequently seen in patients with chest-wall deformities. Complete right bundle branch block is characterized by a QRS width of > 0.12 s. The Wilson type has broad, rounded S-waves, whereas the S-waves have no specific structure in classical right bundle branch block. T-waves are altered in both forms (Fig. 119).

Incomplete left bundle branch block with a QRS width between 0.10 and 0.12 s is occasionally seen in left ventricular hypertrophy, but it is also seen in coronary artery disease and myocardial disorders.

Complete left bundle branch block with a QRS width of > 0.12 s is often found in dilated cardiomyopathy. It is rarely found without concomitant cardiac disease, whereas right bundle branch block is often found in healthy subjects. This is especially true for the physiological form of incomplete right bundle branch block, but also for complete right bundle branch block of the Wilson type. While in complete right bundle branch block the right fascicle and in complete left bundle branch block the left anterior and the posterior fascicles of the conduction system are blocked, all three fascicles are affected in "trifascicular" block. Isolated interruption of the left anterior fascicle is recognized on the ECG as marked rotation of the frontal plane QRS axis to the left while posterior fascicular block leads to marked right axis deviation.

If there is a sudden change in the QRS axis to extreme left or right axis deviation, interruption of the left anterior or left posterior fascicle may be assumed. A slow shift in the electrical axis may be the consequence of hypertrophy or of unusual cardiac position. If there is complete right bundle branch block in a patient with extreme left or right axis deviation and no other explanation is evident, bifascicular block may be diagnosed: interruption of the right fascicle and of the left anterior or left posterior fascicle. As a next step, trifascicular block, and complete AV conduction block may eventually develop. But as this is not frequent, pacemaker therapy is not usually indicated for chronic bifascicular block alone.


# 12.7 WPW, LGL, and long QT syndromes

In the Wolff-Parkinson-White (WPW) syndrome, the QRS complex often shows a slurring of the upstroke, the delta wave (Fig. 120). The QRS complex is therefore prolonged in a way similar to bundle branch block. The PR interval is shortened. These changes are due to premature ventricular activation caused by an accessory conduction pathway connecting the atrium and the ventricle. Whereas, normally, there is only one connection via the His bundle, in the WPW syndrome there are one or more additional electrically conducting myocardial bridges. These bridges, called Kent bundles, cause different forms of the WPW syndrome according to their location. Type A WPW has positive QRS complexes and delta waves in $V_1$ to $V_3$; it can be easily distinguished from Type B which shows negative potentials in these leads.

While the WPW syndrome may occasionally be an isolated electrocardiographic anomaly, it will in other patients lead to severe tachyarrhythmias due to the electrical impulse moving in a circuit made up of the atrium, AV node, ventricle, and back up the Kent bundle to the atrium. Such a tachycardia is called a "circus movement tachycardia".

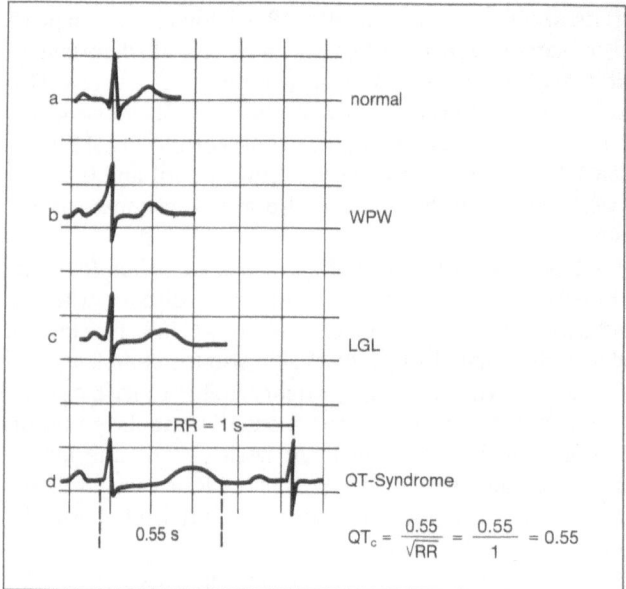

**Fig. 120.** Normal ECG (**a**); Wolff-Parkinson-White (WPW) syndrome (**b**); Lown-Ganong-Levin (LGL) syndrome (**c**) and long QT-syndrome (**d**).

Besides drug therapy, namely with Type-IA agents, amiodarone, or ajmaline, or surgical section, radio-frequency energy destruction of the conducting tissues is now possible using a catheter electrode.

In the Lown-Ganong-Levine (LGL) syndrome, the PR interval is also shortened, but the QRS complex looks normal. The anomaly is caused by accessory atrioventricular tracts which bypass the AV node. About half of the patients show a tendency for tachycardias, which again are caused by circus movement activation.

The long QT syndrome is a term for cardiac arrhythmias occurring in association with a prolongation of the QT interval. Usually the QT interval is less than 500 ms when the heart rate is 60/min. For rates other than 60/min, the QT-value is corrected using the formula:

Corrected QT time ($QT_c$) = measured QT interval divided by the square root of RR interval (s)

$$QT_c = \frac{QT}{\sqrt{RR}} .$$

With values for $QT_c$ above 500 ms cardiac arrhythmias are more likely to develop; these may be life-threatening. The syndrome may be congenital, it is often associated with acute myocardial infarction, but it may also be caused by electrolyte disorders, digitalis overdose or from antiarrhythmics with QT-prolonging effects (such as quinidine).

Therapy is directed towards the cause. Most of the common antiarrhythmics should not be used because they induce further QT prolongation. A therapeutic trial using antiarrhythmics of the lidocaine type (Type IB) or β-blockers may be considered. Left stellate ganglion blockade may be a further therapeutic maneuver for preventing tachyarrhythmias. The potential efficacy of this procedure may be tested by pharmacological blockade prior to surgical intervention.

# 13 Cardiac failure

## 13.1 Definition, classification

Cardiac failure is a syndrome which occurs in the wake of various cardiac disorders. It is defined as an inability of the heart to meet the body's blood supply needs.

A significant aim of treatment in any cardiac disorder is to prevent the development of cardiac failure. This holds true for systemic arterial hypertension and also for coronary artery disease. Most cardiac valvular disorders or congenital lesions may now be corrected prior to the development of cardiac failure. However, in disorders of the myocardium and in primary pulmonary hypertension, the development of cardiac failure often cannot be avoided.

Classical cardiac failure is associated with cardiac enlargement due to dilatation of the cardiac chambers, with a diminished cardiac output and an increased filling pressure (LVEDP > 15 mmHg). The cardiac output decreases below 4 l/min/1.73 m$^2$ or 2.5 l/min/m$^2$, the arteriovenous oxygen difference exceeds 30%, and the saturation of mixed venous blood in the pulmonary artery decreases below 65%.

Predominant failure of the left ventricle causes decreased left ventricular stroke output and pulmonary venous congestion; right ventricular failure, on the other hand, results in systemic venous congestion. Symptoms of left heart failure may also occur due to a disturbed inflow into the left ventricle as a result of mitral stenosis or hypertrophic cardiomyopathy. Right-heart failure may be caused by a filling disturbance due to constrictive pericarditis. Pre-cardiac obstruction, e.g., with thrombosis of the vena cava, may cause symptoms similar to right-heart failure.

Symptoms of right- and left-ventricular failure may coexist in many cases. This holds especially true for disorders of the left heart, where hemodynamic disorders will rapidly affect the right heart via the pulmonary circulation.

Congestion is not so obvious in some patients, but there are symptoms of a reduced cardiac output. One then speaks of "forward failure" in contrast to "backward failure".

Exercise-induced heart failure is defined as a disorder where the symptoms or signs of heart failure occur only with physical exercise, but not at rest.

## 13.2 Clinical manifestations

Dyspnea is the classical symptom of left-heart failure. This occurs predominantly with physical exercise such as walking up a hill or stairs, but it may also occur at night, especially in the early morning hours, due to increased intravascular fluid. Patients will note improvement by standing upright or sitting with their legs dependent. In severe cases, frank pulmonary edema may occur.

With pulmonary venous congestion, rales may be auscultated; initially these are soft inspiratory rales only, but with severe congestion and in pulmonary edema, the rales may be so loud that they will be heard from a distance. In some patients, especially with left-heart failure due to acute myocardial infarction, a purely interstitial pulmonary edema may occur which is associated with dyspnea, but with few rales.

Left-heart foreward failure predominantly leads to an impaired stroke output and, consequently, a decreased circulation to the brain. Patients complain of dizziness and syncopal attacks, particularly during physical exercise. These symptoms are seen for example in left-heart failure occurring with severe aortic stenosis or hypertrophic cardiomyopathy.

Right-heart failure may occur with minor complaints, if it is predominantly a congestive failure. The patient experiences fluid overload of the lower extremities as a first symptom. Physical examination shows ankle edema and pretibial edema in both legs of comparable severity – if there is no additional unilateral venous disorder. Patients constantly lying in bed occasionally show fluid overload at the sacrum first. If edema is due to cardiac cause, there is always congestion of the liver and neck veins. This can be identified by studying the neck veins with the patient in the upright sitting position. Pressure on the enlarged liver may increase the neck vein congestion. Edema caused by venous insufficiency should not be misinterpreted as heart failure. When venous disease is the cause, the edema is not associated with liver enlargement and, frequently, there is a difference between both legs. A careful history usually reveals previous phlebitis.

Abdominal fluid overload is a late sign of right-heart failure. Prominent ascites is often caused by portal congestion. Ascites is often the main symptom in constrictive pericarditis.

Pleural effusion is a sign of congestive heart failure, usually of right-heart failure, and additional left-heart failure. The pleural space is drained via the veins of the systemic and the pulmonary circulation.

In congestive heart failure there is usually an increase in intravascular blood volume. Polycythemia occurs in cardiac failure due to pulmonary hypertension. In contrast, patients with mostly forward failure show a relatively decreased blood volume and anemia. Therapy must thus be geared to account for these differences.

In severe heart failure there is usually tachycardia due to an overactive sympathetic nervous system, the skin is pale and the blood pressure low. The first heart sound is soft due to impaired LV contraction, and a third heart sound can be recognized. With severe ventricular dilatation there may be a murmur of mitral or tricuspid insufficiency, secondary to chamber enlargement.

The ECG is usually abnormal, without specific signs related to heart failure. The decreased cardiac output can be identified using the indicator dye-dilution method or by measurement of oxygen saturation in the mixed venous blood in the pulmonary artery. Dilatation of the cardiac chambers can be seen on echocardiography. Radiologically visible pulmonary congestion is a reliable sign of left-heart failure. Early forms of cardiac insufficiency may be differentiated by determining the heart volume from echo or x-ray in the supine position.

The severity of heart failure and its prognosis correlate with the elevation of plasma adrenalin.

172

# 13.3 Therapy

Heart failure usually necessitates bedrest – but bedrest may also be detrimental as in virtually all other cardiac circulatory disorders or diseases. In the case of severe dyspnea, elevation of the upper part of the body and lowering the legs may be helpful; this is especially true for pulmonary edema. General measures for therapy of chronic heart failure include normalization of the body weight and restriction of salt intake. The underlying disease which led to cardiac failure should be treated if at all possible.

Drug therapy usually includes digitalis. There are exceptions, such as acute left-heart failure in patients having myocardial infarction where the onset of digitalis activity is too slow. In cardiac arrhythmias the possible arrhythmogenic effect of digitalis has to be taken into account. Formerly, rapid loading of digitalis glycosides was performed, but today, slower loading is usually preferred to minimize toxicity. In chronic heart failure, one usually starts with the maintenance dose, but one should realize that peak activity of digoxin and digitoxin will take 1 to 4 weeks, respectively.

Diuretics are indicated in congestive heart failure. Potassium-sparing agents or combinations are used to avoid potassium depletion, except in patients with renal insufficiency where there is a tendency for hyperkalemia.

Vasodilators were introduced as an additional therapeutic option. With these agents one aims to reduce cardiac afterload. This type of approach is especially effective if heart failure is associated with hypertension, but it may also be used with normal and even decreased blood pressure. Agents such as prazosin, nifedipine, and nitrates have proven disappointing for improving functional capacity. However, ACE-(angiotensin-converting-enzyme) inhibitors are more effective in many cases. ACE-inhibitors block angiotensin synthesis, but they also seem to have additional properties (e.g. inhibit smooth muscle cell proliferation).

When heart failure is truly refractory to drug therapy, patients may be candidates for heart transplantation.

# 14 Cardiovascular disorders and sports

## 14.1 Relation between structure and function of the heart, adaptation to increased exercise

There is a close relationship between cardiac structure and function. Endurance or interval exercise training is a strong physiologic stimulus for the heart to increase in size. The cardiac weight may increase from 300 g to 500 g in an athlete. The heart volume may increase from approximately 600 ml to more than 1200 ml, but this is not only caused by an increase in muscle mass (hypertrophy), but also by an increase in cardiac blood volume (dilatation). The increase in volume attained by physical exercise regresses within a few months if training is stopped. Persisting cardiomegaly in former athletes is caused either by undiagnosed cardiac disease or it is due to a constitutionally large heart. In sports activities where physical exercise capacity can be correlated with cardiac size – such as in cycling, long-distance running, rowing – athletes who are born with a strong and large heart are more likely to achieve maximum performance.

Adaptation to maximum physical capacity encompasses the entire cardiovascular system, including the peripheral circulation, the lungs, and the blood, as well as the skeletal muscle and other organs (e.g., endocrine glands such as the pancreas and adrenals). The increased metabolism induces an increase in liver volume. The autonomic nervous system shows an increase in vagal tone, which is responsible for typical athlete-associated anomalies such as AV block, bradycardia, and hypotension.

## 14.2 Measurement of physical exercise capacity, exercise methods, and measurement targets

Measurement of "physical capacity" has to be modified according to the kind of sport under study. Whereas, for example, muscle strength is of decisive importance for weight lifting, oxygen delivery and utilization are most important in endurance-type sports.

In other types of sporting activities the ability for coordination or mobility are of major importance. The usual measurements of physical exercise capacity cannot reflect other physical aptitudes for specific kinds of sporting activities. For example, the subject's weight may play a role if the sport is weight-dependent (running) rather than relatively weight-independent (wrestling), (see also 3.10).

Maximum oxygen consumption is a good measure of cardiopulmonary exercise capacity. It is measured in ml $O_2$/min at a standard condition (BTPS = body temperature

37°, pressure 760 mm Hg, saturated = saturated in water vapor). Beyond the range of maximum oxygen uptake there is lactate excess and, consequently, a decrease in blood pH. There is a close, almost linear relationship between physical capacity (in watts) and oxygen consumption. The correlation is only non-linear if the exercise efficiency changes. This occurs, for example, during treadmill ergometry, if the patient turns from walking to running at the same speed; the same physical capacity in watts is related to a different oxygen uptake because walking and running are not equally efficient. Thus, for measurements of physical exercise capacity, the corresponding $O_2$-uptake has to be measured if different kinds of exercise are to be compared. For each of the different types of exercise testing there is a different relationship between $O_2$-uptake and workload. However, by taking the different correlations into account, exercise testing with a bicycle ergometer in the sitting or recumbent position, step climbing and the treadmill can be compared. Furthermore, one can relate the biological capacity to the body surface area which approximates lean body mass. In this way, one can best compare exercise responses in persons of different body sizes and weight.

In the USA, analogous comparisons are drawn using METS (metabolic equivalent, temperature 37°C, saturated). This parameter is related to the basal metabolic rate or is calculated, as an approximate value, in relation to the body weight, as 1 MET equal to 3.5 ml $O_2$/kg/min.

# 14.3 Risks of sport

Sudden death may occur during sporting activities; almost every physician will be involved in such a case. Is death caused by exercising or just a coincidence? Unexpected deaths during sporting activities occur in trained top-class athletes, but are more likely in persons who engage in sport only occasionally. Autopsies usually reveal a previously unrecognized organic cardiac disorder: most frequently, coronary artery disease, but also cardiomyopathies (mostly the hypertrophic form), valvular disorders, especially of the aortic valve, and congenital coronary anomalies.

The fact that sudden death may be directly associated with physical exercise has been confirmed by life-threatening episodes during exercise testing. During diagnostic ergometry – usually in patients suspected of having coronary artery disease – ventricular fibrillation occurs at a rate of 1:2000–10000 (see also 4.2.2, page 48). Without treatment by a physician and defibrillation these rhythm disturbances are usually lethal. Therefore, in persons who have unrecognized organic disease, physical activity can in rare instances lead to sudden death. Usually, this is caused by a tachyarrhythmia such as ventricular fibrillation. Immediate cardiac massage is often lifesaving if started promptly after circulatory arrest.

## 14.4 Sports for the healthy

Sports have both physical and mental components. Physically, the cardiovascular effect is a major aspect. Effective training is achieved with heart rates above 130/min with correction for age: about 160 for the 15–20 year-old, and 120 in the 50 year-old.

Sports with endurance or interval elements show the greatest cardiovascular effects, and for these types of sports the exercise heart rate is a quantitative measure of the degree of circulatory stress. But other organ systems are affected as well; especially locomotion, with its age, sex and overuse problems. If a certain type of sport is recommended, these factors need to be carefully considered.

The psychic dimension of sport is subjective; it is associated with the experience of adventure, willpower, and self-affirmation. There is a feeling of happiness and satisfaction resulting from adequate physical activity.

In an age of information-overload the rather "boring" or repetitive types of sports like hiking, jogging, skiing, roller-skating, ice-skating, cycling, and rowing are especially suitable and should be recommended. Hiking in the mountains requires setting aside more time, but is excellent exercise. Jogging needs a systematic and very slow increase in load, but can be enjoyed by the majority of people. Athletic rowing with a sliding seat necessitates a knowledge of the technique, but it carries fewer problems with regard to an overloading of any one part of the locomotor system.

Sports which require high levels of concentration such as table tennis or tennis should in general not be recommended as a means to keep fit, unless they form part of a more comprehensive program. Skiing and surfing and the like necessitate concentration as well, but they are usually not competitively practiced, and they produce both a training effect and pleasure. The physician should be wary of recommending abstinence from sport.

## 14.5 Physical rehabilitation therapy, sport and atherosclerosis, sport in modern society

Physical activity may be used as a therapeutic device in functional and organic disorders. A direct therapeutic effect is possible when there has been deconditioning due to decreased mobility. The management of hypertension and the hyperkinetic heart syndrome may also be effectively supported by physical rehabilitation therapy. Patients with coronary disease exercising in training groups benefit from both the indirect and direct effects of sporting activities. The elimination of anxiety and recovery of self-confidence play an important indirect role, and the group helps minimize overzealous efforts. As a direct benefit, physical training allows a more economical use of the muscles and the circulation. However, it is unrealistic to expect a directly positive effect on the development of atherosclerosis and on the formation of coronary collaterals. Those coronary patient groups whose exercises are supervised by a physician have gained widespread acceptance, such that their number has increased considerably.

Physical rehabilitation therapy, in a suitable form, should be recommended for most cardiac disorders. It is important that the patient learns to find suitable types of activity and the right amount of exertion. More can be expected from individual observation of the patient during physical exercise than from the application of arbitrary standards. Besides the knowledge of a specific heart rate which should not be exceeded it is important for the coronary patient to aquire in self-recognition of arrhythmias, angina or angina equivalents, and dyspnea.

Sports and physical activity generally contribute to health and should be recommended. Infants and youngsters should be given the chance to enjoy the pleasures of physical activity. Common sense and an understanding of physiology should be used to select the right degree and individually suited type of activity. The physical activity is probably appropriate if there is a sensation of comfort following it and if normal bodily functions such as sleep, appetite, mood, and energy are affected positively. The right degree of physical activity improves one's power of concentration and stimulates feelings of happiness and satisfaction.

# References for further reading

1. Netter FH (1971) FF Yonkman (ed) The Ciba Collection of Medical Illustrations, Vol 5: Heart. Ciba Corp., New York
2. Krayenbuhl HP, Kübler W (1981) Kardiologie in Klinik und Praxis, Bde. 1+2. Thieme, Stuttgart New York
3. ten Cate FJ (1985) Hypertrophic Cardiomyopathy – Clinical Recognition and Management. Dekker, New York Basel
4. Becker HJ, Kober G, Kaltenbach M (1984) EKG-Repetitorium. Deutscher Ärzte-Verlag, Köln
5. Kaltenbach M (1974) Die Belastungsuntersuchung von Herzkranken. Boehringer, Mannheim
6. Kaltenbach M, Roskamm H (1980) Vom Belastungs-EKG zur Koronarangiographie. Springer, Berlin Heidelberg New York
7. Zuckermann R (1965) Herzauskultation. Edition Leipzig. Leipzig
8. Buchner CH, Steim H, Dragert W (1972) Herzrhythmusstörungen. Boehringer, Ingelheim
9. Kaltenbach M, Schneider W (1980) Krankheiten des Herzens und des Kreislaufs. In: Kuhn HA, Schirmeister J (Hrsg) Innere Medizin. Springer, Berlin Heidelberg New York
10. Braunwald E (1988) Heart Disease. A Textbook of Cardiovascular Medicine. W. B. Saunders, Philadelphia London Toronto
11. Hurst JW, Logue RB, Schlant RC, Sonnenblick EH, Wallace AG, Wenger NK (1990) The Heart. Sixth Edition. McGraw Hill, New York
12. Roskamm H (ed) (1984) Koronarerkrankungen. Handbuch der Inneren Medizin. Bd. 9: Herz und Kreislauf, Teil 3. Springer, Berlin Heidelberg New York Tokyo
13. Vlietstra RE, Holmes DR Jr (1987) PTCA. Percutaneous Transluminal Coronary Angioplasty. FA Davis, Philadelphia
14. Holmes DR Jr, Vlietstra RE (1989) Interventional Cardiology. FA Davis, Philadelphia

*Current contributions to the topic in:*

Zeitschrift für Kardiologie
European Heart Journal
Circulation
Journal of the American College of Cardiology
British Heart Journal
American Journal of Cardiology
International Journal of Cardiology

# Subject Index

## A

ACE inhibitor  85, 137, 149, 173
ACVB, see bypass
AIDS  93
ajmaline bitartrate  160, 164, 170
akinesia  85
akinetic area  82
alcohol  135, 162
alpha (receptor) blocker  147, 150
amiodarone  160, 170
amyloidosis  137, 143
aneurysm
−, aortic  96 f., 99
−, dissecting  96 f.
−, ventricular  84
aneurysmectomy  84
angina pectoris  16, 37 f., 43, 47 f., 59 ff., 141, 147, 177
−, crescendo  74
−, exercise-induced  59 f.
−, Prinzmetal  60
− at rest  60
−, silent  75
−, stable  59
− therapy  63 ff.
−, unstable  59 f.
angiocardiogram  125
angio(cardio)graphy (see also coronary angiography)  102, 106, 123
angioplasty, see balloon angioplasty
angioscopy  60
ankylosing spondylitis  92, 98 f.
antibiotics  90 ff.
− prophylaxis  92
anticoagulants  81, 137
anticoagulation  68, 107, 150
antiproliferative drugs  36
antistreptolysin titer  92
antithrombotic drugs  68

aortic coarctation  9, 118, 123 ff., 147
− pressure measurement  9, 124
aortic
− auscultation  10, 111
− ECG  23, 111
− insufficiency  90, 92, 98 f., 102, 110 ff., 146
− phonocardiogram  23, 109, 111
− stenosis  30, 39, 89, 98 f., 107 ff., 114, 141, 172
aortitis
−, luetic  96, 99
−, Takayasu's disease  96
aortography  33, 60, 109, 112, 124
arterial occlusive disease  38, 96
arterial pulses, peripheral  6
arterial stenosis, blood-pressure measurement  9
arteriosclerosis, see atherosclerosis
arterio-venous fistula  23
artery
−, carotid  11 f., 111
−, central, elasticity  111, 146
−, dorsalis pedis  7
−, femoral  7
−, iliac  7
−, intercostal  124
−, internal mammary  66, 124
−, popliteal  7
−, posterior tibial  6 f.
−, radial  7 f.
−, renal  11 f.
−, internal thoracic  66
ascites  115, 172
aspirin  37, 80 f., 88, 92
asystole  79
atherectomy  33
atheroma (see also atherosclerosis)  36, 42, 59 f., 88
−, complicated  74
−, uncomplicated  74

atherosclerosis  36 ff., 96, 176
atrial fibrillation  156, 161 ff.
atrial septal defect  105, 118 ff.
−, coronary sinus defect  118
−, ostium-primum defect  118 ff.
−, ostium-secundum defect  118
−, sinus-venosus defect  118
atrial tachycardia  164
atrioventricular canal  118
atropine  80, 167
auscultation areas  11, 13
Austin-Flint murmur  23
AV block  157 f., 165 ff., 174
−, Mobitz type  158, 166
−, Wenckebach type  158, 166

## B

"backward failure"  171
balloon angioplasty  33, 36, 59, 66 f., 81, 86 f., 110, 147
balloon pump, intraaortic  80 f., 84
balloon valvuloplasty  105, 110
Bayes theorem  56
beta (receptor) blocker  62 f., 65 f., 88, 138, 142, 147, 152 ff.
bicuspid aortic valve  98, 107
bidirectional shunting  118
bifascicular block  169
bioprothesis  107, 110
bisferiens pulse  141
blood pressure  145 ff.
−, exercise  8, 49
− hypertensive crisis  149
− measurement  8 f., 49
− normal range  8
body surface area  34 f.
Bougie-method  68
bradycardia  75, 80, 146 f., 157, 174
bundle branch block  168

bypass 72 f., 107
–, internal mammary artery
  66 f., 72
– surgery 66 f., 86


# C

calcium antagonist 37, 60,
  62 f., 64 ff., 88, 137, 147, 150
– diltiazem 64, 147
– gallopamil 147
– nifedipine 64, 144, 147,
  149, 173
– verapamil 64, 142, 147,
  154, 164
calcium channel blocker, see
  calcium antagonist
capillary pressure measurement,
  see blood pressure measurement
capillary pressure method 9,
  124
capillary pulsation 111
captopril 80
cardiac aneurysm 84, 87
cardiac arrhythmia 2, 62,
  79 f., 85, 93, 135, 141, 151,
  156 ff., 173, 177
– classification 156
– extrasystole 62, 159
– –, atrial 101, 161 ff.
– –, supraventricular 112,
  135, 161 f., 164
– –, ventricular 135, 152,
  157
cardiac fibrillation
– –, atrial 101, 135, 141,
  156 f., 161
– –, ventricular 49 f., 76,
  79 f., 85, 94, 109, 141,
  156, 159 ff., 175
– salvos 159
– tachycardia 93, 147, 154,
  156 f., 159 ff., 172
– –, ventricular 85, 135, 156,
  158 ff.
cardiac catherization 33 f., 94,
  102
cardiac dullness 8, 93
cardiac failure, see heart failure
cardiac murmur, see heart murmur
cardiac muscle mass 139, 174
cardiac neurosis 62 f.
cardiac output 102, 140, 151,
  153, 171

–, measurement 25 f., 31 f.
cardiac silhouette 27, 101,
  106, 137
cardiac sound, see heart sound
cardiac tamponade 94
cardiac transplantation 85,
  138, 173
cardiac trauma 94
cardiac volume 27 ff., 46, 85,
  101, 111 f., 119, 137, 172,
  174
– normal value 29
cardiac weight 29, 135, 174
cardiomyopathy 133 ff.
–, dilated 133 ff., 137, 156,
  169
–, hypertrophic 31 f., 62, 113,
  133, 141, 156, 171, 175
–, nonobstructive 143
–, restrictive 133, 143 f.
carotid artery 11 f., 111
carotid pulse curve 22, 107,
  141
– in aortic insufficiency 111
– in aortic stenosis 109
– cock's-comb shape 109
– normal pressure curve 109
– pressure half-time 109
catecholamines 16, 60, 62,
  142, 147
cellulitis 63
cephalosporin 90
cerebrovascular disease 1, 37
cerebral hemorrhage 124
cerebral infarction, stroke 2
chest fluoroscopy 27
chest pain, cardiac 47, 62 f.
–, non-cardiac 62 f.
chest roentgenogram 27
chest trauma 94
chest-wall deformities 169
cholesterol level 43 ff.
chordae tendinae rupture 90,
  105
chorea minor 92
cigarette smoking 3, 37, 43,
  45 f., 88
cineangiogram 66, 76, 78
cine x-ray films 33
clonidine 147, 154
cold stimulus 60
collaterals 38 f., 42, 74, 176
computed tomography 32, 124
conduction disturbance 16,
  135, 139
constitutional type 6
contraceptives, hormonal 43

contraction, impaired 135
coronary angiography (see also
  coronary arteriography) 57,
  61, 63, 67, 69 f., 71, 73, 77,
  80, 82 f., 141
coronary arteries 39
– anatomy 40
– classification 39
– distribution types 41
– patency rate 72
– stenosis 42, 57
coronary arteriography (see
  also coronary angiogra-
  phy) 33, 57 ff., 108 f., 135
coronary artery disease, see coronary heart disease
coronary heart disease 17, 22,
  30 f., 37 ff., 46 ff., 50, 52,
  55, 137, 145, 156
– mortality rate 2
– prognosis 30, 46 f., 52
– risk factors 43 ff.
coronary insufficiency (see also
  heart failure, myocardial failure) 37, 39, 74, 107
coronary reserve 60, 85
coronary score 44, 46, 58 f.
coronary artery spasm 60 f.
Corrigan's sign 111
creatine phosphokinase
  (CPK) 78 f.
cyanosis 100, 131, 150


# D

defibrillator 168
defibrillation 50, 94, 161, 175
delta wave 169 f.
diabetes mellitus 45, 64
diaphragm, lowered 7
digitalis 85, 106, 137, 142,
  159, 164, 170, 173
– and ECG 17
digital substraction angiography 31, 124
diptheria 93
dip-plateau phenomenon 93
dipyridamole 66
diuretics 85, 106, 149, 159, 173
dobutamine 80
dopamine 80
Doppler (pressure) measurement 9, 48, 101
Doppler echocardio-
  graphy 106, 108, 112, 119,
  123

dorsalis pedis artery, palpation 7
drumstick fingers 150
Ductus Botalli apertus 128
dye-dilution method 25 f., 31, 172
–, cardiac output measurement 25
– curves 119 f., 129
– Fick principle 25
– thermodilution method 25
dyspnea 81, 152
–, exercise-induced 107


E

Ebstein's anomaly 98 f., 116, 118, 132
echocardiography 22 f., 46, 90, 93, 101, 108, 111 f., 119, 123, 132, 135, 139
–, M-mode 23 f., 103
–, two-dimensional 23 f., 85
ECG, see electrocardiography
E. coli bacteria 89
edema 115, 172
Eisenmenger's syndrome 123, 132, 150
ejection fraction 29, 31, 54, 85, 112, 134, 137, 140
electrocardiography 15 ff., 81, 157 ff.
– and catecholamine infusion 16
– and digitalis 17, 53
– electrical heart axis 19, 21
– exercise 16 f., 22, 48 ff., 53, 85 ff.
– extremity leads 18
– His bundle 158
– Holter monitoring 158 f.
– hypertrophy 17, 20 f.
– ischemic changes 16 f., 52 f.
– leads 18 ff.
– in myocardial infarction 17, 76 f., 81, 85
– normal range 15, 19
– p cardiale 21
– p mitrale 21, 101
– p pulmonale 21
– PQ interval 15
– PR interval 15, 165 f., 169
– and pulmonary stenosis 113 f.
– p-wave 15, 17, 22, 101, 161

– QRS-complex 15, 17, 19, 21 f., 161, 168 f.
– QT interval 15, 161, 167, 170
– QTc interval 15, 161, 170
– QT-syndrome, long 170
– ST-segment 15, 17, 48, 87
– depression 17, 48, 52 f., 76, 137
– elevation 17, 48, 52 f., 60, 76
– sinoatrial conduction 166
–, transesophageal 119
– T-wave changes 17, 52 f., 87
– T-wave peaking 76, 87
– in upright position 17, 165
– vector loop 22
electromechanical dissociation 16
electrophysiological study 158
emboli 149
embolectomic surgery 150
endocardial fibrosis 137, 143
endocarditis 89 ff., 123
–, aortic valve 92
–, bacterial 89 ff., 98 f.
–, antibiotic prophylaxis 90
–, enterococci 90
–, streptococci 90
– vegetations 90
–, fungal 98
–, Loeffler's 92
–, marantic 92
–, rheumatic 89, 91 f., 98 f., 101, 107, 115
–, subacute 89
ergometry, see electrocardiography, exercise
ergonovine 61
exercise ECG, see electrocardiography, exercise
extrasystole, see cardiac arrhythmia


F

Fabry's disease 142 f.
Fallot's tetralogy 113, 118, 129 ff.
– therapy 132
femoral artery, palpation 7
fever 89 f., 93, 146
–, rheumatic 92, 98

fibrinolysis 42, 60, 80 f.
fibrinolytic agents 60
Fick principle 25
filling pressure 49, 65, 76, 81, 137, 171
first-pass metabolism 64
fistula, arterio-venous 23
"forward failure" 171
friction rub 93
furosemide 80


G

gamma camera 54
growth factors 36


H

heart catherization, see cardiac catherization, angio(cardio)graphy, coronary angiography, left-heart catherization, right-heart catherization
heart dullness, see cardiac dullness
heart failure (see also coronary insufficiency, myocardial failure) 80, 85, 124 f., 135, 138, 141, 171 ff.
heart failure cells 100
heart murmur 10, 22 f., 84
– diastolic 100
– presystolic 100
– "machinery" 127
– volume 10
heart rate 31 f., 151 f., 176
– with exercise 49, 51
heart silhouette, see cardiac silhouette
heart sound
–, first 100 f., 172
–, second 100 f., 106, 146, 150
– – splitting 119
–, third 75, 106, 135, 172
heart transplantation, see cardiac transplantation
heart volume, see cardiac volume
heart weight, see cardiac weight
hemochromatosis 137, 143
heparin 60, 80 f.
herpes zoster 63
His bundle ECG 158

Holter monitoring 158 f.
hyperlipidemia 45
hyperkinetic heart syndrome
   49, 51, 62, 151 ff., 158, 176
hyperplasia 139
hyperthyroidism 146, 153,
   158, 164
hypertension 17, 45, 64, 96,
   124 f., 149, 173, 176
–, pulmonary 100, 102, 119,
   121, 123, 149 f., 171 f.
–, renal 146
–, renovascular 146 f.
–, systemic 2, 30, 39, 48, 121,
   124, 145 ff., 171
hypertensive regulatory disorder 50, 151
hypertrophy 30, 32, 62, 100,
   108, 113, 135, 139 f., 145, 172
hyperventilation 60, 155
- syndrome 155
hypokalemia 17, 159
hypotension 93, 141, 154 f.,
   174
hypotonic circulatory disorder
   154 f.

# I

iliac artery, palpation 7
indicator dye-dilution, see dye-
   dilution
intra-arterial thrombus 74
intracostal artery 124
internal mammary artery 66,
   124
internal thoracic artery 66
intracardiac mapping 159
ischemia 32, 85
–, silent 22, 48
ischemia score 47, 52
ischemic heart disease,
   mortality rate 3

# K

Kent bundle 169

# L

left bundle branch block 135,
   160, 168 f.,
left-heart catherization 34,
   123, 129, 137

left-heart failure 100, 135, 150,
   171 ff.
left ventricular hypertrophy 20 f., 106 ff., 112
left-to-right shunt 25 f., 76,
   118 ff., 126, 128
leukocytosis 93
lip cyanosis 100
lidocaine (see also xylocaine)
   80, 170
lipid fractions 45 ff.
lipid-lowering drugs 45, 88
lipids 45 ff.
liver, palpation 7
liver, pulsatile 116
liver congestion 172
Loeffler's endocarditis 92
Lown-Ganong-Levine (LGL)
   syndrome 170
luetic aortic aneurysm 96, 99
lungs, auscultation 10 f.
– percussion 10
lupus erythematosus 92 f.
lymphogranulomatosis 93,
   143

# M

malaria 93
"manager disease" 88
Marfan's syndrome 96, 98 f.
methoxamine 143
methyldopa 147
mexiletine 160
mitral facies 140
mitral opening snap 100
mitral valve disorder 106
mitral (valve) insufficiency
   23, 62, 84, 89, 91, 98 f.,
   105 ff., 116, 139, 141, 172
– auscultation 106
– ECG 23, 106
– in mitral valve prolapse
   62, 89, 98 f., 105
– murmur 75, 135
mitral (valve) stenosis 10, 33,
   99 ff., 115, 149, 156, 171
– ECG 23, 101, 164
– phonocardiogram 23, 101
–, silent 101
molsidomine 64
morphine 80
myocardial antibodies 93
myocardial biopsy 136, 141
– and myocarditis 93 f.
myocardial failure (see also co-

ronary insufficiency, heart
   failure) 100
myocardial fibrosis 135 f.,
   139, 142
myocardial infarction 2, 37,
   42 f., 45 ff., 74 ff., 87, 135,
   156, 170, 172
– ECG changes 76
– medical management 80 f.
– mobilization 88 f.
–, non-transmural 39, 74, 87 f.
–, silent 48, 75
myocardial ischemia (see also
   coronary insufficiency) 48,
   50, 60
myocardial mass 135
myocardial reserve, see
   coronary reserve
myocardial scar 55
myocarditis 93 f.
–, eosinophilic 143
–, florid 137
–, viral 135
myopericarditis 93

# N

neck vein congestion 172
necrosis 75 f.
needle puncture 94
nerve growth factor 139
neurofibromatosis (von Reck-
   linghausens's disease) 139
neuropathy, diabetic 19
nerve irritation 62
nitrate 65, 173
– isosorbide dinitrate 64, 81
– isosorbide mononitrate 64,
   81
– patch 64
– tolerance 64
nitroglycerin 60, 62, 64 f.,
   80 f., 142, 149 f.
nitroprusside 143, 149
non-transmural infarction 39,
   74, 87 f.
nuclear imaging techniques
   31 f., 54 ff.
nuclear magnetic resonance
   (NMR) 32

# O

obesity 45, 145 f.
orciprenaline 16

182

orthostatic disturbance 155
oxygen consumption 174
oxygen therapy, chronic 150

# P

pacemaker 94, 137, 139, 157, 166 f.
palpation 6 f.
panniculitis 63
papillary muscle dysfunction 99, 105 f.
patent ductus arteriosus 33, 89, 118, 125 ff.
– phonogram 23, 127
penicillin 92
pericardial effusion 8, 94 f.
pericardial puncture 94
pericarditis 62, 93 ff.
–, constrictive 94 f., 172
–, Coxsackie 94
–, exudative 93
–, fibrinous 93
–, tuberculous 94
peritonitis 89
phlebitis 172
phlebotomy 150
phonocardiography 22 f.
physical rehabilitation therapy 176 f.
physical training 176
platelet aggregation inhibitors 37, 60
plethora 146
pleural effusion 172
polyarthritis 92
polycythemia 132, 150, 172
popliteal artery 7
positron emission tomography 32
posterior tibial artery 6 f.
posterior tibial pulses 7
post-extrasystolic pause 159
procainamide 160
precordial thump 79
pressure, intracardiac 33, 95, 100, 128
pressure gradient 101, 108 f., 113 ff., 125, 140 ff.
programmed stimulation 158
pulmonary artery 130
pulmonary auscultation 10 f.
pulmonary congestion 75, 81, 100 f., 106, 172
pulmonary flow 119
pulmonary ectesia 123

pulmonary edema 49, 80, 100, 172
pulmonary embolism 149
pulmonary percussion 10
pulmonary plethora 119
pulmonary (valve) insufficiency 99, 113, 115
pulmonary (valve) stenosis 23, 30, 33, 99, 113 ff.
–, infundibular 130
– phonocardiogram 23
pulmonary venous connection, anomalous 118
pulmonary vessels 27
pulse, peripheral 6
pulse pressure 111
pulse rate (see also heart rate) 51, 152
– and exercise 51

# Q

quinidine 160, 162, 170
QT syndrome, long 170

# R

radial artery, palpation 7 f.
radicular irritation 62
radionuclide ventriculography 31 f., 54 f., 85, 112
– regurgitation fraction 112
rales 81, 172
Ratschow's test 7, 48
redistribution 32, 55
rehabilitation 85, 87
rehabilitation program 86
re-infarction 46, 87
renal artery, auscultation 11 f.
renal hypertension 146
renin-angiotensin mechanism, overactive 149
renovascular hypertension 146 f.
respiratory alkalosis 60
resuscitation 79
revascularization 63, 66 ff.
rheumatic fever 89, 91 f., 98
rib notching 124 f.
right bundle branch block 160, 168 f.
right-heart catherization 33, 81, 114, 119, 123, 129, 137, 150, 153

right-heart failure 100, 116, 132, 135, 171 ff.
right-to-left shunt 25 f., 123, 128, 131
right-ventricular failure 119
right-ventricular hypertrophy 20 f., 113 f., 132
rubella infection 113

# S

salicylates 68
sarcoidosis 93, 137, 143
scintillation camera 31 f.
septal rupture 84
serum cholesterol 45
shock, cardiogenic 80
shunt 123
shunt blood 119
shunt volume 119
sick sinus syndrome 158, 166 f.
sinus arrest 147
sinus node recovery time 158, 166
sinus of Valsalva aneurysm 112
"small vessel disease" 62
spleen 90
– palpation 7
splitting of the second heart sound 119
staphylococcal sepsis 89
steal phenomenon 66
steroids 92, 157
Stokes-Adams attack 166
streptococcus, β-hemolytic 92
streptococcus viridans 90
streptokinase 80 f.
stroke volume 29, 31 f., 111, 140
ST-segment, see ECG
sudden (cardiac) death 75, 79, 109, 141, 156, 175
syncope 94, 107, 141
syphilis 96
systolic click 106

# T

tachycardia 93, 146 f., 151, 154, 156 f., 159 ff., 172
–, paroxysmal 157, 161 ff.
Takayasu's disease, see aortitis
telangiectasia 100

thallium scintigraphy   32, 54 ff.
thermistor   25
thermodilution method   25
thrombolysis, see fibrinolysis
thrombolytic drug therapy   81
thrombosis   36, 60, 89, 91, 96, 171
– prophylaxis   60, 68, 107, 137
thrombotic deposits   60
thrombus, intra-arterial   74
Tietze's syndrome   63
tilt-table examination   155
tissue plasminogen activator (rt-PA)   81
transesophageal echocardiography   119
transposition of the great arteries   132
tricuspid atresia   132
tricuspid (valve) insufficiency   23, 98 f., 116 f., 172
–, phonogram   23, 117
tricuspid (valve) stenosis   99, 115 f., 119
trifascicular block   169
typhus   93

**U**

urinary tract infection   89
urokinase   80 f.

**V**

vagal stimulation   60, 164
vancomycin   90
vascular headaches   64
vasoconstrictor   143
vasodilators   60, 85, 106, 137, 142 f., 150, 173
– peripheral   147
valve replacement   90, 105 f., 110, 116
valvular dilatation   113, 115 f.
valvular heart disease   90
valvular insufficiency   32
valvular opening   100
valvular orifice area   101 f.
Valsalva-maneuver   142
valvuloplasty   110
venous occlusion plethysmography   153
venous pulse   116 f.

ventricular arrhythmias, see cardiac arrhythmias
ventricular fibrillation   49 f., 76, 79 f., 85, 94, 109, 141, 156, 159 ff., 175
ventricular score   47
ventricular septal defect   23, 89, 118, 122 f., 132, 149
– phonogram   23, 122
ventricular tachycardia   156, 159 f.
ventricular volume   31
ventriculogram   72, 77, 84, 142
volume overloading   106
v-wave   104, 106

**W**

watch-glass nails   150
Wenckebach point   166
Whipple's disease   93
Wolff-Parkinson-White (WPW) syndrome   53, 164, 169 f.

184